Biosensors: Science and Technology

Biosensors: Science and Technology

Edited by
Bob Tucker

WILLFORD PRESS
www.willfordpress.com

Published by Willford Press,
118-35 Queens Blvd., Suite 400,
Forest Hills, NY 11375, USA

ISBN: 978-1-68285-376-4

Cataloging-in-Publication Data

Biosensors : science and technology / edited by Bob Tucker.
p. cm.
Includes bibliographical references and index.
ISBN 978-1-68285-376-4
1. Biosensors. 2. Bioelectronics. 3. Detectors. I. Tucker, Bob.
R857.B54 B56 2017
610.28--dc23

For information on all Willford Press publications
visit our website at www.willfordpress.com

Willford Press

Printed in China.

Contents

Preface

This book has been a concerted effort by a group of academicians, researchers and scientists, who have contributed their research works for the realization of the book. This book has materialized in the wake of emerging advancements and innovations in this field. Therefore, the need of the hour was to compile all the required researches and disseminate the knowledge to a broad spectrum of people comprising of students, researchers and specialists of the field.

Biosensors are devices that are used to detect a biological analyte. It is a very important field of study for biotechnology and biomedicine. Biosensor technology is very useful for early detection and study of disease. This book on biosensors discusses the recent advances that have been seen in the field. Popular applications that have already been developed in this field include glucose monitoring devices and drug residue detectors for the food industry. Topics included in this book discuss the advanced research that is taking place in this field. It is a valuable compilation of topics, ranging from the basic to the most complex advancements in the field of biosensors. This book, with its detailed analyses and data, will prove immensely beneficial to professionals and students involved in this area at various levels.

At the end of the preface, I would like to thank the authors for their brilliant chapters and the publisher for guiding us all-through the making of the book till its final stage. Also, I would like to thank my family for providing the support and encouragement throughout my academic career and research projects.

Editor

1

Aryl Diazonium Chemistry for the Surface Functionalization of Glassy Biosensors

Wei Zheng [1], Remko van den Hurk [1], Yong Cao [2], Rongbing Du [2], Xuejun Sun [3], Yiyu Wang [4], Mark T. McDermott [2] and Stephane Evoy [1,*]

[1] Department of Electrical and Computer Engineering, University of Alberta, Edmonton, Alberta, AB T6G 2V4, Canada; wzheng2@ualberta.ca (W.Z.); Remko@ualberta.ca (R.v.d.H.)

[2] Department of Chemistry and National Institute for Nanotechnology, University of Alberta, Edmonton, Alberta, AB T6G 2G2, Canada; yong2@ualberta.ca (Y.C.); rdu@ualberta.ca (R.D.); mmcdermo@ualberta.ca (M.T.M.)

[3] Department of Experimental Oncology, Cross Cancer Institute, University of Alberta, Edmonton, Alberta, AB T6G 1Z2, Canada; xuejun.sun@ualberta.ca

[4] Department of Chemical and Materials Engineering, University of Alberta, Edmonton, Alberta, AB T6G 1H9, Canada; yiyu@ualberta.ca

* Correspondence: sevoy@ualberta.ca

Academic Editor: Ebrahim Ghafar-Zadeh

Abstract: Nanostring resonator and fiber-optics-based biosensors are of interest as they offer high sensitivity, real-time measurements and the ability to integrate with electronics. However, these devices are somewhat impaired by issues related to surface modification. Both nanostring resonators and photonic sensors employ glassy materials, which are incompatible with electrochemistry. A surface chemistry approach providing strong and stable adhesion to glassy surfaces is thus required. In this work, a diazonium salt induced aryl film grafting process is employed to modify a novel SiCN glassy material. Sandwich rabbit IgG binding assays are performed on the diazonium treated SiCN surfaces. Fluorescently labelled anti-rabbit IgG and anti-rabbit IgG conjugated gold nanoparticles were used as markers to demonstrate the absorption of anti-rabbit IgG and therefore verify the successful grafting of the aryl film. The results of the experiments support the effectiveness of diazonium chemistry for the surface functionalization of SiCN surfaces. This method is applicable to other types of glassy materials and potentially can be expanded to various nanomechanical and optical biosensors.

Keywords: biosensors; glasses; optical fibers; nanostrings; diazonium; surface linkers

---

1. Introduction

Biological detection is of importance in many fields such as disease biomarker diagnosis and monitoring, drug discovery, and molecular identification [1–7]. For instance, the multiplexed assaying of proteins enables the understanding and diagnosis of complex diseases where traditional genomic assays are somewhat inadequate. Prions play a significant role in diseases, such as the Creutzfeldt-Jakob disease and transmissible spongiform encephalopathies [8,9]. In turn, peptides, such as the amyloid-beta (Aβ), are recognized causative agent of degenerative conditions such as Alzheimer's disease [9–11]. Protein microarrays enable multiplexed assays and have been employed to quantify cancer cells and biomarkers [12,13]. In addition, protein misfolding cyclic amplification is used for the testing of prions and the diagnosis of related diseases [14–17]. The technique however involves multiple steps and is inappropriate for large scale screening.

Label-free biosensors have been looked upon as alternative platforms for such assays [18,19]. Such biosensors typically integrate a bio-recognition probe with a transduction system, as well as electronic systems such as signal amplifiers, processors, and display. Transduction platforms, such as quartz crystal microbalance (QCM) [20–23], micromechanical resonators [24–30], flow cytometry [18,31–33], amperometry [34–38], surface plasmon resonance (SPR) [39–46], and planar optical waveguides [47–49], have been investigated. In turn, numerous biological probes such as DNA [50], RNA [51], monoclonal [52,53] polyclonal antibodies [54], bacteriophages [35,55–59] and their binding proteins [58,60] have been leveraged to impart specificity to the transduction. Most of these sensing platforms involve the immobilization of the probe/target system onto a metallic or semiconducting surface. The last few years have however seen the emergence of alternate transduction mechanisms that rather involve the interaction of the analyte with an optical field propagating in glassy waveguides [61–70]. More specifically, fiber-optic sensors offer the advantages of miniaturization, multiple detection, low loss remote monitoring, and large information contents [69]. Further, advancement in the nanomachining of glasses [71,72] has enabled the realization glassy sensing nanostrings [73,74] as narrow as 8 nm [75].

The use of stable interfacial moieties offering strong adhesion, biocompatibility, protection against corrosion and long term stability is crucial to the realization of reliable biosensors [76–78]. Chemical bonding is usually preferred over simple physisorption as it provides better coverage and more stable linkage. Electrochemistry is commonly employed to insure optimal coverage and reliability. Electrochemical approaches are however only suitable for conductive and semi-conductive materials and are thus not applicable to the functionalization of insulating glasses. Electrochemistry also requires complex apparatus, can involve harsh chemicals and lead to the deterioration of the biological system [79,80]. Hence, a simpler, milder, versatile and biocompatible process for the linking of biomolecules onto glasses would be required.

A recently reported diazonium salt reduction induced aryl film grafting process represents a potent candidate for such applications [79,80]. This diazonium chemistry involves a single salt redox process, is implemented in aqueous solution at room temperature and does not require complicated equipment. The mild conditions involved insure process compatibility with pre-existing biological layers. Furthermore, diaznonium chemistry forms covalent bonding onto the surface, thus offers high thermal, mechanical and ambient stability. Moreover, this chemical modification is applicable to all types of materials, from metals to insulator, organic to inorganic.

We here report a diazonium salt induced aryl film grafting process to modify a novel SiCN glassy material [28,72,81,82] (Figure 1). Various surfaces, ranging from metal [83], semi-conductor [84] carbon [85,86] and non-conductive materials [79,80] can be modified by the reduction of aryldiazonium salts by either electrochemically or chemically. As shown in Figure 1, the surface modification is based on radical reactions. Reduction of diazonium salts generates reactive aryl radicals, which then bind to SiCN surfaces. This attachment of the aryl film on substrate surface is very stable [83]. The covalent interface bonding on carbon [87–89], graphene [90,91], silicon [92,93], copper [94], and gold [95–97] surfaces has thus been reported.

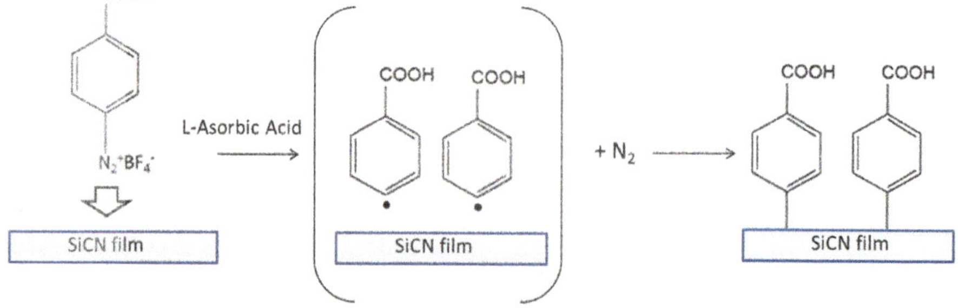

Figure 1. Diagram of diazonium aryl functionalization of SiCN surfaces.

In a prior report, we employed such grafting process for the functionalization of resonant SiCN nanostrings [98]. In that work, the grafting was employed to covalently attach anti-rabbit IgG as a molecular probe. Specific enumeration of rabbit IgG was successfully performed through observation of downshifts of the resonant frequencies. In the work reported here, a similar grafting process is rather used to enable a sandwhich assay. More specifically, rabbit IgG binding assays are performed on the diazonium treated SiCN surface. Fluorescently-labelled rabbit IgG and gold nanoparticles (AuNPs) conjugated with rabbit IgG were used individually as markers to demonstrate the absorption of anti-rabbit IgG and further verify the successful use of aryl films for the functionalization of SiCN surfaces (Figure 2).

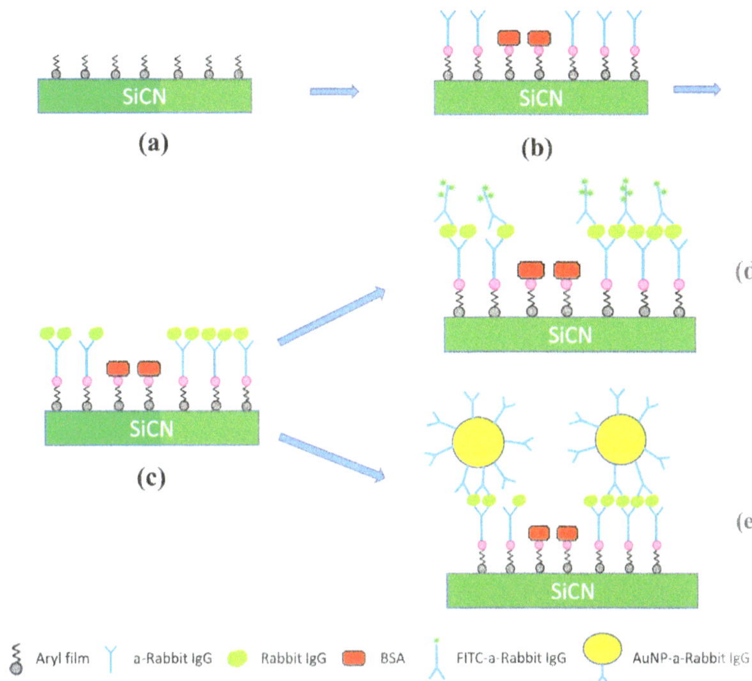

Figure 2. Schematic diagram of rabbit IgG sandwich assay onto SiCN surfaces. (**a**) grafting of aryl groups, as described in Figure 1; (**b**) activation of carboxyl groups and attachment of anti-rabbit IgG and BSA blocking layer; (**c**) specific capture of rabbit IgG; (**d**) tagging using FITC-labelled anti-rabbit IgG; (**e**) tagging using gold nanoparticles functionalized with anti-rabbit IgG.

2. Results and Discussion

2.1. *SiCN Film Composition*

Figure 3 displays an X-ray photoelectron spectroscopy (XPS) survey of a typical SiCN film. Significant binding energy peaks are observed for silicon, carbon and nitrogen. Data analysis yields the quantitative elemental composition of the films (Table 1). The atomic Si:C:N composition ratio was roughly 4:3:3.

Table 1. Element composition analysis of SiCN film.

Element	Atomic Concentration %	Mass Concentration %
N 1s	29.69	21.94
C 1s	30.87	19.57
Si 2p	39.46	58.49

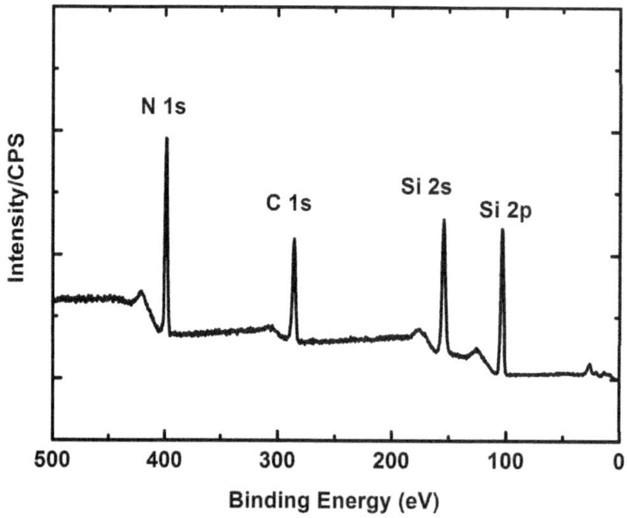

Figure 3. XPS survey of SiCN film.

2.2. SEM and EDX of AuNPs

Figure 4 shows scanning electron microscope (SEM) images of AuNPs on sample A1 (Figures 3B and 4A) and control chip C1 (Figure 4C,D). The images show a dense and roughly uniform distribution of AuNPs over the surface. Almost no AuNP were observed on the control chip C1. It is noteworthy that these results were obtained using high concentrations of anti-rabbit IgG-conjugated AuNPs. To exclude the possibility of non-specific binding by saturation, a 1:3 dilution of anti-rabbit IgG conjugated AuNPs solution was applied to sample chip B1 and control chip D1. The results are shown in Figure 4. Sample B1 shows a roughly uniform coverage of AuNP but at a lower distribution density compared to that of A1. Very small amounts of AuNP are present on control chip D1, again pointing to a negligible level of non-specific binding to the surface. This minimal amount of non-specific binding is likely caused by the interaction between the polyclonal goat anti-rabbit IgG and the goat IgG. The interaction of the AuNPs themselves to the IgG molecules on the substrate may however be caused by other factors. No AuNP are shown under magnification of 20,000x. The contrast of AuNP density between samples and negative controls observed in both experiments (*i.e.*, Figures 4 and 5) therefore points to a high selectivity of binding of anti-rabbit IgG conjugated AuNPs onto the surface.

Figure 6 compares the density of AuNPs on chips A1 and B1. Under 50,000x and 200,000x magnification, the ratio of AuNP of A1 to B1 is around 3:1 which is consistent with the relative concentrations of anti-rabbit IgG conjugated AuNP solutions concentration employed in the two experiments. Figure 7 shows the EDX analysis of SiCN substrate immobilized with sandwich rabbit IgG structure. The point analysis of the particle (panel B) shows significant peaks for elements gold, silicon, carbon and nitrogen, which further supports the attachment of AuNPs onto the SiCN substrate. The elements map shows their relative proportions on and off the particle. In spite of background noise of sparse gold distribution of the particle, the contrast of gold density on and off particle is high enough to conclusively establish the presence of discrete AuNPs on the surface (panel C). Panels D, E, F show less silicon, a bit more carbon and almost the same amount of nitrogen on the particle, which agrees with the fact that anti-rabbit IgG conjugated AuNPs contains carbon and nitrogen, but no silicon. The shape of elements mapping are slightly distorted due to the electron astigmation at high magnification but they still reflects the concentrations of elements distribution effectively.

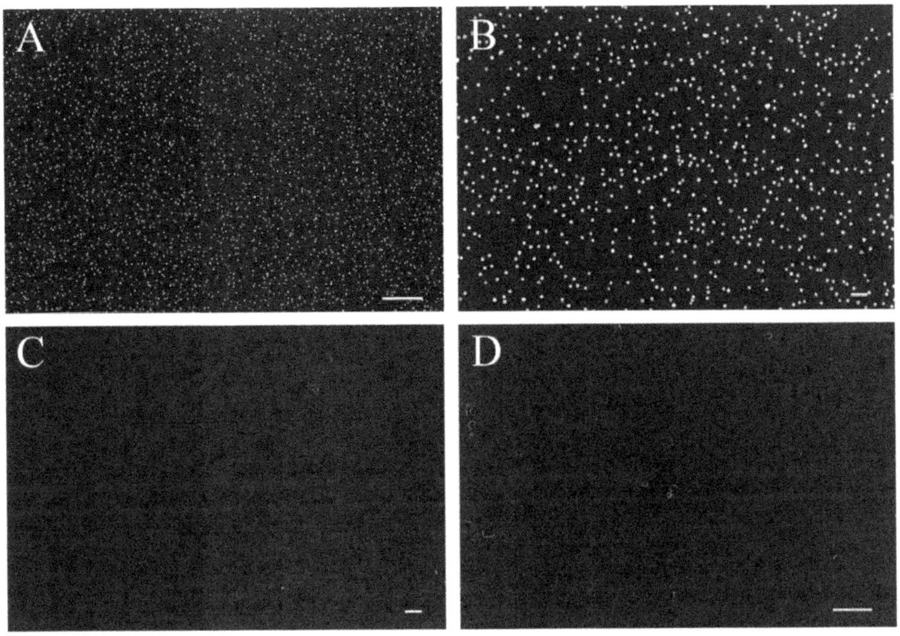

Figure 4. Comparison of presence of AuNP on the surface of sample chip A1 and negative control chip C1: (**A**) AuNP distribution on chip A1 under 10,000x magnification, scale bar length is 1 μm; (**B**) AuNP distribution on chip A1 under 20,000x magnification, scale bar length is 200 nm; (**C**) AuNP distribution on chip C1 under 10,000x magnification, scale bar length is 1 μm; (**D**) AuNP distribution on chip C1 under 20,000x magnification, scale bar length is 200 nm.

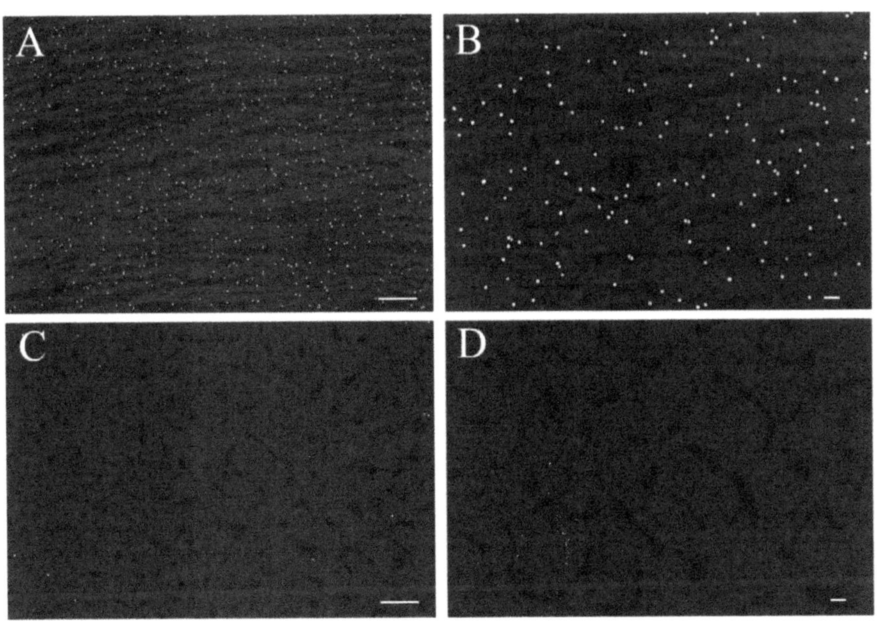

Figure 5. Comparison of presence of AuNPs on the surface of sample chip B1 and negative control chip D1: (**A**) AuNP distribution on chip B1 under 10,000 times magnification, scale bar length 1 μm; (**B**) AuNP distribution on chip B1 under 20,000 times magnification, scale bar length 200 nm; (**C**) AuNP distribution on chip D1 under 10,000 times magnification, scale bar length is 1 μm; (**D**) AuNP distribution on chip D1 under 20,000 times magnification, scale bar length is 200 nm.

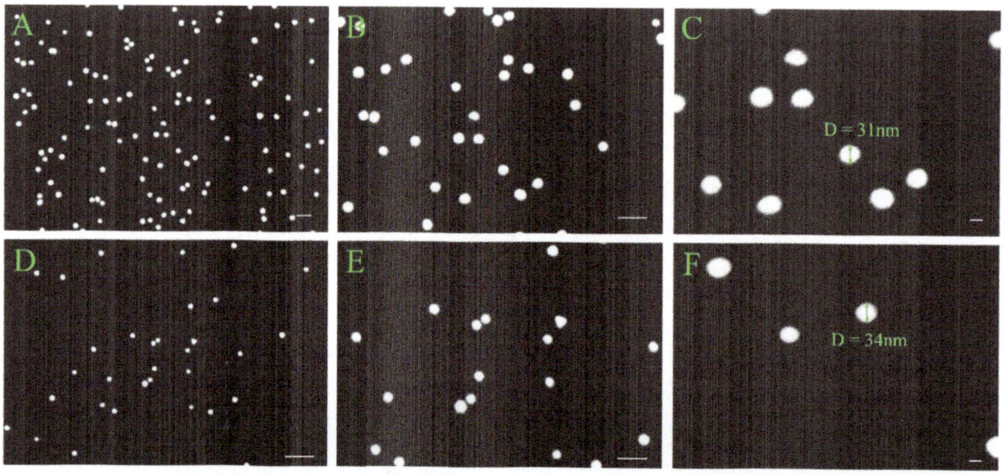

Figure 6. Comparison of presence and density of AuNP on the surface of chips A1 and B1 under high magnification: (**A**) AuNP distribution on chip A1 under 50,000 times magnification, scale bar stands for 100 nm; (**B**) AuNP distribution on chip A1 under 100,000 times magnification, scale bar stands for 100 nm; (**C**) AuNP distribution on chip A1 under 200,000 times magnification, scale bar stands for 20 nm; (**D**) AuNP distribution on chip B1 under 50,000 times magnification, scale bar stands for 200 nm; (**E**) AuNP distribution on chip B1 under 100,000 times magnification, scale bar stands for 100 nm; (**F**) AuNP distribution on chip B1 under 200,000 times magnification, scale bar stands for 20 nm.

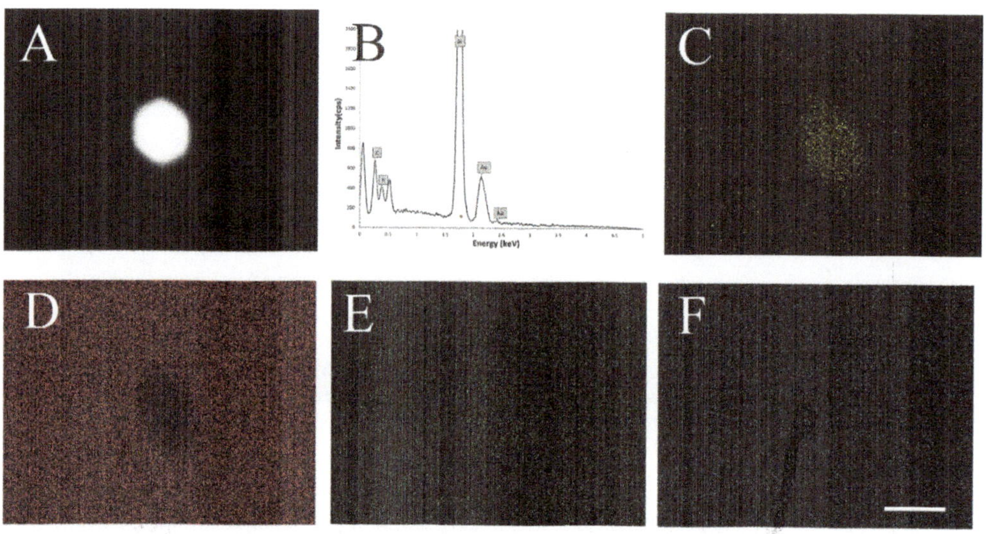

Figure 7. EDX analysis of substrate immobilized with AuNP: (**A**) SEM image of AuNP; (**B**) EDX spectrum of a point of the particle, showing peaks of gold, silicon, carbon and nitrogen; (**C**) EDX map of distribution and relative intensity of gold in scanned area; (**D**) EDX map of distribution and relative intensity of silicon in scanned area; (**E**) EDX map of distribution and relative intensity of carbon in scanned area; (**F**) EDX map of distribution and relative intensity of element nitrogen in scanned area. Scale bar stands for 50 nm.

2.3. Fluorescence Imaging

As seen in Figure 8, the fluorescein-5-Isothiocyanate (FITC) fluorescent marker was present only in chips A2 and B2 but not in negative control chips C2 and D2. The FITC fluorescent intensity is clearly stronger in A2 than it is in B2, while almost no difference exists between C2 and D2. Table 2 tabulates the mean fluorescent intensity and signal to noise ratio for those samples. The signal to noise ratios of 185 and 105 under FITC dilution of 1:200 and 1:400, respectively, conclusively establishes the selective absorption of FITC-conjugated anti-rabbit IgG to the target molecule rabbit IgG. The fluorescence intensity of A2 is 47% larger than that of B2, suggesting non-saturation binding of FITC conjugated anti-rabbit IgG to substrate. The intensities from negative control samples C2 and D2 are almost the same for both FITC concentration, further pointing to an almost inexistent binding of FITC conjugated anti-rabbit IgG to substrate. Hence, these results conclusively establish that the chemical bonding of probe molecule anti-rabbit IgG to the aryl film on SiCN substrate induced by diazonium modification has been accomplished.

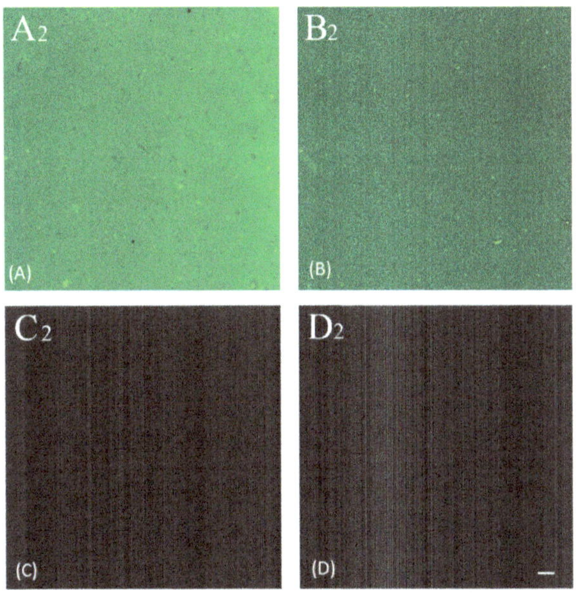

Figure 8. Comparison of presence of FITC on the surface of sample chip A2, B2 and control chip C2, D2: (**A**) FITC distribution on chip A2; (**B**) FITC distribution on chip B2; (**C**) FITC distribution on chip C2; (**D**) FITC distribution on chip D2. Scale bar stands for 2 μm.

Table 2. Mean optical intensity of FITC on the surface of sample chip A2, B2 and control chip C2, D2.

Sample	Intensity (AU)	Signal to Noise Ratio	Dilution Ratio of FITC Conjugated Anti-Rabbit IgG
A2 C2	37,967 205	185	1:200
B2 D2	25,791 245	105	1:400

3. Materials and Methods

3.1. SiCN Film Deposition

A previously reported deposition technique was employed to deposit the thin film [28,72]. More specifically, a single-crystal (100) silicon wafer was subjected to a 15 min piranha clean (3:1 H_2SO_4:H_2O_2) to eliminate surface organics, and immediately followed by a 3 min buffered oxide etch (BOE, 10:1 HF:NH_4F) to strip the native oxide. The SiCN film was deposited onto the clean silicon wafer by plasma enhanced chemical vapor deposition (PECVD). First, the PECVD chamber (Trion Orion) was pre-conditioned at a mixed gases flow of 25 sccm DES, 40 sccm NH_3, 55 sccm N_2 at a temperature of 300 °C, a pressure of 500 mTorr, and a power of 50 W for 1200 s. The silicon wafer was then loaded in the reactor. The chamber was purged by 55 sccm N_2 at a pressure of 500 mTorr and a temperature of 300 °C for 10 s. The chamber was prepared for the deposition by a mixed gases flow of 25 sccm DES, 40 sccm NH_3, 55 sccm N_2 at a temperature of 300 °C, a pressure of 500 mTorr for 10 s. A SiCN thin film was deposited with at a mixed gases flow of 25 sccm DES, 40 sccm NH3, 55 sccm N2 at a temperature of 300 °C, a pressure of 500 mTorr, and a power of 50 W for 125 s. The wafer was then annealed in a 3-zone Minibrute tube furnace at 525 °C for 2 h.

3.2. *XPS Element Analysis*

Surface XPS analyses were performed to characterize the elemental composition of the deposited film, namely the ratio of silicon, carbon and nitride. The XPS was performed in a Kratos Axis Ultra spectrometer using a monochromatic Al Kα source (hν = 1486.6 eV). Instrument base pressure was lower than 5×10^{-8} Pa. The survey scans were acquired out with a pass energy of 160 eV.

3.3. *Diazonium Modification of SiCN*

Aryl diazonium salt was synthesized from the corresponding anilines using a previously reported procedure [86]. Briefly, 0.1 moles 4-Aminobenzoic acid (Sigma-Aldrich) was dissolved in 50 mL floroboric acid (48%, Sigma-Aldrich) and then cooled in an ice water bath. After cooling the solution to 0 °C, Sodium nitrite (10 g, Sigma-Aldrich) dissolved in DI water (20 mL) was added drop by drop with stirring. The reaction mixture was further cooled in ice water bath and stirred for another 1 h. The resultant precipitate was filtered in a Buchner funnel and washed with cold anhydrous ether (Sigma-Aldrich).

The SiCN surface was modified by diazonium salt reduction induced aryl film grafting process as per the following procedure. A piranha and BOE etch similar to the one described previously was first employed to clean the SiCN surface from organic contaminants. Indeed, the SiCN films were batch deposited on multiple wafers at a time, with individual wafers often stored for months prior to use. A re-cleaning of the SiCN film surface prior to aryl grafting was thus deemed compulsory in the light of this extensive storage. Following this cleaning, the SiCN chips were incubated in 2:1 volume ratio of 0.05 M 4-carboxybenzenediazonium tetrafluoroborate ($COOH{-}C_6H_4{-}N_2BF_4$) and 0.05 M L-ascorbic acid (VC) (Sigma-Aldrich) for 60 min. The chips were then successively rinsed in water, ethanol, and acetone followed by a 5 min sonication in dimethylformamide (DMF) (Sigma-Aldrich). The presence of grafted aryl film onto the SiCN film after sonication in DMF was verified with XPS analysis. For such verification, a Br terminated diazonium salt 4-bromobenzenediazonium tetrafluoroborate was rather used. Bromium was used as elemental marker as it is otherwise absent from the SiCN film surface. Related XPS spectra clearly indicated the presence of the Br groups following the sonication step in DMF, confirming the stability of the grafting [98].

Carboxyl groups were activated by incubating the chips in a 1:1 volume ratio of 0.4 M EDC (N-(3-dimethylaminopropyl)-N′-ethylcarbodiimide hydrochloride) (Sigma-Aldrich) and 0.1 M NHS (N-hydroxysuccinimide) (Sigma-Aldrich) solution for 30 min.

3.4. *Gold Nanoparticle Labelled Sandwich Rabbit IgG Assay*

In this AuNP labelled sandwich rabbit IgG assay, anti-rabbit IgG was used as the recognition bioreceptor, rabbit IgG was the target and anti-rabbit IgG conjugated AuNP served as detection markers.

3.4.1. Immobilization of AuNP Labelled Sandwich Rabbit IgG

Immobilization of recognition bioreceptor: Four SiCN chips (A1, B1, C1, D1) baring activated carboxyl groups were incubated in 100 μg/mL goat anti-rabbit IgG solution (polyclonal, Sigma-Aldrich) at room temperature for 2 h. The chips were rinsed with PBST (Phosphate Buffered Saline Tween-20) and then incubated in 5% BSA (bovine serum albumin) at room temperature for 1 h to block non-specific binding sites. The chips were then rinsed once again in PBST.

Immobilization of target: Two chips (A1 and B1) were immobilized with the detection target by incubating in 200 μg/mL rabbit IgG solution (polyclonal, Sigma-Aldrich) at room temperature for 1 h. As parallel control experimnent, the other two chips (C1 and D1) were incubated in 200 μg/mL goat IgG solution (polyclonal, Sigma-Aldrich) at room temperature for 1 h. The chips were then rinsed once again in PBST.

Immobilization of detection marker: Chips A1 and C1 were immersed in 40 nm AuNP (4.5×10^{11} /mL) conjugated anti-rabbit IgG solution (10 μg/mL, Ted Pella) at room temperature for 1 h. Chips B1 and D1 were immersed in 1:3 diluted solution of 40 nm AuNP conjugated anti-rabbit IgG at room temperature for 1 h. Following incubation, the chips were water rinsed and dried under nitrogen flow. Table 3 summarizes the conditions under which each sample was prepared.

Table 3. Description of Samples.

Sample	Control Type	Dilution Ratio	Label
A1	positive	1:1	AuNP
B1	positive	1:3	AuNP
C1	negative	1:1	AuNP
D1	negative	1:3	AuNP
A2	positive	1:200	FITC
B2	positive	1:400	FITC
C2	negative	1:200	FITC
D2	negative	1:400	FITC

3.4.2. SEM and EDX

A high resolution field emission scanning electron microscopy (Zeiss Sigma FE-SEM) was used to observe the presence of the gold nanoparticles on the surface of chips A1, B1, C1 and D1. Images were obtained at magnifications ranging from 10,000x to 200,000x using an acceleration voltage of 15 KV, and using a secondary electron (SE) in-lens and backscattered electron (BSE) detector. An energy-dispersive X-ray detection instrument (EDX) was used to identify the elemental composition of surfaces of chips A1, B1, C1 and D1. An Oxford Instruments X-Max^N 150 mm^2 Silicon Drift Detector (SDD) detector was used for such point analysis and mapping of elemental spatial distributions.

3.5. *FITC Labelled Sandwich Rabbit IgG Assay*

The FITC labelled sandwich rabbit IgG assay was similar to the AuNP labelled sandwich rabbit IgG assay with the exception that FITC conjugated anti-rabbit IgG was used as the detection marker.

3.5.1. Immobilization of FITC Labelled Sandwich Rabbit IgG

The procedure for immobilization of bioreceptor and target is similar to the one described in section 4.4.1. Four diazonium modified SiCN chips (A2, B2, C2, D2) were incubated in 100 μg/mL goat anti-rabbit IgG solution (polyclonal, Sigma-Aldrich) for 2 h, and 5% BSA (bovine serum albumin) for 1 h at room temperature. Chips A2 and B2 were incubated in 200 μg/mL rabbit IgG solution (polyclonal, Sigma-Aldrich) for 1 h whereas chips C2 and D2 were subject to 200 μg/mL goat IgG solution (polyclonal, Sigma-Aldrich) as control for 1 h at room temperature. Chips A2 and C2 were immersed in 1:200 diluted FITC conjugated anti-rabbit IgG solution (Sigma-Aldrich) while Chips B2 and D2 were immersed in 1:400 diluted FITC conjugated anti-rabbit IgG solution at room temperature for 1 h.

3.5.2. Confocal Microscopy Imaging

Chips A2, B2, C2, D2 were individually imaged on a Zeiss LSM 710 Laser scanning confocal microscope mounted on an Axio-observer inverted microscope (ZEN 2011, Jena, Germany) with a plan Apochromat 20x (NA 0.8) dry lens. Fluorescence signal was collected with a 488 nm laser and with an emission wavelength ranging from 492 nm to 590 nm. Images were digitized at 16 bit with a Nyquist sampling rate using a pinhole size of one airy unit. The average intensity of individual images were calculated using the imageJ software (National Institutes of Health).

Acknowledgments: This work was supported by that Natural Sciences and Engineering Research Council of Canada through its Discovery Grant program, as well as by the National Research Council of Canada via the National Institute for Nanotechnology. The authors acknowledge the University of Alberta Nanofab staff for their technical support, more specifically Shihong Xu and Les Schowalter.

Author Contributions: All authors contributed to the conception and design of the experiments; Wei Zheng deposited the SiCN films and Rongbing Du performed the reagent synthesis; Wei Zheng, Rongbing Du, and Yong Cao performed the surface functionalization; Wei Zheng analyzed the data with assistance of Xuejun Sun and Yiyu Wang; Wei Zheng wrote the paper, which was edited and reviewed by all authors.

Conflicts of Interest: The authors declare no conflict of interest. The founding sponsors had no role in the design of the study; in the collection, analyses, or interpretation of data; in the writing of the manuscript, and in the decision to publish the results.

Abbreviations

The following abbreviations are used in this manuscript:

NEMS	Nano-electromechanical Systems
AuNP	Gold nanoparticle
SEM	Scanning electron microscopy
XPS	X-ray photoelectron microscopy
PBST	Phosphate Buffered Saline Tween-20
PECVD	Plasma enhanced chemical vapor deposition
FITC	Fluorescein-5-Isothiocyanate

References

1. Haes, A.J.; Chang, L.; Klein, W.L.; Van Duyne, R.P. Detection of a biomarker for alzheimer's disease from synthetic and clinical samples using a nanoscale optical biosensor. *J. Am. Chem. Soc.* **2005**, *127*, 2264–2271. [CrossRef] [PubMed]
2. Tothill, I.E. Biosensors for cancer markers diagnosis. *Semin. Cell Dev. Biol.* **2009**, *20*, 55–62. [CrossRef] [PubMed]
3. Giuliano, K.A.; Taylor, D.L. Fluorescent-protein biosensors: New tools for drug discovery. *Trends Biotechnol.* **1998**, *16*, 135–140. [CrossRef]
4. Keusgen, M. Biosensors: New approaches in drug discovery. *Naturwissenschaften* **2002**, *89*, 433–444. [CrossRef] [PubMed]
5. Cooper, M.A. Optical biosensors in drug discovery. *Nat. Rev. Drug Discov.* **2002**, *1*, 515–528. [CrossRef] [PubMed]
6. Gartia, M.R.; Braunschweig, B.; Chang, T.-W.; Moinzadeh, P.; Minsker, B.S.; Agha, G.; Wieckowski, A.; Keefer, L.L.; Liu, G.L. The microelectronic wireless nitrate sensor network for environmental water monitoring. *J. Environ. Monit.* **2012**, *14*, 3068–3075. [CrossRef] [PubMed]
7. Liao, J.C.; Mastali, M.; Gau, V.; Suchard, M.A.; Møller, A.K.; Bruckner, D.A.; Babbitt, J.T.; Li, Y.; Gornbein, J.; Landaw, E.M. Use of electrochemical DNA biosensors for rapid molecular identification of uropathogens in clinical urine specimens. *J. Clin. Microbiol.* **2006**, *44*, 561–570. [CrossRef] [PubMed]
8. Edgeworth, J.A.; Farmer, M.; Sicilia, A.; Tavares, P.; Beck, J.; Campbell, T.; Lowe, J.; Mead, S.; Rudge, P.; Collinge, J.; *et al.* Detection of prion infection in variant creutzfeldt-jakob disease: A blood-based assay. *Lancet* **2011**, *377*, 487–493. [CrossRef]
9. Jucker, M.; Walker, L.C. Pathogenic protein seeding in alzheimer disease and other neurodegenerative disorders. *Ann. Neurol.* **2011**, *70*, 532–540. [CrossRef] [PubMed]
10. Stohr, J.; Watts, J.C.; Mensinger, Z.L.; Oehler, A.; Grillo, S.K.; DeArmond, S.J.; Prusiner, S.B.; Giles, K. Purified and synthetic alzheimer's amyloid beta (a beta) prions. *PNAS* **2012**, *109*, 11025–11030. [CrossRef] [PubMed]
11. Rushworth, J.V.; Ahmed, A.; Griffiths, H.H.; Pollock, N.M.; Hooper, N.M.; Millner, P.A. A label-free electrical impedimetric biosensor for the specific detection of alzheimer's amyloid-beta oligomers. *Biosens. Bioelectron.* **2014**, *56*, 83–90. [CrossRef] [PubMed]

12. Sreekumar, A.; Nyati, M.K.; Varambally, S.; Barrette, T.R.; Ghosh, D.; Lawrence, T.S.; Chinnaiyan, A.M. Profiling of cancer cells using protein microarrays: Discovery of novel radiation-regulated proteins. *Cancer Res.* **2001**, *61*, 7585–7593. [PubMed]
13. Woodbury, R.L.; Varnum, S.M.; Zangar, R.C. Elevated hgf levels in sera from breast cancer patients detected using a protein microarray elisa. *J. Proteome Res.* **2002**, *1*, 233–237. [CrossRef] [PubMed]
14. Saborio, G.P.; Permanne, B.; Soto, C. Sensitive detection of pathological prion protein by cyclic amplification of protein misfolding. *Nature* **2001**, *411*, 810–813. [CrossRef] [PubMed]
15. Castilla, J.; Saa, P.; Soto, C. Detection of prions in blood. *Nat. Med.* **2005**, *11*, 982–985. [CrossRef] [PubMed]
16. Chen, B.A.; Morales, R.; Barria, M.A.; Soto, C. Estimating prion concentration in fluids and tissues by quantitative pmca. *Nat. Methods* **2010**, *7*, U519–U547. [CrossRef] [PubMed]
17. Moudjou, M.; Sibille, P.; Fichet, G.; Reine, F.; Chapuis, J.; Herzog, L.; Jaumain, E.; Laferriere, F.; Richard, C.A.; Laude, H.; *et al.* Highly infectious prions generated by a single round of microplate-based protein misfolding cyclic amplification. *mBio* **2013**, *5*. [CrossRef] [PubMed]
18. Abdel-Hamid, I.; Ivnitski, D.; Atanasov, P.; Wilkins, E. Flow-through immunofiltration assay system for rapid detection of e. Coli o157:H7. *Biosens. Bioelectron.* **1999**, *14*, 309–316. [CrossRef]
19. Lazcka, O.; Del Campo, F.J.; Munoz, F.X. Pathogen detection: A perspective of traditional methods and biosensors. *Biosens. Bioelectron.* **2007**, *22*, 1205–1217. [CrossRef] [PubMed]
20. Fung, Y.S.; Wong, Y.Y. Self-assembled monolayers as the coating in a quartz piezoelectric crystal immunosensor to detect salmonella in aqueous solution. *Anal. Chem.* **2001**, *73*, 5302–5309. [CrossRef] [PubMed]
21. Chang, Y.P.; Liu, W.C.; Tseng, M.C.; Chu, Y.H. Ionic liquids tailored for reaction-based gas sensing on quartz crystal microbalance. *Rev. Anal. Chem.* **2015**, *34*, 77–86. [CrossRef]
22. Wang, Z.; Yang, M.; He, J.; Yang, Q. Progress of different sensing materials modified qcm gas sensors. *Prog. Chem.* **2015**, *27*, 251–266.
23. Guo, H. Progress of quartz crystal microbalance in chiral analysis. *J. Nanosci. Nanotechnol.* **2014**, *14*, 1884–1897. [CrossRef]
24. Ilic, B.; Czaplewski, D.; Zalalutdinov, M.; Craighead, H.G.; Neuzi, P.; Campagnolo, C.; Batt, C. Single cell detection with micromechanical oscillators. *J. Vac. Sci. Technol. B* **2001**, *19*, 2825–2828. [CrossRef]
25. Ilic, B.; Yang, Y.; Craighead, H.G. Virus detection using nanoelectromechanical devices. *Appl. Phys. Lett.* **2004**, *85*, 2604–2606. [CrossRef]
26. Poshtiban, S.; Singh, A.; Fitzpatrick, G.; Evoy, S. Bacteriophage tail-spike protein derivitized microresonator arrays for specific detection of pathogenic bacteria. *Sens. Actuators B Chem.* **2013**, *181*, 410–416. [CrossRef]
27. Campbell, G.A.; Medina, M.B.; Mutharasan, R. Detection of staphylococcus enterotoxin b at picogram levels using piezoelectric-excited millimeter-sized cantilever sensors. *Sens. Actuators B Chem.* **2007**, *126*, 354–360. [CrossRef]
28. Fischer, L.M.; Wright, V.A.; Guthy, C.; Yang, N.; McDermott, M.T.; Buriak, J.M.; Evoy, S. Specific detection of proteins using nanomechanical resonators. *Sens. Actuators B Chem.* **2008**, *134*, 613–617. [CrossRef]
29. Quitoriano, N.J.; Belov, M.; Evoy, S.; Kamins, T.I. Single-crystal, si nanotubes, and their mechanical resonant properties. *Nano. Lett.* **2009**, *9*, 1511–1516. [CrossRef] [PubMed]
30. Bausells, J. Piezoresistive cantilevers for nanomechanical sensing. *Microelectron. Eng.* **2015**, *145*, 9–20. [CrossRef]
31. Abdel-Hamid, I.; Ghindidlis, A.L.; Atanasov, P.; Wilkins, E. Development of a flow-through immunoassay system. *Sens. Actuators B* **1998**, *49*, 202–210. [CrossRef]
32. Adan, A.; Alizada, G.; Kiraz, Y.; Baran, Y.; Nalbant, A. Flow cytometry: Basic principles and applications. *Crit. Rev. Biotechnol.* **2016**, *36*. [CrossRef] [PubMed]
33. Mross, S.; Pierrat, S.; Zimmermann, T.; Kraft, M. Microfluidic enzymatic biosensing systems: A review. *Biosens. Bioelectron.* **2015**, *70*, 376–391. [CrossRef] [PubMed]
34. Gau, J.J.; Lan, E.H.; Dunn, B.; Ho, C.M.; Woo, J.C. A MEMS based amperometric detector for *E. coli* bacteria using self-assembled monolayers. *Biosens. Bioelectron.* **2001**, *16*, 745–755. [CrossRef]
35. Gervals, L.; Gel, M.; Allain, B.; Tolba, M.; Brovko, L.; Zourob, M.; Mandeville, R.; Griffiths, M.; Evoy, S. Immobilization of biotinylated bacteriophages on biosensor surfaces. *Sens. Actuators B Chem.* **2007**, *125*, 615–621. [CrossRef]

36. Xu, Y.; Xie, X.; Duan, Y.; Wang, L.; Cheng, Z.; Cheng, J. A review of impedance measurements of whole cells. *Biosens. Bioelectron.* **2016**, *77*, 824–836. [CrossRef] [PubMed]
37. Chillawar, R.R.; Tadi, K.K.; Motghare, R.V. Voltammetric techniques at chemically modified electrodes. *J. Anal. Chem.* **2015**, *70*, 399–418. [CrossRef]
38. Amatore, C.; Delacotte, J.; Guille-Collignon, M.; Lemaître, F. Vesicular exocytosis and microdevices-microelectrode arrays. *Analyst* **2015**, *140*, 3687–3695. [CrossRef] [PubMed]
39. Taylor, A.D.; Yu, Q.; Chen, S.; Homola, J.; Jiang, S. Comparison of *E. coli* O157:H7 preparation methods used for detection with surface plasmon resonance sensor. *Sens. Actuators B* **2005**, *107*, 202–208. [CrossRef]
40. Liu, X.; Hu, Y.; Zheng, S.; Liu, Y.; He, Z.; Luo, F. Surface plasmon resonance immunosensor for fast, highly sensitive, and in situ detection of the magnetic nanoparticles-enriched Salmonella enteritidis. *Sens. Actuators B Chem.* **2016**, *230*, 191–198. [CrossRef]
41. Arya, S.K.; Singh, A.; Naidoo, R.; Wu, P.; McDermott, M.T.; Evoy, S. Chemically immobilized t4-bacteriophage for specific escherichia coli detection using surface plasmon resonance. *Analyst* **2011**, *136*, 486–492. [CrossRef] [PubMed]
42. Singh, A.; Arya, S.K.; Glass, N.; Hanifi-Moghaddam, P.; Naidoo, R.; Szymanski, C.M.; Tanha, J.; Evoy, S. Bacteriophage tailspike proteins as molecular probes for sensitive and selective bacterial detection. *Biosens. Bioelectron.* **2010**, *26*, 131–138. [CrossRef] [PubMed]
43. Butet, J.; Brevet, P.F.; Martin, O.J.F. Optical second harmonic generation in plasmonic nanostructures: From fundamental principles to advanced applications. *Acs. Nano.* **2015**, *9*, 10545–10562. [CrossRef] [PubMed]
44. Langer, J.; Novikov, S.M.; Liz-Marzán, L.M. Sensing using plasmonic nanostructures and nanoparticles. *Nanotechnology* **2015**, *26*. [CrossRef] [PubMed]
45. Nguyen, H.H.; Park, J.; Kang, S.; Kim, M. Surface plasmon resonance: A versatile technique for biosensor applications. *Sensors* **2015**, *15*, 10481–10510. [CrossRef] [PubMed]
46. Wang, P.; Bo, L.; Semenova, Y.; Farrell, G.; Brambilla, G. Optical microfibre based photonic components and their applications in label-free biosensing. *Biosensors* **2015**, *5*, 471–499. [CrossRef] [PubMed]
47. Buswell, S.C.; Wright, V.A.; Buriak, J.M.; Van, V.; Evoy, S. Specific detection of proteins using photonic crystal waveguides. *Opt. Express* **2008**, *16*, 15949–15957. [CrossRef] [PubMed]
48. Mukundan, H.; Kubicek, J.Z.; Holt, A.; Shively, J.E.; Martinez, J.S.; Grace, K.; Grace, W.K.; Swanson, B.I. Planar optical waveguide-based biosensor for the quantitative detection of tumor markers. *Sens. Actuators B Chem.* **2009**, *138*, 453–460. [CrossRef]
49. Schmitt, K.; Schirmer, B.; Hoffmann, C.; Brandenburg, A.; Meyrueis, P. Interferometric biosensor based on planar optical waveguide sensor chips for label-free detection of surface bound bioreactions. *Biosens. Bioelectron.* **2007**, *22*, 2591–2597. [CrossRef] [PubMed]
50. Liao, W.C.; Ho, J.A.A. Attomole DNA electrochemical sensor for the detection of escherichia coli o157. *Anal. Chem.* **2009**, *81*, 2470–2476. [CrossRef] [PubMed]
51. Joung, H.A.; Lee, N.R.; Lee, S.K.; Ahn, J.; Shin, Y.B.; Choi, H.S.; Lee, C.S.; Kim, S.; Kim, M.G. High sensitivity detection of 16s rrna using peptide nucleic acid probes and a surface plasmon resonance biosensor. *Anal. Chim. Acta* **2008**, *630*, 168–173. [CrossRef] [PubMed]
52. Taylor, A.D.; Yu, Q.M.; Chen, S.F.; Homola, J.; Jiang, S.Y. Comparison of *E coli* o157:H7 preparation methods used for detection with surface plasmon resonance sensor. *Sens. Actuators B Chem.* **2005**, *107*, 202–208. [CrossRef]
53. Oh, B.K.; Lee, W.; Chun, B.S.; Bae, Y.M.; Lee, W.H.; Choi, J.W. The fabrication of protein chip based on surface plasmon resonance for detection of pathogens. *Biosens. Bioelectron.* **2005**, *20*, 1847–1850. [CrossRef] [PubMed]
54. Taylor, A.D.; Ladd, J.; Yu, Q.M.; Chen, S.F.; Homola, J.; Jiang, S.Y. Quantitative and simultaneous detection of four foodborne bacterial pathogens with a multi-channel spr sensor. *Biosens. Bioelectron.* **2006**, *22*, 752–758. [CrossRef] [PubMed]
55. Balasubramanian, S.; Sorokulova, I.B.; Vodyanoy, V.J.; Simonian, A.L. Lytic phage as a specific and selective probe for detection of staphylococcus aureus—A surface plasmon resonance spectroscopic study. *Biosens. Bioelectron.* **2007**, *22*, 948–955. [CrossRef] [PubMed]
56. Wan, J.H.; Johnson, M.L.; Guntupalli, R.; Petrenko, V.A.; Chin, B.A. Detection of bacillus anthracis spores in liquid using phage-based magnetoelastic micro-resonators. *Sens. Actuators B Chem.* **2007**, *127*, 559–566. [CrossRef]

57. Singh, A.; Arutyunov, D.; Szymanski, C.M.; Evoy, S. Bacteriophage based probes for pathogen detection. *Analyst* **2012**, *137*, 3405–3421. [CrossRef] [PubMed]
58. Singh, A.; Arutyunov, D.; McDermott, M.T.; Szymanski, C.M.; Evoy, S. Specific detection of campylobacter jejuni using the bacteriophage nctc 12673 receptor binding protein as a probe. *Analyst* **2011**, *136*, 4780–4786. [CrossRef] [PubMed]
59. Tawil, N.; Sacher, E.; Mandeville, R.; Meunier, M. Surface plasmon resonance detection of *E. coli* and methicillin-resistant s. Aureus using bacteriophages. *Biosens. Bioelectron.* **2012**, *37*, 24–29. [CrossRef] [PubMed]
60. Chibli, H.; Ghali, H.; Park, S.; Peter, Y.A.; Nadeau, J.L. Immobilized phage proteins for specific detection of staphylococci. *Analyst* **2014**, *139*, 179–186. [CrossRef] [PubMed]
61. Ray, S.; Mehta, G.; Srivastava, S. Label-free detection techniques for protein microarrays: Prospects, merits and challenges. *Proteomics* **2010**, *10*, 731–748. [CrossRef] [PubMed]
62. Cho, H.; Lee, B.; Liu, G.L.; Agarwal, A.; Lee, L.P. Label-free and highly sensitive biomolecular detection using sers and electrokinetic preconcentration. *Lab Chip* **2009**, *9*, 3360–3363. [CrossRef] [PubMed]
63. Xu, D.X.; Densmore, A.; Delâge, A.; Waldron, P.; McKinnon, R.; Janz, S.; Lapointe, J.; Lopinski, G.; Mischki, T.; Post, E.; *et al.* Folded cavity soi microring sensors for highsensitivity and real time measurement ofbiomolecular binding. *Opt. Express* **2008**, *16*, 15137–15148. [CrossRef] [PubMed]
64. Xu, D.X.; Vachon, M.; Densmore, A.; Ma, R.; Delâge, A.; Janz, S.; Lapointe, J.; Li, Y.; Lopinski, G.; Zhang, D.; *et al.* Label-free biosensor array based on silicon-on-insulator ring resonators addressed using a WDM approach. *Opt. Lett.* **2010**, *35*, 2771–2773. [CrossRef] [PubMed]
65. Liu, G.L.; Lee, L.P. Nanowell surface enhanced raman scattering arrays fabricated by soft-lithography for label-free biomolecular detections in integrated microfluidics. *Appl. Phys. Lett.* **2005**, *87*, 074101. [CrossRef]
66. Furuki, M.; Kameoka, J.; Craighead, H.G.; Isaacson, M.S. Surface plasmon resonance sensors utilizing rnicrofabricated channels. *Sens. Actuators B Chem.* **2001**, *79*, 63–69. [CrossRef]
67. Cui, Y.; Wei, Q.Q.; Park, H.K.; Lieber, C.M. Nanowire nanosensors for highly sensitive and selective detection of biological and chemical species. *Science* **2001**, *293*, 1289–1292. [CrossRef] [PubMed]
68. Wang, X.D.; Wolfbeis, O.S. Fiber-optic chemical sensors and biosensors (2008–2012). *Anal. Chem.* **2013**, *85*, 487–508. [CrossRef] [PubMed]
69. Mehrvar, M.; Bis, C.; Scharer, J.M.; Moo-Young, M.; Luong, J.H. Fiber-optic biosensors—Trends and advances. *Anal. Sci.* **2000**, *16*, 677–692. [CrossRef]
70. Wang, Y.-M.; Pang, X.-F.; Zhang, Y.-Y. Recent advances in fiber-optic DNA biosensors. *J. Biomed. Sci. Eng.* **2009**, *2*, 312–317. [CrossRef]
71. Sekaric, L.; Carr, D.W.; Evoy, S.; Parpia, J.M.; Craighead, H.G. Nanomechanical resonant structures in silicon nitride: Fabrication, operation and dissipation issues. *Sens. Actuators A Phys.* **2002**, *101*, 215–219. [CrossRef]
72. Fischer, L.M.; Wilding, N.; Gel, M.; Evoy, S. Low-stress silicon carbonitride for the machining of high-frequency nanomechanical resonators. *J. Vac. Sci. Technol. B* **2007**, *25*, 33–37. [CrossRef]
73. Verbridge, S.S.; Craighead, H.G.; Parpia, J.M. A megahertz nanomechanical resonator with room temperature quality factor over a million. *Appl. Phys. Lett.* **2008**, *92*. [CrossRef]
74. Southworth, D.R.; Barton, R.A.; Verbridge, S.S.; Ilic, B.; Fefferman, A.D.; Craighead, H.G.; Parpia, J.M. Stress and silicon nitride: A crack in the universal dissipation of glasses. *Phys. Rev. Lett.* **2009**, *102*. [CrossRef] [PubMed]
75. Mohammad, M.A.; Dew, S.K.; Evoy, S.; Stepanova, M. Fabrication of sub-10 nm silicon carbon nitride resonators using a hydrogen silsesquioxane mask patterned by electron beam lithography. *Microelectron. Eng.* **2011**, *88*, 2338–2341. [CrossRef]
76. Grieshaber, D.; MacKenzie, R.; Voros, J.; Reimhult, E. Electrochemical biosensors-sensor principles and architectures. *Sensors* **2008**, *8*, 1400–1458. [CrossRef]
77. Gopel, W.; Heiduschka, P. Interface analysis in biosensor design. *Biosens. Bioelectron.* **1995**, *10*, 853–883. [CrossRef]
78. Credou, J.; Volland, H.; Dano, J.; Berthelot, T. A one-step and biocompatible cellulose functionalization for covalent antibody immobilization on immunoassay membranes. *J. Mater. Chem. B* **2013**, *1*, 3277–3286. [CrossRef]

79. Mevellec, V.; Roussel, S.; Tessier, L.; Chancolon, J.; Mayne-L'Hermite, M.; Deniau, G.; Viel, P.; Palacin, S. Grafting polymers on surfaces: A new powerful and versatile diazonium salt-based one-step process in aqueous media. *Chem. Mater.* **2007**, *19*, 6323–6330. [CrossRef]
80. Mesnage, A.; Esnouf, S.; Jegou, P.; Deniau, G.; Palacin, S. Understanding the redox-induced polymer grafting process: A dual surface-solution analysis. *Chem. Mater.* **2010**, *22*, 6229–6239. [CrossRef]
81. Guthy, C.; Das, R.M.; Drobot, B.; Evoy, S. Resonant characteristics of ultranarrow SiCN nanomechanical resonators. *J. Appl. Phys.* **2010**, *108*, 014306. [CrossRef]
82. Guthy, C.; Belov, M.; Janzen, A.; Quitoriano, N.J.; Singh, A.; Wright, V.A.; Finley, E.; Kamins, T.I.; Evoy, S. Large-scale arrays of nanomechanical sensors for biomolecular fingerprinting. *Sens. Actuators B Chem.* **2013**, *187*, 111–117. [CrossRef]
83. Shewchuk, D.M.; McDermott, M.T. Comparison of diazonium salt derived and thiol derived nitrobenzene layers on gold. *Langmuir* **2009**, *25*, 4556–4563. [CrossRef] [PubMed]
84. El Hadj, F.A.; Amiar, A.; Cherkaoui, M.; Chazalviel, J.N.; Ozanam, F. Study of organic grafting of the silicon surface from 4-nitrobenzene diazonium tetrafluoroborate. *Electrochim. Acta* **2012**, *70*, 318–324. [CrossRef]
85. Young, J.; Su, Y.; Lee, S.; Pak, C.; Kim, H. Enhanced durability of linker-containing carbon nanotube functionalized via diazonium reaction. *Electrochim. Acta* **2015**, *154*, 63–69.
86. Solak, A.O.; Eichorst, L.R.; Clark, W.J.; McCreery, R.L. Modified carbon surfaces as "organic electrodes" that exhibit conductance switching. *Anal. Chem.* **2003**, *75*, 296–305. [CrossRef] [PubMed]
87. Combellas, C.; Kanoufi, F.; Pinson, J.; Podvorica, F.I. Time-of-flight secondary ion mass spectroscopy characterization of the covalent bonding between a carbon surface and aryl groups. *Langmuir* **2005**, *21*, 280–286. [CrossRef] [PubMed]
88. Assresahegn, B.D.; Brousse, T.; Bélanger, D. Advances on the use of diazonium chemistry for functionalization of materials used in energy storage systems. *Carbon* **2015**, *92*, 362–381. [CrossRef]
89. Menanteau, T.; Benoît, C.; Breton, T.; Cougnon, C. Enhancing the performance of a diazonium-modified carbon supercapacitor by controlling the grafting process. *Electrochem. Commun.* **2016**, *63*, 70–73. [CrossRef]
90. Bouša, D.; Pumera, M.; Sedmidubský, D.; Šturala, J.; Luxa, J.; Mazánek, V.; Sofer, Z. Fine tuning of graphene properties by modification with aryl halogens. *Nanoscale* **2016**, *8*, 1493–1502. [CrossRef] [PubMed]
91. González, M.C.R.; Orive, A.G.; Salvarezza, R.C.; Creus, A.H. Electrodeposition of gold nanoparticles on aryl diazonium monolayer functionalized hopg surfaces. *Phys. Chem. Chem. Phys.* **2016**, *18*, 1953–1960. [CrossRef] [PubMed]
92. Stewart, M.P.; Maya, F.; Kosynkin, D.V.; Dirk, S.M.; Stapleton, J.J.; McGuiness, C.L.; Allara, D.L.; Tour, J.M. Direct covalent grafting of conjugated molecules onto si, gaas, and pd surfaces from aryidiazonium salts. *J. Am. Chem. Soc.* **2004**, *126*, 370–378. [CrossRef] [PubMed]
93. Bengamra, M.; Khlifi, A.; Ktari, N.; Mahouche-Chergui, S.; Carbonnier, B.; Fourati, N.; Kalfat, R.; Chehimi, M.M. Silanized aryl layers through thiol-yne photo-click reaction. *Langmuir* **2015**, *31*, 10717–10724. [CrossRef] [PubMed]
94. Hurley, B.L.; McCreery, R.L. Covalent bonding of organic molecules to cu and al alloy 2024 t3 surfaces via diazonium ion reduction. *J. Electrochem. Soc.* **2004**, *151*, B252–B259. [CrossRef]
95. Laurentius, L.; Stoyanov, S.R.; Gusarov, S.; Kovalenko, A.; Du, R.; Lopinski, G.P.; McDermott, M.T. Diazonium-derived aryl films on gold nanoparticles: Evidence for a carbon–gold covalent bond. *Acs Nano* **2011**, *5*, 4219–4227. [CrossRef] [PubMed]
96. Chevalier, C.L.; Landis, E.C. Electrochemical attachment of diazonium-generated films on nanoporous gold. *Langmuir* **2015**, *31*, 8633–8641. [CrossRef] [PubMed]
97. Neal, S.N.; Workie, B.; McCandless, B.E.; Mohamed, A.A. Gold-organic thin films from the reductive grafting of diazonium gold(III) salts. *J. Electroanal. Chem.* **2015**, *757*, 73–79. [CrossRef]
98. Zheng, W.; Du, R.B.; Cao, Y.; Mohammad, M.A.; Dew, S.K.; McDermott, M.T.; Evoy, S. Diazonium chemistry for the bio-functionalization of glassy nanostring resonator arrays. *Sensors* **2015**, *15*, 18724–18741. [CrossRef] [PubMed]

2

Measurement of Rapid Amiloride-Dependent pH Changes at the Cell Surface Using a Proton-Sensitive Field-Effect Transistor

Daniel Schaffhauser [1], Michael Fine [2], Miyuki Tabata [1], Tatsuro Goda [1] and Yuji Miyahara [1,*]

[1] Institute of Biomaterials & Bioengineering, Tokyo Medical and Dental University, Bldg 21-4-403B, 2-3-10 Kanda-Surugadai, Chiyoda, Tokyo 101-0062, Japan; danielschaffhauser@gmail.com (D.S.); tabata.bsr@tmd.ac.jp (M.T.); goda.bsr@tmd.ac.jp (T.G.)

[2] Department of Physiology, UT Southwestern Medical Center, 5323 Harry Hines Blvd., Dallas, TX 75390, USA; michael.fine@utsouthwestern.edu

* Correspondence: miyahara.bsr@tmd.ac.jp

Academic Editors: Mark A. Reed and Mathias Wipf

Abstract: We present a novel method for the rapid measurement of pH fluxes at close proximity to the surface of the plasma membrane in mammalian cells using an ion-sensitive field-effect transistor (ISFET). In conjuction with an efficient continuous superfusion system, the ISFET sensor was capable of recording rapid changes in pH at the cells' surface induced by intervals of ammonia loading and unloading, even when using highly buffered solutions. Furthermore, the system was able to isolate physiologically relevant signals by not only detecting the transients caused by ammonia loading and unloading, but display steady-state signals as would be expected by a proton transport-mediated influence on the extracellular proton-gradient. Proof of concept was demonstrated through the use of 5-(*N*-ethyl-*N*-isopropyl)amiloride (EIPA), a small molecule inhibitor of sodium/hydrogen exchangers (NHE). As the primary transporter responsible for proton balance during cellular regulation of pH, non-electrogenic NHE transport is notoriously difficult to detect with traditional methods. Using the NHE positive cell lines, Chinese hamster ovary (CHO) cells and NHE3-reconstituted mouse skin fibroblasts (MSF), the sensor exhibited a significant response to EIPA inhibition, whereas NHE-deficient MSF cells were unaffected by application of the inhibitor.

Keywords: ISFET; pH; proton; CHO; MSF; ammonia; amiloride; EIPA; NHE

---

1. Introduction

Proton-dependent membrane transport plays a significant role in many physiological processes, such as pH regulation in blood and tissue, maintenance of cellular volume, glycolysis or as a co-requisite for the transport and absorption of amino acids, peptides and iron [1,2]. These processes generate changes in extracellular proton gradients that are difficult to detect as the length of proton flux is largely determined by the buffering capacity of the extracellular bulk solution [3]. Improvement of the pH signal strength can thus be achieved through reduction of the buffering strength of the extracellular bulk solution or by measuring the pH in close proximity to the cell membrane. However, apart from the proton's ability to diffuse through water much faster than other ions, it has been discovered that protons are able to migrate still faster along the outside of lipid bilayers with relative ease. Several experiments have demonstrated how protons travel across large portions of a membrane before diffusing into the bulk solution. One study on the purple membrane of *H. salinarium* involved the use of Pyranine as a fluorescent pH indicator where the time constant for transfer of a proton along the membrane surface was shown to be almost six times faster than the one to the bulk solution [4]. In another study, double patch clamping was used to measure proton flux between two integral gramicidin channels, where it was found that protons could migrate along the membrane up to a distance of 200 μm [5]. Subsequently, a mathematical model for proton diffusion along biological membranes was developed by Medvedev and Stuchebrukhov which also included the influence of the buffering strength of the bulk solution on the surface proton retardation [6]. Using these principals of proton behavior along the surface of cell, we demonstrated in previous experiments that it is possible to monitor pH-dependent transport through membrane proteins heterologously expressed in large *Xenopus laevis* oocytes using an ion-sensitive field-effect transistor (ISFET) designed for proton detection [7]. Furthermore, we demonstrated that we could achieve so even when using strongly buffered solutions under constant superfusion. We took advantage of the large surface area of an oocyte and isolated a section of the membrane tightly against the sensor's surface, restricting the interface from the buffered superfusion. Under these conditions, pH-sensing was still possible, suggesting significant proton coupling between the exposed and isolated membrane sections as one would expect if protons freely "hopped" along the surface of the cell before diffusing into bulk solution. For this method, the ISFET utilized a high proton affinity Ta_2O_5 gate insulator generating significant specificity for proton detection with little interference from other ions [8]. As modeled in Figure 1, we identify the possible pathways of protons near and inside the cell. These pathways are essentially created via proton sources and sinks, all characterized by their ability to buffer protons reasonably well. In the present study, these sources and sinks are created by the inner and outer surfaces of the plasma membrane, the bulk solution and the sensor itself.

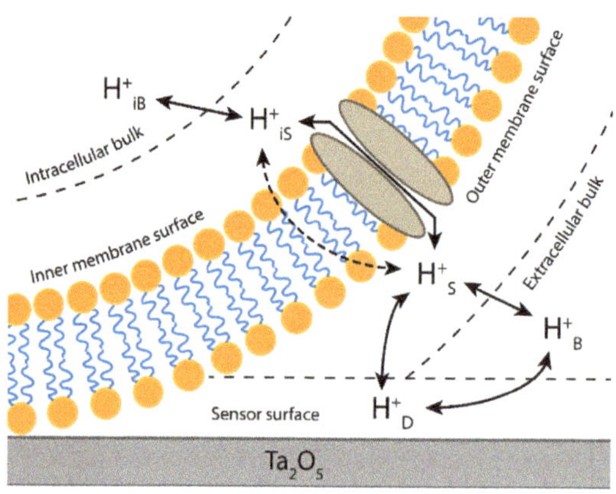

Figure 1. Simplified model of the proton pathways near the plasma membrane and the sensor surface. Proton translocation across the membrane is possible either through an active transporter protein or gated channel (**solid arrow**) or via direct diffusion across the lipid-bilayer (**dotted arrow**). In reality, charged ions and protons are unlikely to diffuse across the lipid-bilayer. However, some molecules can freely diffuse across the bilayer in their uncharged state. If these molecules associate with free protons, they can leave behind or sequester protons as they diffuse back and forth across the membrane changing the net proton balance without actual proton translocation.

Based on our previous experimental findings and success with the ISFET sensor, we developed a system for the measurement of pH at the surface of immobilized mammalian cells. It has previously been demonstrated on tumor cells that it is possible to measure their extracellular proton gradient during transient perfusion using an Al_2O_3 ISFET and after permeabilization with TX100 [9]. However, only relatively slow changes in pH could be measured. In our study, we monitored rapid pH fluxes of continuously superfused cells utilizing ammonia to briefly acidify the intracellular environment and stimulate the release of protons into the extracellular space through the sodium-coupled transport of sodium/hydrogen exchangers (NHEs). The high membrane permeability of uncharged ammonia allows the transmembranal proton balance to be altered temporarily by alternating intervals of ammonia loading and unloading [10]. During unloading, uncharged ammonia diffuses freely across the membrane into the extracellular space leaving behind a proton resulting in a net acidification of the intracellular environment. The resulting acidification of the cell is subsequently compensated through outward NHE transport of excess protons. The activation of NHEs is dependent on an inward transmembrane sodium gradient as the energy source and inhibited by the amiloride derivative 5-(*N*-ethyl-*N*-isopropyl)amiloride (EIPA) [11]. Amiloride and its derivatives are biophysical substitutes for sodium and thus inhibit NHE through competitive binding in the sodium binding pocket [12,13]. Being a diuretic, amiloride is therapeutically used to treat a number of medical conditions such as hypertension or congestive heart failure [14–17]. We opted for EIPA due to its increased affinity for NHE over other sodium-coupled transporters and high effectiveness in blocking NHE in the low-micromolar range, thus lowering the probability of interference with the sensor signal [18]. After careful optimization of the experimental parameters, it was possible to record strong pH-dependent signals near the cellular membrane, with the ability to resolve fast transients occurring during the ammonia loading and unloading intervals. EIPA-sensitive signals were indeed recorded in Chinese hamster ovary (CHO) cells and NHE3-reconstituted mouse skin fibroblasts (MSF), whereas NHE-deficient MSF were largely devoid of any EIPA response.

2. Materials and Methods

2.1. System Setup

The sensor consisted of an *n*-channel field-effect transistor (FET) with Ta_2O_5 as a gate insulator of 40 nm thickness and no metalization (ISFETCOM Co. Ltd., Hidaka, Japan). The sensor was commercially available for industrial pH applications provided in a complete package consisting of a fiberglass substrate and a polyimide cover with a window to prevent wetting of the drain and source contacts. Integration of the sensor with the solutions handling system was achieved by adhering a glass ring to the sensor top, effectively forming a reservoir of approximately 0.1 mL. A perfusion pipette containing a bundle of silica capillary tubes was mounted onto a manual two-axis positioning stage, in order to facilitate alignment of the pipette with the sensor. The individual capillary tubes were connected to a system comprising a six-fold syringe pump and three-way electrically actuated valves for channel selection. A tube for aspiration was fixed to the pipette with its opening approximately 2 mm away from the opening of the pipette. An additional syringe pump was connected to the aspiration tube to create a sink for the superfusion system. A reference electrode consisting of a chlorinated silver wire was inserted into the aspiration tube, functioning as a means for grounding the bulk solution. A schematic representation of the complete assembly is shown in Figure 2a. The assembly was mounted onto an aluminum base plate comprising mounting holes for the positioning stage onto which the pipette was mounted and a precisely machined rectangular recession for reproducible alignment of the sensor with the pipette (Figure 2b). A temperature sensor with continuous readout capability was mounted onto the base plate to ensure that the experiment was conducted at the desired temperature of 37 °C, achieved by placing the entire apparatus into an enclosed incubator. For sensor readout, the FET was operated as a source-drain follower, as described earlier [19]. The drain to source voltage was set to 0.5 V and the drain current was set to 0.5 mA. A high-resolution data-acquisition system with 50/60 Hz rejection was connected for recording the voltage between drain and reference (LabJack U6-Pro, LabJack Corp., Lakewood, CO, USA). User control and automation of the experiment was achieved through our proprietary software written in Visual Basic NET.

2.2. Cell Culture

Chinese hamster ovary (CHO) cells were maintained in Dulbecco's Modified Eagle Medium: Nutrient Mixture F-12 (DMEM/F12) (ThermoFisher Scientific, Waltham, MA, USA) supplemented with 10% fetal bovine serum (FBS) (Atlanta Biologicals, Norcross, GA, USA), non-essential amino acids, 4 mM L-Glutamine, 10 mg/L sodium pyruvate and 100 units per mL of the antibiotics penicillin and streptavidine (Sigma-Aldrich, St. Louis, MO, USA). Cells were cultured in a humidified 37 °C cell-culture incubator with 5% CO_2. Mouse skin fibroblasts (MSF) were maintained and supplemented as described above using DMEM as the base medium. Passaging of cells was performed at approximately 80% confluence. For each passage and prior to experimentation, cells were washed in Dulbecco's phosphate-buffered saline (ThermoFisher Scientific, Waltham, MA, USA) and trypsinized in a Ca^{2+}- and Mg^{2+}-free solution for 5 min using a trypsin concentration of 0.25% weight per volume (Gibco).

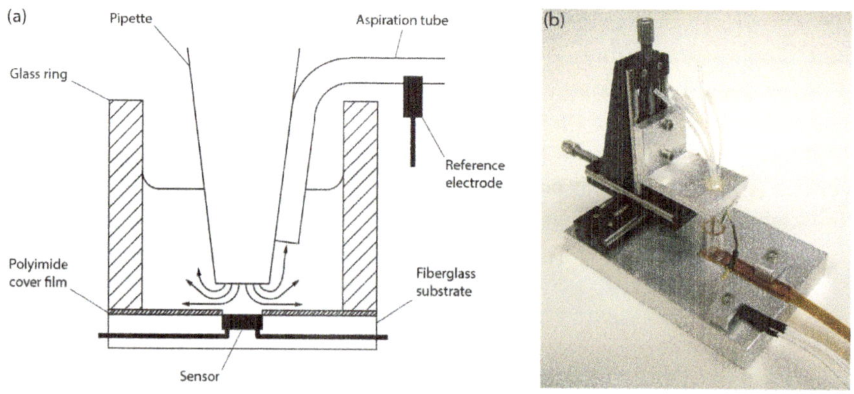

Figure 2. (**a**) Graphical representation of the integration concept; (**b**) Photographic image of the unconnected setup.

2.3. Solutions and Reagents

An isotonic solution similar to Ringer's solution containing 140 mM NaCl, 4 mM KCl and 1 mM $MgCl_2$, adjusted to a pH of 7.4, was used as a base solution for all experiments. Buffering of the solutions was achieved through the addition of either 1 mM or 10 mM bis-tris propane (BTP), a buffer known for its very wide buffering range. Sucrose was added to solutions to maintain equiosmolar conditions and prevent any influence of osmosis and cellular shrinking or swelling on the signal. For the solutions containing ammonia, 20 mM of NH_4Cl was added and any pH shift was accounted for by titration with NaOH. In addition, 10 μM EIPA (Sigma-Aldrich) was added to the final buffered solution for NHE-inhibition.

2.4. Sample Preparation and Experimental Procedure

The sensor surface was cleaned using a solution consisting of deionized (DI) water, NH_4OH and H_2O_2 to ensure that no organic material remained attached to the sensor surface. After rinsing with DI water, 100 μL of aqueous 0.01% (*w*/*v*) poly-L-lysine solution (Sigma-Aldrich) was pipetted into the sample reservoir and left for 10 min at room temperature. The reservoir was then rinsed with DI water and dried using N_2 gas. During the sensor incubation with poly-L-lysine, confluent cells were trypsinized and placed back into suspension with serum containing medium at 37 °C. When the sensor was completely dry, 100 μL of the cell suspension was pipetted into the reservoir and the entire assembly was placed in a 37 °C, 5% CO_2 incubator for 3 h, allowing the cells to settle and attach onto the sensor surface. After incubation, the remaining solution was carefully aspirated and replaced with warmed experimental buffer solutions. The assembly was then placed in a small incubator capable of maintaining the experimental temperature of 37 °C. The superfusion system was activated with a constant flow of buffer solution until the signal drift reached acceptably low levels (approximately 1 to 3 min). A superfusion sequence consisting of alternating solutions with and without ammonia was initiated to stimulate the cells' response to changes in intracellular pH (pH_i). In later experiments, EIPA was used during the unloading phase to inhibit the cells' response to intracellular acidification through an NHE blockade.

Figure 3 shows a representative experimental signal generated at the sensor surface during the intervals of ammonia loading and unloading in the absence and presence of EIPA. In the first interval, NH_3 diffuses rapidly across the plasma membrane, releasing protons at the external surface of the membrane. This proton loss results in a localized decrease in extracellular pH (pH_e) that is detected by the sensor as illustrated by the upward transient and elevated steady state. Once uncharged NH_3 diffuses across the bilayer into the cytosol, it rapidly protonates, reducing intracellular free proton concentration and causing an increase in pH_i. As the membrane bilayer is relatively impermeable to charged protons, only the increase in free protons on the outside of the cell is readily detected by the sensor. Due to the fast reaction kinetics and diffusion rates as well as the limited intracellular volume, the reaction quickly reaches steady-state equilibrium, allowing the next interval to start approximately 30 s after initiating the ammonia loading. In the next interval (2), external ammonia is removed, creating a strong chemical gradient from the intracellular to the extracellular space. This drives cytosolic uncharged NH_3 out of the cell through diffusion across the plasma membrane where it sequesters free protons outside the cell, transiently raising pH_e, and, importantly, leaving behind a free proton inside the cell, thus lowering pH_i. This intracellular acidification in turn facilitates the sodium-coupled transport of NHE, counteracting the intracellular acidification via the exchange of internal H^+ with external Na^+. During this phase, the sensor will detect a combination of signals driven primarily at first by the transient diffusion of NH_3 to the outside where it protonates and briefly increases pH_e. This is followed by the slower facilitated transport of NHE exchanging extracellular sodium for intracellular proton resulting in an upward voltage shift (decrease in pH_e) in relation to the initial fast downward voltage shift generated by the transient diffusion of NH_3. In the third interval, the addition of EIPA specifically inhibits the activity of NHE, allowing analysis of its contribution to the detected signal via comparison with the signal of the second interval. The resulting difference between the second and third interval allows for the detailed examination of contribution to extracellular acidification near the membrane by NHE transport.

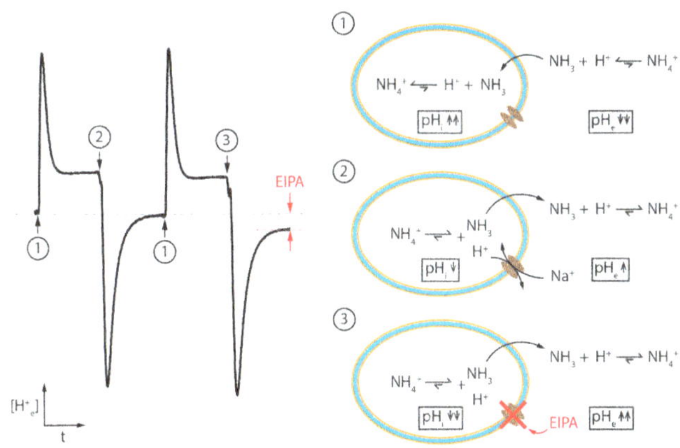

Figure 3. Typical ISFET signals generated during the three individuals intervals. Each interval has a duration of approximately 30 s. The black dotted line indicates the baseline when superfusing with buffered solution. Black arrows indicate the change to the next solution. The red dotted line and red arrows indicate the signal difference caused by the presence of EIPA. The sensor's signal is proportional to the external proton concentration [$H^+{}_e$], and, therefore, inversely proportional to the external pH (pH_e) [7]. Interval 1 is the intracellular alkalinization through exposure to $NH_4{}^+$. Interval 2 is the intracellular acidification through removal of $NH_4{}^+$. This activates NHE, causing the release of intracellular H^+. Interval 3 is similar to interval 2, but with the addition of EIPA, inhibiting the NHE-mediated release of H^+. The result is a reduction in the [$H^+{}_e$] and sensor signal as inhibition of NHE generated a larger increase in near-membrane pH_e compared to that of interval 2. Note that, like interval 2, interval 3 is preceded by interval 1 in order to restore the cells to their initial condition and generate an acidified intracellular environment.

3. Results and Discussion

3.1. *Optimization of the Superfusion*

In order to obtain the best response from the sensor, we adjusted the distance between the tip of the pipette and the center of the active sensor surface. A shorter distance resulted in an improvement of the solution exchange efficiency and therefore faster signals with higher amplitude. However, the shear stress on the cells increased with decreasing distance and thus increased the risk of cell detachment from the sensor surface (Figure 4). An increase in flow rate had similar effects and it became crucial to optimize the superfusion system using both parameters. In the end, we found a good compromise between flow stability, cell stability and minimal use of solution using a flow rate between 1 and 2 μL/s and a distance of approximately 0.2 mm between tip and sensor surface. To put this into perspective, the largest dimension of the active area of the sensor was approximately 0.3 mm (Figure 4). To verify that the cells had not detached during the experiment, microscopic images of each sample were taken before and after individual experiments. Computational fluid analysis (CFD) using the solvers for the Navier–Stokes equation and Fickian diffusion equation in COMSOL confirmed that quick and efficient solution exchange without turbulent flow is provided at these conditions. In the simulation, the solution leaving the pipette reached the sensor in a little over 1 s, which was deemed acceptable considering the duration of the individual superfusion cycles are a minimum of 30 s (Figure 5).

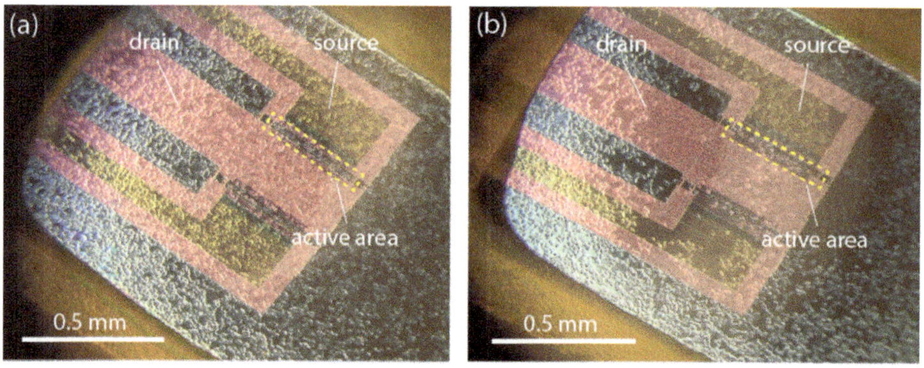

Figure 4. Microscopic photographs of CHO cells attached to the poly-D-lysine coated sensor. The yellow dotted box indicates the active area of the sensor. Images were taken (**a**) before and (**b**) after superfusion. In this case, there was too much shear stress on the cells, causing them to detach during the experiment. Under optimized conditions, there were no significant differences detected between the images taken before and after each experiment.

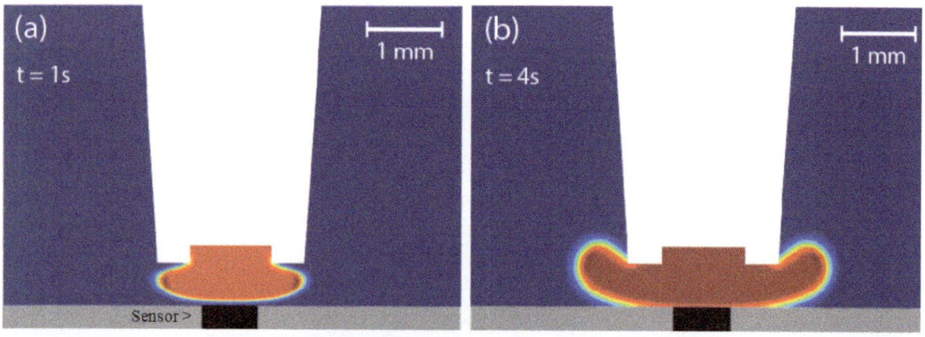

Figure 5. CFD analysis of the flow exiting the pipette (white area) when switching to a new solution. The deep blue area is old solution and the deep red area is new solution. (**a**) shows the distribution of new solution 1 s after switching and (**b**) after 4 s.

3.2. Ammonia Loading and Unloading

We determined the ideal buffer concentration of the superfusion solutions through assessment of the signals recorded during alternating cycles of ammonia loading and unloading. As expected, lower buffer concentrations resulted in signals with higher amplitude but also reduced their responsiveness due to the slower exchange between the bulk solution and the cell surface. Buffer optimization was dependent not only on signal intensity and speed, but on the fact that lower concentrations of buffer increase the susceptibility to changes in pH when other ions like ammonia, with a relatively high pK_a of 9.4, are added and removed.

Figure 6a shows a superfusion sequence using 20 mM NH_4Cl with 10 mM buffer concentration followed by a 1 mM buffer. The behavior of the signal drift is excellent, amounting to approximately +0.2 mV over a time course of 4 min and 20 s. In combination with a very low noise floor, this allows reliable measurement of signals well below 1 mV. As expected, the transient signals have a much lower amplitude at 10 mM than at 1 mM. This is most likely due to the increased proton exchange efficiency between the cell surface and the bulk solution, giving newly generated or consumed protons at the cell surface less probability for being detected by the sensor. The transient signal during the unloading cycle is stronger than during the loading cycle, which can be explained by the accumulation of intracellular NH_3. As these are intact cells, intracellular ammonia can continue to rise as there is no cap on the initial rise of the intracellular pH governing the balance between NH_3 and NH_4^+, whereas ammonia and buffer pH are tightly controlled on the outside of the cell. As NH_3 rapidly diffuses out of the cell, the unloading transient returns to steady-state levels where the rate and signal are primarily controlled by proton flux emanating from the cytosol. Interestingly, the respective steady-state signals differ as well, even though the cell-free control shows no significant difference in the signal between the solutions with and without ammonia (Figure 6b). This effect during the ammonia loading is triggered by a similar mechanism in which cytosolic pH elevation favors protonation of ammonia into NH_4^+. This increases the amount of NH_3 that is available to diffuse into the cell during the steady-state phase as pH is elevated and thus the level of free protons left on the outside of the cell membrane detected by the sensor. A change in the steady-state signal is also observed when the buffer is switched between 1 mM and 10 mM. More protons are detected at 1 mM, which confirms a higher proton concentration near the cell surface than in bulk, as well as an attenuation of the signal at 10 mM due to a higher buffering power of the bulk solution. If there was no difference in the signal, this would implicate that there was either no proton gradient or that such a gradient was not detectable by the sensor. A comparison of the difference in the steady-state signals when switching ammonia reveals that there is different behavior between 1 mM and 10 mM buffer concentration. At 10 mM, there are more protons detected when switching on the ammonia, whereas at 1 mM there is a reduction. We assume that it could be caused by pH regulatory effects of the cells and alterations in transport activity. Loading the cells with uncharged ammonia causes an increase in cytosolic pH due to protonation of the ammonia. This leads to a reduction in activity of NHE, effectively weakening the extracellular proton gradient. This explanation is evident at 1 mM buffer concentration, but at 10 mM, the effect is reversed as the reduction of NHE activity due to elevated cytosolic pH is masked at higher extracellular buffer concentrations. While this could suggest that simple alterations in extracellular buffer may reveal functional output of surface membrane transporters (*i.e.*, decreases in NHE activity) during the ammonia loading phase, it was decided that subsequent analysis of transporter derived proton flux focuses on detecting increases in activity during cellular acidification. To this extent, the unloading phase with 10 mM buffer provided a more physiologically relevant and consistent signal to specifically detect increases in proton flux via NHE.

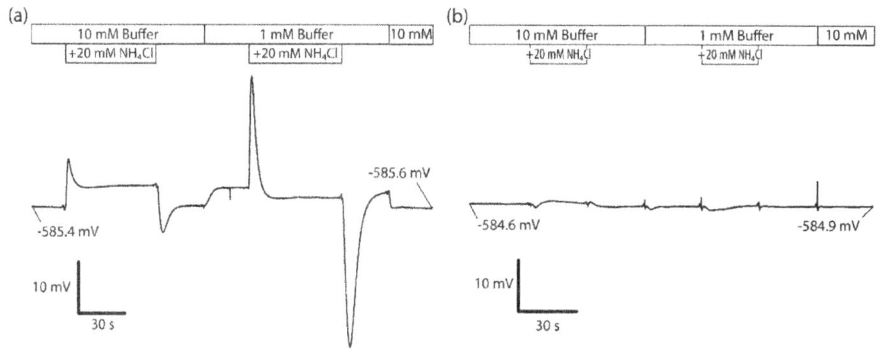

Figure 6. Superfusion sequence utilizing ammonia loading and unloading intervals at 10 mM and 1 mM buffer concentration in the (**a**) presence and (**b**) absence of cells on the sensor.

3.3. Repeated Ammonia Cycles and Dependence on Cell Density

In order to assess how the signal intensity scales with cell density, two representative experiments were compared with differing cell densities. Figure 7a shows a superfusion sequence conducted on sample with approximately 18 cells attached to the active sensor area. Eight cycles of ammonia loading and unloading were performed with the presence of the NHE inhibitor EIPA during the unloading phase of cycles 3, 5 and 7. Although the influence of EIPA will not be discussed in this section, we found it important to optimize performance and generate conditions directly comparable to the proceeding section. Measuring the peak-to-peak intensity between the loading and unloading phases of a cycle, we found that the signal increased approximately 26% from an initial 78 mV to 98 mV over the course of eight cycles. However, the negative peaks from the unloading phases mainly contributed to this increase, whereas the positive peaks from the loading phases remained virtually constant. As the peak loading signal is generated from controlled exposure of exogenous ammonia, the small decrease in the midline and unloading peak may correspond to a change in the cellular physiological state. Ammonia has been reported to have many long term effects on cell culture and repeated exposure to ammonia may decrease the ability of the cell to maximally extrude cytosolic protons, resulting in a slow decrease in the sensor signal [20]. Consequently, the steady-state difference between the loading and unloading phases decreased by approximately 9% from an initial 7.5 mV to 6.9 mV over the course of eight cycles. If the steady-state signals are indeed dependent on the extracellular proton gradient, a decrease of the signal would suggest a decrease of the cells' pH regulatory activity.

Figure 7b shows the same experiment performed on a different sample with a lower cell density of approximately 11 cells on the active area of the sensor. Again, we observed an increase of approximately 24% in peak-to-peak intensity, although with lower amplitudes from an initial 48.5 mV to 60 mV after eight cycles. The steady state signals decreased by approximately 8% from an initial 6.7 mV to 6.2 mV after eight cycles. Comparing the cell densities between the two experiments, a proportional relationship with the peak-to-peak intensities is found: an increase in cell density of approximately 75% resulted in an increase in sensor signal of approximately 63%. In the case of the steady-state signals, however, the increase was only 11%. A quantitative relationship between the transient signals and the steady-state signals cannot be established at this stage. However, the general trend that an increased cell density on the sensor results in increased cell-dependent signal levels remains intact.

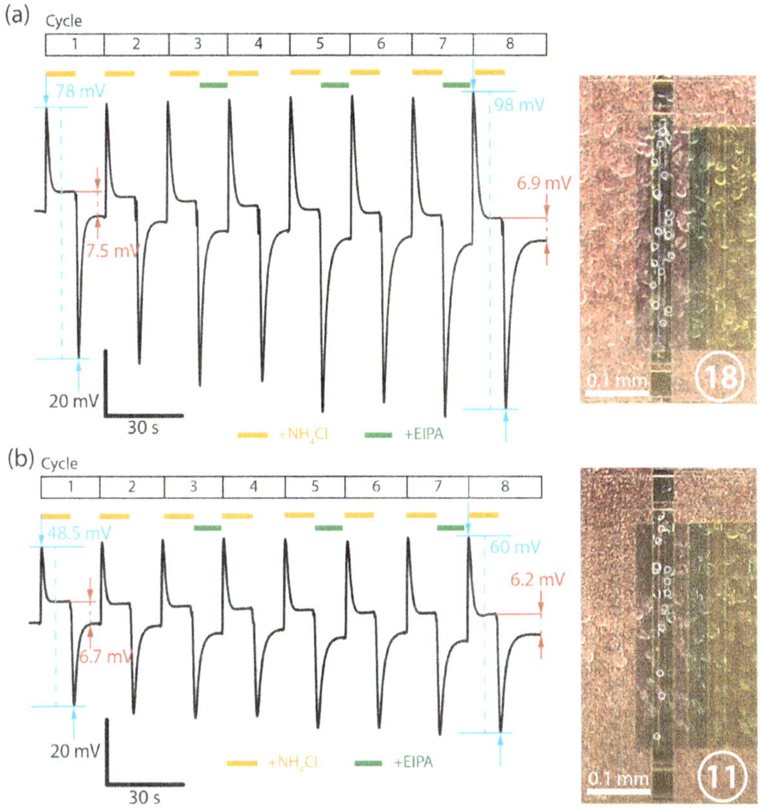

Figure 7. Superfusion sequence of alternating ammonia loading and unloading intervals. Cycles 3, 5 and 7 are unloading intervals in the presence of EIPA. Two representative samples with approximate cell densities of (**a**) 18 cells and (**b**) 11 cells are depicted. White circles mark individual cells.

3.4. Amiloride-Sensitivity

To determine the sensor efficacy for evaluation of physiological transporter activity, we focused on the non-electrogenic transport of protons through the sodium-hydrogen exchanger. EIPA is a member of the amiloride class of diuretics that has been classically used for studies involving NHE transport due to its rapid kinetics and exceptional inhibition across most members of the NHE superfamily [18]. The EIPA-sensitive response from Chinese hamster ovary (CHO) cells, NHE-deficient mouse skin fibroblasts (MSF) and NHE-deficient mouse skin fibroblasts reconstituted with NHE3 was evaluated. In order to obtain the EIPA-sensitive response, the dataset of the ammonia unloading phase was subtracted from the dataset of the ammonia unloading phase in the presence of EIPA (Figure 8a). Figure 8b shows the average EIPA-response of three CHO samples. The signal is composed of two main transients, peaking at +33 mV after 7 s with a rapid drop thereafter, bottoming out at −15 mV after 14 s and finally transitioning into an asymptotic recovery phase. This suggests the presence of two mechanisms: (a) an initial fast transient characterized by an EIPA-dependent decrease in the transient alkalinization of the extracellular space; (b) a slower response in the opposite direction as the cytosol becomes acidic indicating an increase in the near-surface proton flux emanating from the cell. As the second slower response is characterized by a low cytosolic pH gradient, it is clear that this reduced sensor signal is attributed to the inhibition of the canonical mode of transport of NHE, namely the exchange of Na^+ with H^+ as both ions are strongly favored for transport along the chemical gradients. What is less clear is the interpretation of the initial fast transient demonstrating an EIPA-sensitive decrease in extracellular basification. During the first transient, the sensor indicates a strong basification on the extracellular space, which is predominantly non-EIPA-sensitive. This is due to the rapid diffusion of intracellular NH_3 across the bilayer during washout. Once in the extracellular space, NH_3 is rapidly protonated to NH_4^+, generating the basification indicated by the sensor. EIPA should not directly effect the diffusion of ammonia across the bilayer and there should be no signal difference during this phase; however, it is clear that this response is attenuated by the presence of EIPA. One possibility of how EIPA could mitigate this response is through the non-canonical transport of NH_4^+ in exchange for sodium via NHE. It has been demonstrated previously that NH_4^+ can be transported by directly competing with cytosolic proton binding during NHE exchange [11,21–23]. Moreover, extracellular NH_4^+ is unlikely to be deprotonated and detected by the sensor due to its low dissociation constant of around 1% at near physiological pH [23]. This suggests that under EIPA-free conditions there is a partial contribution of NHE toward the basification of the extracellular space as NHE favors the transport of NH_4^+. This transient mode would only be possible during the initial moments of washout when cytosolic pH is high and passive diffusion of NH_3 has not yet led to a rapid drop in both pH and free ammonia levels. The NHE dependent transport of charged ammonia out of the cell slows down the acidification process and allows more uncharged NH_3 to diffuse out of the cell, become protonated and generate an increased drop in sensor signal. Blockage of NHE through EIPA at this time appears to cause extracellular acidification, converse to its normal mode of operation, but is likely due to NHE transport of NH_4^+ being blocked, causing alterations in NH_3 diffusion rates. After the ammonia has been driven out of the cells, free protons remain in the cytosol, activating the main mode of NHE (second transient) and the sensor predominantly detects EIPA-dependent extracellular acidification from proton transport across NHE.

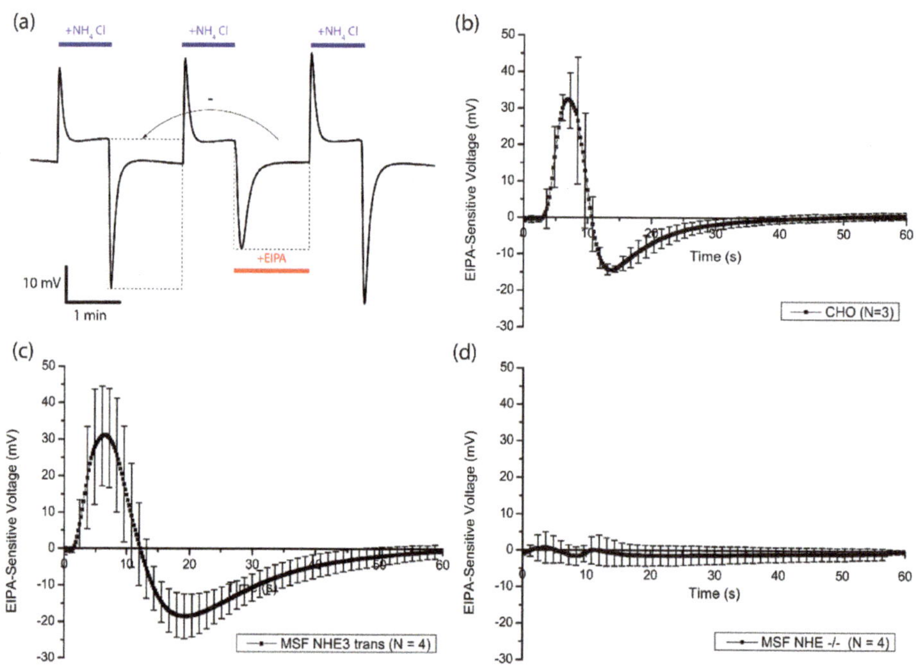

Figure 8. (**a**) superfusion sequence of three cycles of ammonia loading and unloading on CHO cells. The second cycle was performed in the presence of EIPA. Dotted boxes show the data that was used for the subtraction in order to obtain the EIPA-sensitive curves: Averaged curves of (**b**) three CHO samples, (**c**) four NHE3-reconstitued MSF samples and (**d**) four NHE-deficient MSF samples.

The EIPA response in MSF reconstituted with NHE3 showed a similar pattern to the CHO cells, with a comparable peak value for the first transient, but a more pronounced recovery phase thereafter (Figure 8c). As the recovery phase is indicative of proton transport through NHE, differences in this phase are likely due to factors that affect the expression level and function of NHE in a cell-type specific manner as well as physiological characteristics of individual cell types such as surface area to volume ratios and intracellular buffering capabilities. In NHE-deficient MSF, no significant EIPA-response was recorded (Figure 8d), as would be expected from cells with no means for H^+/Na^+ exchange.

4. Conclusions

In this article, we described a system for measuring the pH response of mammalian cells in close proximity to the plasma membrane using an ISFET sensor and a continuous superfusion system. We obtained fast, stable and strong pH signals from CHO cells and MSF using BTP as a buffer agent at 1 mM and 10 mM. Short intervals of ammonia loading and unloading proved to be a viable method for stimulating cellular pH response via intracellular alkalinization through NH_3 loading followed by rapid intracellular acidification during washout. Optical observations before and after experimentation revealed no obvious visual markers for cell membrane stress including membrane shedding, blebs or the formation of large intracellular puncta even after many repetitions of these cycles. However, a gradual shift of the transient signal occurred, possibly as a result of ammonia generating a successive and altered cellular response to pH stress [20]. The amplitude of the signal was also found to be dependent on the cell density at the sensor surface. Furthermore, cell-dependent steady-state signals were detected, suggesting that the ISFET sensor was not only capable of recording transient signals but also the extracellular proton-gradient. Finally, a series of experiments using EIPA as a potent blocking agent for NHE was conducted to isolate the NHE-dependent transport during the unloading of ammonia. We found that CHO cells as well as NHE-deficient MSF reconstituted with NHE3 responded positively to EIPA. NHE-deficient MSF exhibited virtually no response. To our surprise, the positive EIPA-responses consisted of multiple transients whose mechanisms remain to be fully elucidated but appear related to reports indicating the capability of direct ammonium transport through NHE. Nevertheless, this work may lay the foundation for further investigation regarding the evaluating of agents acting on pH-regulatory pathways. The next important steps would include experimentation to obtain dose-response curves and investigation of other proton-sensitive membrane proteins such as ATP-dependent proton-pumps. This would open the possibility for many applications furthering our basic knowledge of the fast transport kinetics of many difficult to evaluate transporters and channels. Due to the method's relative low cost combined with scalability, speed and reliability, these techniques could generate novel applications in drug discovery, screening and diagnostics for a myriad of clinically relevant disciplines.

Acknowledgments: We acknowledge funding and advice provided by Orson Moe and Donald Hilgemann of University of Texas Southwestern Medical Center.

Author Contributions: D.S., M.F. and T.G. conceived and designed the experiments; D.S., T.G. and M.T. performed the experiments; D.S. analyzed the data; Y.M. contributed reagents/materials/analysis tools; D.S. and M.F. wrote the paper.

Conflicts of Interest: The authors declare no conflict of interest.

References

1. Mueckler, M.; Thorens, B. The SLC2 (GLUT) family of membrane transporters. *ABCs Membr. Transp. Health Dis. SLC Ser.* **2013**, *34*, 121–138.
2. Orlowski, J.; Grinstein, S. Diversity of the mammalian sodium/proton exchanger SLC9 gene family. *Pflüg. Arch.* **2003**, *447*, 549–565.
3. Fuster, D.; Moe, O.W.; Hilgemann, D.W. Lipid- and mechanosensitivities of sodium/hydrogen exchangers analyzed by electrical methods. *Proc. Natl. Acad. Sci. USA* **2004**, *101*, 10482–10487. [PubMed]
4. Alexiev, U.; Mollaaghababa, R.; Scherrer, P.; Khorana, H.G.; Heyn, M.P. Rapid long-range proton diffusion along the surface of the purple membrane and delayed proton transfer into the bulk. *Proc. Natl. Acad. Sci. USA* **1995**, *92*, 372–376. [CrossRef] [PubMed]

5. Antonenko, Y.N.; Pohl, P. Coupling of proton source and sink via H^+-migration along the membrane surface as revealed by double patch-clamp experiments. *FEBS Lett.* **1998**, *429*, 197–200. [CrossRef]
6. Medvedev, E.S.; Stuchebrukhov, A.A. Proton diffusion along biological membranes. *J. Phys. Condens. Matter* **2011**, *23*. [CrossRef] [PubMed]
7. Schaffhauser, D.F.; Patti, M.; Goda, T.; Miyahara, Y.; Forster, I.C.; Dittrich, P.S. An Integrated Field-Effect Microdevice for Monitoring Membrane Transport in Xenopus laevis Oocytes via Lateral Proton Diffusion. *PLoS ONE* 2012, *7*, e39238. [CrossRef] [PubMed]
8. Van Hal, R.E.G.; Eijkel, J.C.T.; Bergveld, P. A novel description of ISFET sensitivity with the buffer capacity and double-layer capacitance as key parameters. *Sens. Actuators B Chem.* **1995**, *24*, 201–205. [CrossRef]
9. Lehmann, M.; Baumann, W.; Brischwein, M.; Ehret, R.; Kraus, M.; Schwinde, A.; Bitzenhofer, M.; Freund, I.; Wolf, B. Non-invasive measurement of cell membrane associated proton gradients by ion-sensitive field effect transistor arrays for microphysiological and bioelectronical applications. *Biosens. Bioelectron.* **2000**, *15*, 117–124. [CrossRef]
10. Antonenko, Y.N.; Pohl, P.; Denisov, G.A. Permeation of ammonia across bilayer lipid membranes studied by ammonium ion selective microelectrodes. *Biophys. J.* **1997**, *72*, 2187–2195. [CrossRef]
11. Mahnensmith, R.L.; Aronson, P.S. The plasma membrane sodium-hydrogen exchanger and its role in physiological and pathophysiological processes. *Circ. Res.* **1985**, *56*, 773–788. [CrossRef] [PubMed]
12. Fuster, D.; Moe, O.W.; Hilgemann, D.W. Steady-state Function of the Ubiquitous Mammalian Na/H Exchanger (NHE1) in Relation to Dimer Coupling Models with 2Na/2H Stoichiometry. *J. Gen. Physiol.* **2008**, *132*, 465–480. [CrossRef] [PubMed]
13. Bobulescu, I.A.; Di Sole, F.; Moe, O.W. Na^+/H^+ exchangers: Physiology and link to hypertension and organ ischemia. *Curr. Opin. Nephrol. Hypertens.* **2005**, *14*, 485–494. [CrossRef] [PubMed]
14. Karmazyn, M. Amiloride enhances postischemic ventricular recovery: Possible role of Na^+-H^+ exchange. *Am. J. Physiol. Heart Circ. Physiol.* **1988**, *255*, H608–H615.
15. Karmazyn, M.; Moffat, M.P. Role of Na^+/H^+ exchange in cardiac physiology and pathophysiology: Mediation of myocardial reperfusion injury by the pH paradox. *Cardiovasc. Res.* **1993**, *27*, 915–924. [CrossRef] [PubMed]
16. Hale, S.L.; Kloner, R.A. Effect of combined KATP channel activation and Na^+/H^+ exchange inhibition on infarct size in rabbits. *Am. J. Physiol. Heart Circ. Physiol.* **2000**, *279*, H2673–H2677. [PubMed]
17. Gumina, R.J.; Moore, J.; Schelling, P.; Beier, N.; Gross, G.J. Na^+/H^+ exchange inhibition prevents endothelial dysfunction after I/R injury. *Am. J. Physiol. Heart Circ. Physiol.* **2001**, *281*, H1260–H1266. [PubMed]
18. Masereel, B.; Pochet, L.; Laeckmann, D. An overview of inhibitors of Na^+/H^+ exchanger. *Eur. J. Med. Chem.* 2003, *38*, 547–554. [CrossRef]
19. Casans, S.; Ramirez, D.; Navarro, A. Circuit provides constant current ISFETs/MEMFETs. *EDN* **2000**, *45*, 164.
20. Schneider, M.; Marison, I.W.; von Stockar, U. The importance of ammonia in mammalian cell culture. *J. Biotechnol.* **1996**, *46*, 161–185. [CrossRef]
21. Nagami, G.T. Luminal secretion of ammonia in the mouse proximal tubule perfused *in vitro*. *J. Clin. Investig.* 1988, *81*, 159–164. [CrossRef] [PubMed]
22. Weiner, I.D.; Hamm, L.L. Molecular Mechanisms of Renal Ammonia Transport. *Annu. Rev. Physiol.* **2007**, *69*, 317–340. [CrossRef] [PubMed]
23. Weiner, I.D.; Verlander, J.W. Role of NH_3 and NH_4^+ transporters in renal acid-base transport. *Am. J. Physiol. Ren. Physiol.* **2011**, *300*, F11–F23. [CrossRef] [PubMed]

3

Semi-Quantitative Method for Streptococci Magnetic Detection in Raw Milk

Carla Duarte [1,2,*], Tiago Costa [3], Carla Carneiro [2], Rita Soares [1], Andrei Jitariu [1,4], Susana Cardoso [1,5], Moisés Piedade [3], Ricardo Bexiga [2] and Paulo Freitas [1,6]

1 INESC–MN Instituto de Engenharia de Sistemas e Computadores—Microsistemas e Nanotecnologias, Rua Alves Redol 9, 1000-029 Lisbon, Portugal; ritasoares18@hotmail.com (R.S.); ajitariu@phys-iasi.ro (A.J.); scardoso@inesc-mn.pt (S.C.); Paulo.Freitas@inl.int (P.F.)

2 CIISA at Faculdade de Medicina Veterinária, Universidade de Lisboa, Av. da Universidade Técnica, 1300-477 Lisbon, Portugal; carla.n.carneiro@gmail.com (C.C.); ricardobexiga@fmv.ulisboa.pt (R.B.)

3 INESC-ID Instituto de Engenharia de Sistemas e Computadores—Investigação e Desenvolvimento, Rua Alves Redol 9, 1000-029 Lisbon, Portugal; tiagomlcosta@gmail.com (T.C.); msp@inesc-id.pt (M.P.)

4 Visiting from the National Institute of Research and Development for Technical Physics, 47 Mangeron Blvd, Iasi 700050, Romania

5 Instituto Superior Técnico, Physics Department, Av. Rovisco Pais, 1049-001 Lisbon, Portugal

6 International Iberian Nanotechnology Laboratory (INL), Av. Mestre José Veiga, 4715-330 Braga, Portugal

* Correspondence: duarte.margarida72@gmail.com

Academic Editor: Domenico Caputo

Abstract: Bovine mastitis is the most costly disease for dairy farmers and the most frequent reason for the use of antibiotics in dairy cattle; thus, control measures to detect and prevent mastitis are crucial for dairy farm sustainability. The aim of this study was to develop and validate a sensitive method to magnetically detect *Streptococcus agalactiae* (a Group B streptococci) and *Streptococcus uberis* in raw milk samples. Mastitic milk samples were collected aseptically from 44 cows with subclinical mastitis, from 11 Portuguese dairy farms. Forty-six quarter milk samples were selected based on bacterial identification by conventional microbiology. All samples were submitted to PCR analysis. In parallel, these milk samples were mixed with a solution combining specific antibodies and magnetic nanoparticles, to be analyzed using a lab-on-a-chip magnetoresistive cytometer, with microfluidic sample handling. This paper describes a point of care methodology used for detection of bacteria, including analysis of false positive/negative results. This immunological recognition was able to detect bacterial presence in samples spiked above 100 cfu/mL, independently of antibody and targeted bacteria used in this work. Using PCR as a reference, this method correctly identified 73% of positive samples for streptococci species with an anti-*S. agalactiae* antibody, and 41% of positive samples for an anti-GB streptococci antibody.

Keywords: magnetoresistive sensors; magnetic nanoparticle (NP); *Streptococcus agalactiae*; *Streptococcus uberis*; milk; immunogenic recognition; microfluidic

1. Introduction

Bovine mastitis, the inflammation of the mammary gland most often with infectious origin, is the most costly disease for dairy farmers and the most frequent reason for the use of antibiotics in dairy cattle; thus, control measures to prevent mastitis are crucial for farm sustainability. The identification of contagious bacteria that cause mastitis is necessary to control the disease in the herd, reduce the risk of chronic infections, and target antimicrobial therapy. *Streptococcus agalactiae* (a Lancefield Group B Streptococci) and *Streptococcus uberis* (no Lancefield group) are major mastitis pathogens [1] that can be transmitted from cow to cow in the milking parlor in a contagious way [2]. Their identification is currently performed most often through conventional bacteriology, by growth of bacteria in culture media, isolation, and identification based on phenotypic features. This methodology is time-consuming, with results taking between 48 and 72 h to be obtained, and can lead to no-growth results corresponding to false negatives. In these cases, phenotypic identification is being supplemented with genotypic methods, such as polymerase chain reaction (PCR) [3], for more accurate identification of bacteria associated with intramammary infections.

The suitability of a detection method for routine diagnosis as "cow-side use" depends mainly on the time to produce results, sensitivity, and specificity. Immunological identification of mastitis pathogens has been reported [4,5]. These authors suggested that the diagnosis of clinical mastitis cases could be considerably enhanced if samples showing no growth on culture media could be subjected to an enzyme-linked immunosorbent assay (ELISA), because of the antibodies' observed ability to detect soluble, as well as insoluble, antigens, independently of intact bacterial cell presence in milk. The basis for a true positive result in immunological analysis is the confidence on the specificity of the selected antibody. As mentioned in previous work [6], Western blotting assays using a polyclonal anti-GB streptococci antibody evidenced two stained immunogenic proteins in *Streptococcus uberis* cell wall proteins' pattern besides the expected immunogenic protein set of *Streptococcus agalactiae*. According to Groschup and colleagues [7], some *Streptococcus uberis* strains can also react with Lancefield group B serum.

The use of portable platforms to detect bacteria has been optimized [8] allowing for cell separation, identification and counting to be achieved in a compact and modular format. This feature can be combined with magnetic detection, where magnetoresistive (MR) sensors can be integrated within microfluidic channels to detect magnetically-labeled cells, being promising as one emerging technology for magnetic biodetection [9,10].

The aim of this study was to develop and validate a sensitive method for magnetic detection of *Streptococcus agalactiae* and *Streptococcus uberis* in raw milk samples. For both magnetic detection and conventional microbiology methods, sensitivity, specificity, and positive predictive value (PPV) were calculated in comparison with the PCR reference method.

2. Materials and Methods

2.1. Method Principles

This dynamic detection is based on the detection of the fringe field created by magnetic particles attached to the bacterial cells. By selecting the suitable antibodies, it is possible to perform immunological recognition of Group B Streptococci (including *Streptococcus agalactiae*) and of *Streptococcus uberis* immunogenic proteins (Figure 1A,B). A polyclonal anti-GB Streptococci IgG (8435-2000, AbD Serotec, Kidlington, UK) and one monoclonal anti-*Streptococcus agalactiae* IgM (MA1-10871, Thermo Fisher, Waltham, USA), were used separately. The antibodies were expected to attach to protein A of Nanomag®-D-spio 50 nm particles (79-20-501, MicromodPartikeltechnolo-gie GmbH, Rostock, Germany), by the Fc fraction in immunoglobulins G and by the joining chain (J chain) in immunoglobulins M (Figure 1C). Antibodies and bacterial cell dimensions are shown in Figure 1.

The bio-functionalization of nanoparticles was achieved by the addition of 7.27 μL from the nanoparticles' original vial to 0.53 μL of polyclonal anti-GB streptococci antibody (1 mg/mL) (or to 5.5 μL of monoclonal anti-*Streptococcus agalactiae* antibody (0.5 mg/mL)) in 492.2 μL (or 487.2 μL) of PBS. The incubation step required 1 h at room temperature (RT) and continuous agitation. Final functionalized particles were magnetically isolated by a MS column (130-042-201 Miltenyi, Bergisch Gladbach, Germany) according to MACS MiltenyiBiotec protocol and eluted with phosphate-buffered saline (PBS) + 0.5% bovine serum albumin (BSA) + 2mM ethylene diamine tetra acetic acid (EDTA) buffer after removal of the MS column from the magnet. A volume of 2 μL of this final suspension was added to each PBS or milk sample.

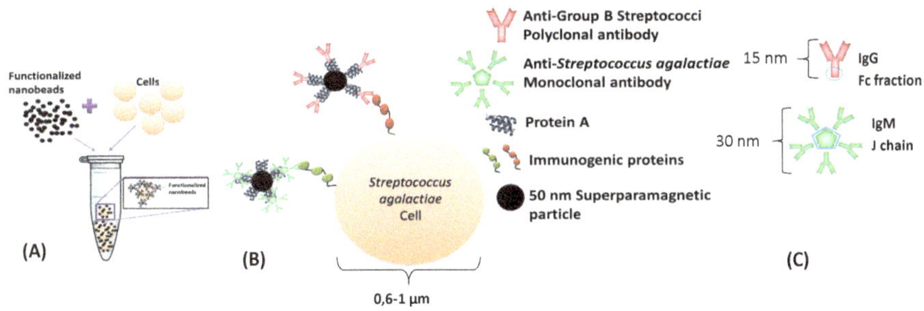

Figure 1. Schematic of immuno-magnetic detection of cells. (**A**) Incubation of functionalized NPs with bacterial cells; and (**B**) biological affinities between different functionalized NPs with bacterial cell wall immunogenic proteins; (**C**) Predictable protein A binding site to each antibody.

2.2. Biosensor Fabrication

Following a previously reported work for magnetic particle detection [10,11], an integrated cytometer platform was used, consisting of magnetoresistive sensors, readout/acquisition electronics and a microfluidic channel where the milk was injected. The device geometry and physical principles of operation are described in Fernandes [6], and are based on spin valves (SV) deposited by ion beam deposition on a Nordiko 3000 tool with the following structure: Si/Al_2O_3 60/Ta1.5/$Ni_{80}Fe_{20}$ 2.5/$Co_{90}Fe_{10}$ 2.0/Cu 2.1/$Co_{90}Fe_{10}$ 2.0/$Mn_{76}Ir_{24}$ 6.0/Ta 5.0 [12,13] (thickness in nm, compositions in atomic %), patterned with 3 µm × 100 µm active dimensions (measured between the AlSiCu 300 nm thick contact leads), according to Figure 2. Passivation was done with a 300 nm thick Si_3N_4 layer deposited by PECVD (Electrotech Delta chemical vapor deposition system). Sensors were annealed at 250 °C for 15 min, in vacuum, and cooled under a 1 Tesla magnetic field.

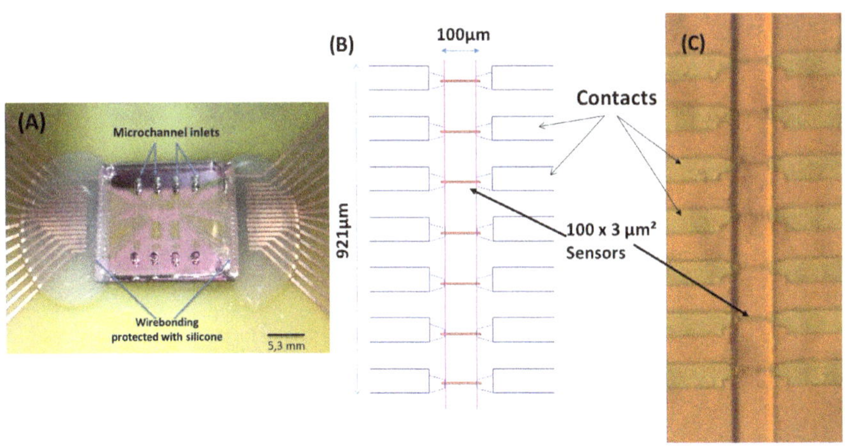

Figure 2. (**A**) Final device with the magnetoresistive chip bonded to the polydimethylsiloxane (PDMS) microchannels. The sensor's wirebonding are protected with silicone. (**B**) Spinvalve (SV) sensor distribution along the microchannels; and (**C**) microscope photo of the fabricated SVs with the PDMS microchannel over them (20× amplification).

The SV sensors' electrical transport characterization (resistance *versus* DC magnetic field) provided information on the magnetoresistance, defined as $MR = (R_{max} - R_{min})/R_{min}$ (where R_{max} and R_{min} are the maximum and minimum resistance levels). The sensor sensitivity is defined as the slope of the curve over the linear range of operation and ranges 0.15%–0.17%/Oe for the sensors measured across the wafer.

The magnetic detection mechanism used nanoparticles which had a superparamagnetic signature, therefore requiring an external magnetic field to activate their magnetization. This was done with an external vertical field created by a permanent magnet (NdFeB, 20-10-01STIC, Supermagnete, Gottmadingen, Germany) mounted below the printed circuit board (PCB). After magnet alignment below this sensor, the effect of the small components in the plane of the sensors was visible in their sensitivity decrease to 0.074%/Oe. The magnetic field strength at the microfluidic channel center was ~31 mT, so the individual nanoparticles were magnetized with a magnetic moment of 2.0×10^{-18} A·m^2. Upon magnetization, the nanoparticles created a magnetic field fringe field at the sensor surface; therefore, the particle presence was detected through the changes in the sensor resistance (or voltage, as shown in Figure 5).

2.3. *Microfluidic Channel Fabrication*

The microchannels (Figure 2B) were fabricated in polydimethylsiloxane (PDMS), with 100 μm (length) × 50 μm (height), following the method described in Fernandes and colleagues' work [6].

The integration of the magnetoresistive chip with the PDMS microchannels was achieved through irreversible bonding of the Si_3N_4 and PDMS surfaces. Both surfaces were exposed to ultraviolet/ozone (UVO Cleaner, Jelight Company Inc., Irvine, CA, USA) for 15 min and then mounted face-to-face and manually aligned to be kept at RT, overnight. The ensemble was then mounted in a PCB, where the sensors were wire-bonded and the wires protected with silicone (Figure 2A).

The raw milk samples' constant flowing through the microchannel section of 50 μm height and 100 μm length was challenging because of its density and colloidal behavior. A surfactant addition to milk samples, namely Tween 20, was used to achieve higher dispersion of fat globules (0.1–10 μm), allowing lower interfacial tension and its dimension reduction [14]. On the other hand, we adopted the milk preparation method of dairy industries for milk homogenization, using agitation (vortex) and higher temperatures (60 °C) to decrease fat globules' dimensions and allow their uniform distribution in the sample.

2.4. *Readout Electronics*

The multi-channel PCB designed to interface 15 spin valve sensors was connected to an amplifier with an operating gain of 5000×, and high-pass and low-pass filters of 300 Hz and 10 kHz, respectively. Each channel included a configurable DC current source, from 0.25 mA to 2 mA [15].

In this work, only one sensor per channel was monitored. One syringe pump was attached to the system, and was the only device not operating under DC batteries (thus, introducing the 50 Hz noise from the main power grid). The sensor output signals were recorded over time by using a connection to an acquisition setup composed by a 16 bit analog-to-digital converter (ADC board DT9836-12-2-BNC), at 50 kHz acquisition frequency. The resulting digital signals were then post-processed in a software developed in Matlab, to apply a low pass digital filter with cut-off frequency of 2 kHz, allowing real-time noise characterization and data-storing into the hard drive for further analysis (Figure 3). The sensors used for this work showed a noise level of 2.5–4 μV (peak-to-peak). During the experiments, the pump operation increased the noise level to 3–4.5 μV.

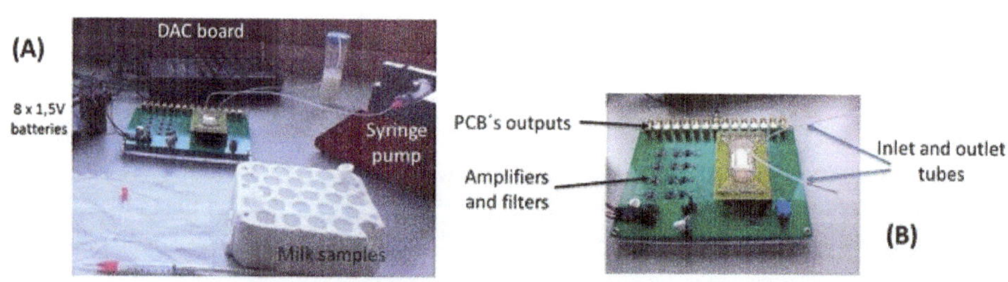

Figure 3. (**A**) Acquisition setup assembly; and (**B**) multi-channel PCB connected to external electronics.

2.5. Magnetic Detection Method Calibration

A blank sample (only PBS or sterile raw milk) and a negative control sample (PBS or sterile raw milk, with 2 μL of functionalized NPs) were always measured prior to the measurements with contaminated milk, giving the background signal of the system.

A first calibration assay was then made with *Streptococcus agalactiae*/pAb anti-GB streptococci spiked on PBS sample.

Finally, *Streptococcus agalactiae*/pAb anti-GB streptococci; *Streptococcus uberis*/pAb anti-GB streptococci and *Streptococcus agalactiae*/mAb anti-*Streptococcus agalactiae* were spiked in sterile milk samples and the correspondent calibration curves made. Each concentration point was the result of three different assays' measurements.

The calibration range between 0.1 and 20 cfu/μL was established taking into account the detection limit for conventional microbiology of 500 cfu/mL (0.5 cfu/μL).

2.6. Bacterial Cells

Streptococcus agalactiae (strain CECT 183) and *Streptococcus uberis* (strain CECT 994) cells were grown separately onto Columbia agar supplemented with 5% sheep blood (bioMérieux, 43021, Marcy l'Étoile, France) and incubated at 37 °C, overnight. A single colony of each isolate was selected and re-suspended in 4 mL of tripticase soy broth over 24 h at 37 °C. Subsequently, the bacterial cells were collected through centrifugation (15 min, 17 °C, 2700 rpm) and re-suspended in PBS (pH 7.2) to allow optical density measurement (at 600 nm) (BECKMAN DU-68 Spectrophotometer) and for colony-forming unit (cfu) estimation. A bacterial suspension with a known concentration of 10^4 cfu/μL was the starting point to get seven different bacterial concentrations for each species, in PBS or in raw milk samples: 0.1; 0.3; 0.5; 1; 2; 10, and 20 cfu/μL.

2.7. Sterile Milk Samples

Raw milk used for the definition of calibration curves experiments was collected aseptically from healthy cows. Conventional microbiological tests were performed according to NMC protocols [16], to confirm no bacterial growth. Briefly, a raw milk sample (10 μL) was plated on a Columbia agar plate and on MacConkey agar plate (CM0007, Oxoid, Hampshire, UK) and both were incubated at 37 °C for 48 h. The absence of growth on both plates was considered to be equivalent to the presence of no viable bacteria in the milk.

Each sample for biosensor testing had a 500 μL volume consisting of 2 μL of a suspension of functionalized NPs, 98 μL of PBST, and 400 μL of one of seven bacterial suspensions with pre-defined bacterial concentrations in PBS or sterile raw milk. The incubation of these samples was performed at RT for 3 h, under agitation.

All raw milk samples were submitted to a pre-treatment of 15 min at 60 °C in a dry bath incubator (Grant, model QBD2, Leicestershire, UK) and 15 min of continuous centrifugation in a vortex mixer (Labnet International Inc., Edison, NJ, USA) after adding bacteria and PBST. Only then, 2 μL of functionalized NPs suspension were added for final incubation step.

2.8. Mastitic Milk Samples

Mastitic milk samples were collected aseptically from 44 cows originating in 11 Portuguese dairy farms. Animals were selected based on the presence of subclinical mastitis, defined by evidence of a somatic cell count over 1,000,000 cells/mL. Mammary quarters to sample were selected in these cows based on a strong positive reaction on the California Mastitis Test. Bacteria identification in mastitic milk samples was performed according to NMC protocols [16].

These mastitic milk samples were distributed in two groups of $n = 31$ samples each for biosensor analysis, of which 16 were tested by both antibodies (anti-GB streptococci and anti-*Streptococcus agalactiae*). The selection of quarter milk samples was based on bacteriological results which included

Staphylococcus aureus ($n = 1$), *Streptococcus agalactiae* ($n = 13$), *Streptococcus uberis* ($n = 11$), *Streptococcus* spp. ($n = 4$), coagulase-negative staphylococci (CNS) ($n = 2$), *Enterococcus* spp. ($n = 7$), *Escherichia coli* ($n = 3$), Yeasts ($n = 3$) and *Prototheca* ($n = 2$). All mastitic milk samples were also submitted to PCR analysis.

2.9. PCR Reference Method Analysis

PCR analysis was performed by an external laboratory (VACUNEK, SL) with the PathoProof Mastitis Complete-16® (Thermo Scientific), a development of the PCR assay initially described in [17], which allows for the detection of 16 bovine mastitis pathogens. This method is semi-quantitative, classifying the amount of bacterial cells in mastitic milk samples as "high", "average", or "low".

2.10. Biosensor Analysis

A volume of 400 μL of mastitic milk was collected and mixed with 98 μL of PBST. Each 498 μL sample was submitted to a pre-treatment of heating (15 min at 60 °C) and homogenization (15 min in vortex). After these steps, a volume of 2 μL of a functionalized NPs suspension was added to reach a final volume of 500 μL to be submitted to incubation (RT, 3 h, under agitation) and further biosensor analysis.

Trials were performed with each antibody set consisting of 31 mastitic samples in different assays. Therefore, the biosensor analysis was validated 62 times. Each trial day began with sensor's noise level measurement (Figure 4-1) and each sample was injected at a flow rate of 50 μL/min, through a PDMS microchannel (Figure 4-2). The microchannel was always cleaned between samples with PBST followed by deionized water, both at a 90 μL/min flow rate (Figure 4-4), until reaching noise level values again, denoting a magnetic-free microchannel filling. A blank sample and a negative control sample were measured whenever a new MR sensor was used and always before mastitic samples analysis.

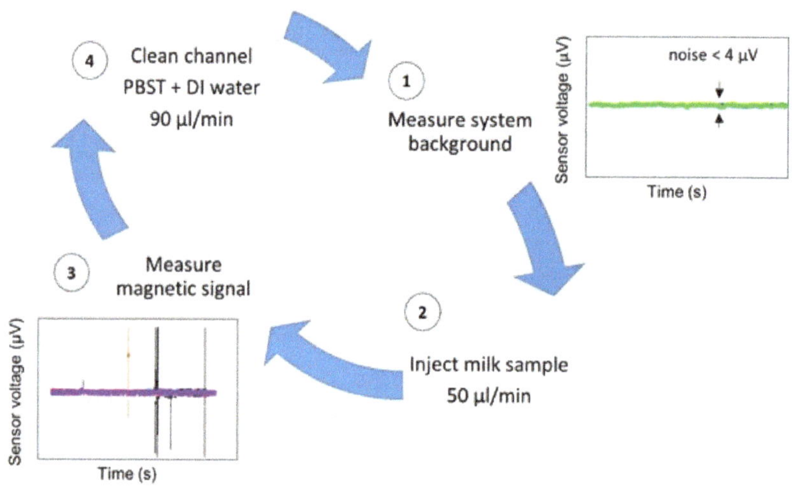

Figure 4. Biosensor analysis procedure steps.

Samples with functionalized NPs on PBS or sterile milk (negative controls) evidenced signal less than 50 μV (Figure 5A). Mastitic milk samples without the targeted bacteria (proved by PCR) and tested with NPs functionalized with chosen antibodies, also evidenced signal less than 50 μV (Figure 5B). Samples used for calibration assays spiked with bacterial cells on sterile milk showed magnetic signal upper than 50 μV (Figure 5C–E).

The classification of mastitic milk samples by the biosensor was based on bacterial detection (presence or absence). Consequently, the "positive" samples were those with at least one magnetic peak above 50 μV, therefore higher than the signal found in negative control samples and in mastitic milk samples without targeted bacteria. Next, this "positive" sample magnetic peak should evidence a bipolar or unipolar shape similar to the ones found in samples used for calibration trials as shown in Figure 5C–E.

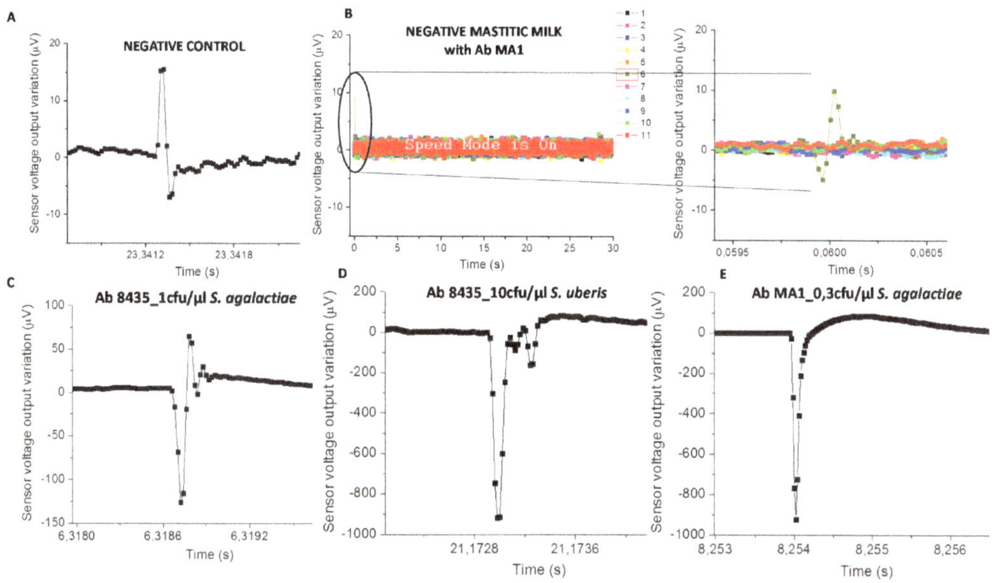

Figure 5. Sensor output for (**A**) negative control with the higher amplitude of 23 μV; (**B**) mastitic milk (without *S. agalactiae* according to the PCR) with NPs functionalized with mAb anti-*S. agalactiae* which presents an amplitude peak of 15 μV (9076AD sample code). The higher amplitude peaks found for each pair of bacteria-antibody were; (**C**) 193.6 μV in raw milk with anti-GB streptococci and 1 cfu/μL of *S. agalactiae*; (**D**) 917.5 μV in raw milk with anti-GB streptococci and 10 cfu/μL of *S. uberis*; and (**E**) 923.7 μV in raw milk with anti-*S. agalactiae* and 0.3 cfu/μL of *S. agalactiae*.

Biosensor analysis was a dynamic detection where a heterogeneous milk sample flowed inside the microchannel. Magnetically labelled bacterial cells were mixed randomly in milk leading to the impossibility of predicting its position above the sensor over time. Consequently, the magnetic peaks' shape and time resulting from biosensor analysis were expected to be different between samples (Figure 5).

2.11. Data Analysis

Isolates were considered to be correctly identified by magnetic detection if the same species was found by the reference method, or if the magnetic detection did not identify the species it was targeting and PCR identified one of the other bacteria. For example, a correct identification referred to a *S. agalactiae* being identified magnetically in a sample that PCR had identified as *S. agalactiae*, but also when not identifying as *S. agalactiae* a sample that through PCR was identified as *Staphylococcus* spp. Regarding conventional microbiology, isolates were considered to be correctly identified if the same species was found as with the reference method. Misidentification was considered when the magnetic detection and conventional microbiology identified a different species than the reference method. For example, a sample that was identified as *Staphylococcus* spp. by PCR and that was identified as *S. agalactiae* by magnetic detection, or a sample that was identified as *S. agalactiae* by PCR and not identified as such by magnetic detection. For both magnetic detection and conventional microbiology methods, sensitivity, specificity, and positive predictive value were calculated in comparison with PCR species identification. Sensitivity was calculated as the proportion of the true positive isolates that were correctly identified with the magnetic detection or microbiological tests, e.g., the proportion of

S. agalactiae isolates based on PCR analysis that were identified as such by magnetic detection and microbiology testing. Specificity was calculated as the proportion of the true negatives that were correctly identified with the magnetic detection and the microbiological tests, e.g., the proportion of isolates other than *S. agalactiae* based on PCR analysis that were identified as something other than *S. agalactiae* by magnetic detection and by microbiological testing. Finally, PPV was calculated as the proportion of isolates identified as a specific species based on magnetic detection or on microbiological testing that truly represented that particular species, e.g., the proportion of isolates that were identified as *S. agalactiae* by magnetic detection or microbiological testing that had been identified as *S. agalactiae* based on PCR analysis.

3. Results

3.1. *Evaluation of Biosensor's Bacterial Quantification*

The calibration trial outcome is shown in Figure 6. The peak´s number per signal amplitude were calculated, showing no evidence of linear correlation with increasing bacterial concentration. The milk samples with the anti-GB streptococci antibody revealed the most exuberant signal with *S. uberis* when compared with the other two bacteria-antibody pairs (Figure 6). Only the *Streptococcus agalactiae*/pAb anti-GB streptococci pair showed no evidence of peaks higher than 200 μV. Despite that, these MR sensors could detect *Streptococcus agalactiae* and *Streptococcus uberis* in milk samples from 0.1 cfu/μL (100 cfu/mL).

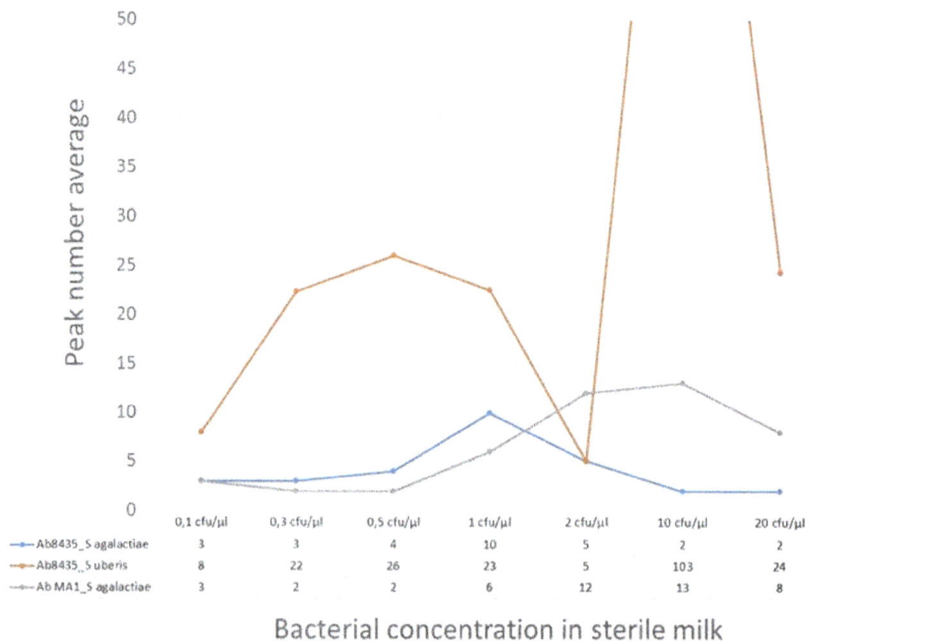

Figure 6. Calibration trial results for milk samples with seven bacterial concentrations (*S. agalactiae* or *S. uberis*) and functionalized NPs with pAb anti-GB streptococci (Ab8435) and mAb anti-*S. agalactiae* (Ab MA1). Peak number average for each bacteria-antibody pair are counted.

The calibration curve for PBS samples with bacteria was obtained for the *Streptococcus agalactiae*/pAb anti-GB streptococci pair. It showed evidence that different bacterial concentrations, as in sterile milk, also presented similar amplitude peaks (under 200 μV). Performing experimental data fitting to simulations for cell quantity estimation by peak, we obtained different results depending on considered functionalized NPs number per cell and cell cluster positioning above the MR sensor (height z) (Figure 7B,C).

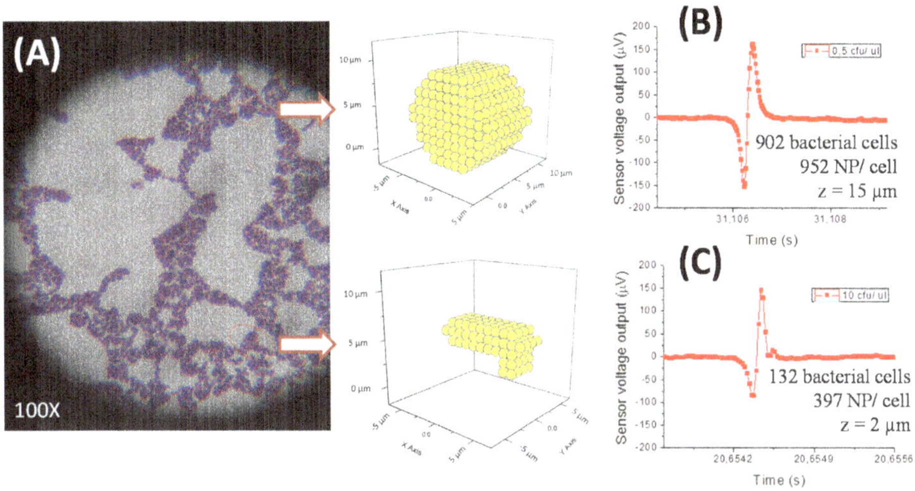

Figure 7. *Streptococcus agalactiae* cells microscopic image where a spherical cluster and an elongated cluster are evidenced (**A**). Experimental data fitting of the highest amplitude peaks obtained in PBS samples with different *S. agalactiae* concentrations (0.5 cfu/µL: 162 µV (**B**) and 10 cfu/µL: 146 µV (**C**)) during calibration curve settlement.

3.2. Validation of Magnetic Detection

Forty-six mastitic milk samples with known bacteriology results, obtained through conventional microbiology were analyzed by PCR. A total of 160 identifications were performed by PCR for all 46 milk samples analyzed with mAb anti-*S. agalactiae* and mAb anti-GB streptococci. The most frequently isolated species based on the PCR were *Staphylococcus* spp., *E. coli*, and yeasts, followed by *S. uberis* and *S. agalactiae*. As a result of the high sensitivity of the PCR methodology, an average of four different pathogens were detected per mastitic milk sample, not allowing for the true causative agent of mastitis to be determined. Therefore, it was decided to use the conventional bacteriology results as the basis for the true identification, confirmed by the PCR (Table 1).

Table 1. Identification of isolates in mastitic milk samples with both magnetic detection (mAb anti-*Streptococcus agalactiae*; pAb anti-GB streptococci) and with conventional microbiology, compared to PCR analysis as the reference method.

		Magnetic Detection						**Microbiological Tests**		
		Anti-*Streptococcus agalactiae*			**Anti-GB Streptococci**					
Mastitic Milk Isolates		**Correctly Identified**			**Correctly Identified**			**Correctly Identified**		
	n	n	%	MI [1]	n	%	MI	n	%	MI
S. aureus	1	0	0.0	0	1	100.0	0	0	0.0	1
S. agalactiae	13	7	70.0	3	2	25.0	6	13	100.0	0
S. uberis	11	3	33.3	6	5	62.5	3	8	72.7	3
Streptococcus spp.	4	0	0.0	3	2	50.0	2	1	25.0	3
Staphylococcus spp.	2	0	0.0	0	1	50.0	1	2	100.0	0
Enterococcus spp.	7	3	75.0	1	1	33.3	2	0	0.0	7
Escherichia coli	3	0	0.0	1	1	50.0	1	3	100.0	0
Yeasts	3	0	0.0	2	1	100.0	0	2	66.7	1
Prototheca	2	0	0.0	2	1	50.0	1	2	100.0	0
TOTAL	46	13	41.9	18	15	48.4	16	31	67.4	15

Correctly identified = True Positives + True Negatives; [1] MI (misidentified) = False Negatives + False Positives.

The magnetic detection with the anti-*Streptococcus agalactiae* antibody tested 31 mastitic milk samples from the total of 46 analyzed by conventional microbiology, which 10 and 13 were identified as *S. agalactiae* (Table 1), respectively. However, from these 31 samples tested, 11 were identified as *S. agalactiae* by PCR and only one was not identified as such by microbiology, but as *S. uberis*. The magnetic detection with the anti-*S. agalactiae* antibody identified 8 *S. agalactiae* isolates correctly in 11 (72.7%) milk samples with this species when compared to PCR. Five mastitic milk samples did not lead to an identification by this polyclonal antibody because they did not present *S. agalactiae* according to the PCR analysis (true negatives) (Table 2). Misidentification was observed for 18 of 31 (58%) isolates in the 31 mastitic milk samples tested with the anti-*Streptococcus agalactiae* antibody (Table 1). Only three misidentified *S. agalactiae* isolates were found in milk samples with this species analyzed by PCR, evidencing a failure of recognition by this monoclonal antibody (Table 1). Adding to that, five mastitic milk samples with *S. uberis* and/or *S. dysgalactiae* and 10 mastitic milk samples without any Streptococci species according to the PCR analysis, were misidentified by biosensor analysis as having *S. agalactiae* and were all classified as false positives (Table 2). Overall a 73% sensitivity, 25% specificity, and 35% PPV were found for magnetic detection with the anti-*Streptococcus agalactiae* antibody. The highest sensitivity value represents the proportion of the true positives (8) that were correctly identified with this monoclonal antibody (Table 2).

Table 2. Sensitivity, specificity, and positive predictive value of the magnetic detection and the conventional microbiology, using PCR analysis as the reference method.

	Magnetic Detection		Microbiological Tests
	Anti- *Streptococcus agalactiae*	Anti-GB Streptococci	
True Positives	8	7	31
True Negatives	5	8	0
False Negatives	3	10	0
False Positives	15	6	15
Sensitivity	73%	41%	100%
Specificity	25%	57%	-
[1]PPV	35%	54%	67%

[1]PPV = Positive Predictive Value

Using the polyclonal anti-GB streptococci in magnetic detection, the 31 mastitic samples tested included 16 identified equitably as eight *S. agalactiae* and eight *S. uberis* by conventional microbiology (Table 1). However, PCR analysis identified two more samples as *S. uberis* in the 31 analyzed by this antibody, amounting 18 bacterial target possibilities. The magnetic detection with the anti-GB streptococci antibody correctly identified seven streptococci isolates present in 18 (38.9%) milk samples with *S. agalactiae* and/or *S. uberis* according to PCR analysis. The microorganisms that were not identified as GB streptococci or *S. uberis* (13/31) by the reference method in mastitic milk samples, were magnetically detected as GB streptococci and/or *S. uberis* in those samples (five false positives) or else, undetected as true negatives (8) (Table 2). Misidentification was observed for 16 isolates in the 31 (51.6%) mastitic samples tested. Eleven misidentified *S. agalactiae* and *S. uberis* isolates were found in milk samples analyzed by PCR with these two streptococci, evidencing a failure of recognition by this polyclonal antibody (Table 1). Overall a sensitivity of 41%, a specificity of 57%, and a PPV of 54% were found for magnetic detection with the anti-GB streptococci antibody. The highest specificity value represents the proportion of the true negatives (8) that were correctly identified with this polyclonal antibody (Table 2).

With regards to microbiological testing for all 46 samples considered, the highest agreement in microorganism identification, in comparison with PCR analysis, was found to be 100% for *S. agalactiae*, *Staphylococcus* spp., *E. coli*, and *Prototheca*, as showed in percentage data of correct identification (Table 1). However, incomplete microbiological identifications of 67.4% (31/46) and a misidentification of 32.6% (15/46) were observed (Table 1). Microbiological tests evidenced a PPV value of 67% and a sensitivity of 100% to identify mastitis pathogens in milk samples, showing that conventional microbiology correctly identified true negatives (Table 2).

4. Discussion

Sensitivities of 73% and 41% and specificity values of 25% and 57% were obtained for magnetic identification of streptococci species with an anti-*Streptococcus agalactiae* antibody and an anti-GB streptococci antibody, respectively. The higher PPV value (54%) evidenced for magnetic detection with the anti-GB streptococci antibody may reinforce the bonding avidity between this polyclonal antibody and the only two immunogenic cell wall proteins of *S. uberis*, compared to 10 or more antigens known in *S. agalactiae*.

Comparing sensitivity and specificity values of this magnetic detection with another study that used immunological detection of mastitis pathogens through an ELISA for detecting *S. aureus* in milk [18], higher sensitivity (69%–90%) and specificity values (61%–97%) [4] were observed. ProStaph test (Proscience Corp, Albertson, NY, USA) had a detection limit of 10^4–10^5 cfu/mL, when the minimum bacterial presence detected by the present immunological recognition was 100 cfu/mL, independently of the antibody and targeted bacteria used.

The microbiological misidentification ratio of 32.6% observed in our study was due to 15 wrong identifications compared with PCR analysis. The use of PCR for the identification of mastitis pathogens may have the advantage [19] of leading to decreased false negative results, but it may also be clinically challenging. PCR's higher sensitivity leads to the identification of all milk sample pathogens and contaminants alike [20], being difficult to assign mastitis causality to a particular microorganism. This was also observed in our study, with the average number of microorganisms identified per milk sample being one.

Regarding the validation of the magnetic detection method, some false positive results could be explained by NPs' agglomeration by the mastitic milk matrix heterogeneity, sporadic low cleaning efficiency of the channel's inlet chamber, and also due to electrical conductivity of mastitic milk samples. Bovine mastitis leads to changes in ion concentration of milk due to increased vascular permeability, resulting from inflammatory response, leading to modifications in electrical conductivity of milk [21]. The conductance in milk causes sensor's resistivity variation translated by higher background noise. Despite a detergent (Tween 20) being in milk samples to reduce fat globules dimensions, to distribute the bacterial cells in the milk, to improve nanoparticles mobilization and to allow for a more homogeneous milk matrix, the optimization trials (not described in this paper) showed the need for a compromise between Tween 20 quantity and magnetic peak discrimination. Different volumes of PBST in 500 µL of milk samples were used. The higher volumes ($\geq$100 µL) showed evidence of bubbles inside the microchannel which hampered milk flowing, caused nanoparticle agglomeration, and did not help magnetic peak discrimination between control samples (milk with only NPs) and samples with bacteria. On the other hand, false negatives may have occurred because of three circumstances. Firstly, the binding yield variations between antibodies and NPs and/or failure in bacterial cells magnetic labelling could narrow bacterial cells identification. This fact should be recognized as possible because IgM and nanoparticles dimensions are closer, so it will be more difficult to have the same number of attached IgM when comparing with NPs functionalization with smaller IgG. Secondly, according to Henriksen's study [22], it is possible that the rotating nature of the magnetic dipole field of NPs magnetized by an external magnetic field, can induce signal cancelation. Therefore, the fields from two differently-placed NPs can partially cancel each other. Finally, microchannel current height (50 µm) could be reduced to improve sensor's detection by forcing bacterial cells dragging over it, but mastitic milk trials showed that milk clots hamper sample flow and height decrease leads to microchannel obstruction, pointing to a compromise between the sensor's detection and sample fluidity.

With regard to bacterial quantification data, this magnetic detection method showed some microbiological and immunological constraints. Bacterial cells group together randomly depending on growth conditions [23]. Each bacteria may express a different number of cell wall proteins, including the immunogenic ones [24]. Together, these facts limit the knowledge of how many immunogenic proteins there are per cell and consequently, how many proteins will be recognized by each specific antibody used. On the other hand, the chemical and colloidal changes of milk components in a state of inflammatory response [14], as occurs with mastitis, prevent and reduce bacterial magnetic labeling efficacy [25]. Consequently, it was not possible to predict peak profiles (number, shape) for each bacterial concentration.

Although the sensitivity of the magnetic detection method is important, many additional factors must be considered, including rapidity, easy to use, flexibility, portability, and costs [26]. This dynamic methodology showed it was possible for a mastitic milk sample to be processed until a final result was obtained in five hours, but was not suitable for processing a large number of samples (maximum of 10–12 per day). It also showed technical simplicity when established, and ease of scoring and interpreting the results. Despite the lower sensitivities obtained, both antibodies used were capable to detect bacterial cells in real milk samples. However, other antibodies could be used for further identification of different bovine mastitis pathogens, reinforcing this method flexibility.

Further studies could be done for biosensor's performance improvement as higher number of analyzed samples per day by using all seven SV of each microchannel and use all of them per die. Another opportunity for better bacterial magnetic signal acquisition could be the dilution of milk samples in water or bacterial isolation from mastitic milk to be further analyzed in PBS, reducing conductance problems.

5. Conclusions

A lab-on-a-chip magnetoresistive cytometer, with microfluidic sample handling, was successfully used to demonstrate the minimal detection of 100 cfu/mL of bacterial cells in raw milk. Milk samples were mixed with a solution combining specific antibodies and magnetic nanoparticles, before the analysis. This paper describes the methodology used for detection of bacteria, including analysis of false positive/negative results.

Comparison with PCR results showed sensitivities of 73% and 41%, specificity values of 25% and 57%, and PPV values of 35% and 54% for magnetic identification of streptococci species with an anti-*S. agalactiae* antibody and an anti-GB streptococci antibody, respectively.

Magnetic detection of milk samples showed some microbiological and immunological constraints. Since bacterial cells have high variability on the number of immunogenic proteins per cell, the number of labeled sites through the antibody is also not well defined. This affects the quantification of the magnetic method. As a consequence, it was not possible to quantify the peak profile (number, shape) for each bacterial concentration. The method, however, allows the determination of their presence, and quantification may be done within lower/upper threshold limits. Simulations of the sensor output as a function of the nanoparticle distribution over the cells (using colonies/clusters configurations compatible with the experimentally observed under microscopy) can provide an indication of minimum and maximum numbers. Further work should be done towards a more accurate quantification based on simulations.

Accuracy in bacterial quantification was affected by false positive results, leading to overestimation of bacteria numbers caused by nanoparticle agglomeration by the mastitic milk matrix heterogeneity and/or microchannel blocking. Additionally, undetected bacteria due to false negatives may be due to binding yield variations between antibodies and nanoparticles and/or failure in bacterial cells magnetic labelling.

This biosensor can be submitted to further improvements which may include incorporation of a milk pre-treatment step into the microfluidic platform and also further studies on electronics to allow multiplex analysis of several samples at the same time. Currently, this biosensor requires an external computer for system operation and displaying test results, so a fully integrated system into a single device could also be made.

Acknowledgments: Work partially supported by the project FCT -EXCL/CTM-NAN/0441/2012 and by the CIISA-46 project UID/CVT/00276/2013. INESC-MN acknowledges FCT funding through the IN-Associated laboratory (Pest-OE/CTM/LA0024/2011). Andrei Jitariu acknowledges the financial support from European Commission in the framework of the Grant Agreement No. 316194-NANOSENS, FP7-REGPOT-2012-2013-1.

Author Contributions: Carla Duarte conceived and designed the experiments; Carla Duarte, Carla Carneiro and Rita Soares performed the experiments; Carla Duarte, Andrei Jitariu, Ricardo Bexiga and Paulo Freitas analyzed the data; Ricardo Bexiga, Susana Cardoso, Moisés Piedade contributed reagents/materials/analysis tools; Carla Duarte, Tiago Costa, Susana Cardoso, Ricardo Bexiga and Paulo Freitas wrote the paper.

Conflicts of Interest: The authors declare no conflict of interest.

Abbreviations

mAb	monoclonal antibody
pAb	polyclonal antibody
ADC	analogue to digital converter
DC	direct current
Fc fraction	fragment crystallizable region of an immunoglobulin G
GB	Group B
Ig	immunoglobulin
MS	magnetic separation
PBST	phosphate buffer saline with 0.05% (v/v) of Tween 20
Oe	Oersted. CGS unit of magnetic field H strength
T	Tesla. SI unit for magnetic induction B strength.

References

1. Bradley, A.J. Bovine Mastitis: An Evolving Disease. *Vet. J.* **2002**, *164*, 116–128. [PubMed]
2. Zadoks, R.N.; Middleton, J.R.; McDougall, S.; Katholm, J.; Schukken, Y.H. Molecular Epidemiology of Mastitis Pathogens of Dairy Cattle and Comparative Relevance to Humans. *J. Mammary Gland Biol. Neoplasia* **2011**, *16*, 357–372. [PubMed]
3. Raemy, A.; Meylan, M.; Casati, S.; Gaia, V.; Berchtold, B.; Boss, R.; Wyder, A.; Graber, H.U. Phenotypic and genotypic identification of streptococci and related bacteria isolated from bovine intramammary infections. *Acta Vet. Scand.* **2013**, *55*. [CrossRef]
4. Hicks, C.R.; Eberhart, R.J.; Sischo, W.M. Comparison of microbiologic culture, an enzyme-linked immunosorbent assay, and determination of somatic cell count for diagnosing *Staphylococcus aureus* mastitis in dairy cows. *J. Am. Vet. Med. Assoc.* **1994**, *204*, 255–260. [PubMed]
5. Bourry, A.; Poutrel, B. Bovine mastitis caused by *Listeria monocytogenes*: Kinetics of antibody responses in serum and milk after experimental infection. *J. Dairy Sci.* **1996**, *79*, 2189–2195. [CrossRef]
6. Fernandes, A.C.; Duarte, C.M.; Cardoso, F.A.; Bexiga, R.; Cardoso, S.; Freitas, P.P. Lab-on-chip cytometry based on Magnetoresistive sensors for bacteria detection in milk. *Sensors* **2014**, *14*, 15496–15524. [CrossRef] [PubMed]
7. Groschup, M.H.; Hahn, G.; Timoney, J.F. Antigenic and genetic homogeneity of *Streptococcus uberis* strains from the bovine udder. *Epidemiol. Infect.* **1991**, *107*, 297–310. [CrossRef] [PubMed]
8. Driskell, J.D.; Tripp, R.A. Emerging technologies in nanotechnology-based pathogen detection. *Clin. Microb. Newsl.* **2009**, *31*, 137–144. [CrossRef]
9. Lazcka, O.; Del Campo, F.J.; Muñoz, F.X. Pathogen detection: A perspective of traditional methods and biosensors. *Biosens. Bioelectron.* **2007**, *22*, 1205–1217. [CrossRef] [PubMed]
10. Loureiro, J.; Andrade, P.Z.; Cardoso, S.; da Silva, C.L.; Cabral, J.M.; Freitas, P.P. Magnetoresistive chip cytometer. *Lab Chip* **2011**, *11*, 2255–2261. [CrossRef] [PubMed]
11. Freitas, P.P.; Cardoso, F.A.; Martins, V.C.; Martins, S.A.M.; Loureiro, J.; Amaral, J.; Chaves, R.C.; Cardoso, S.; Fonseca, L.P.; Sebastião, A.M.; *et al.* Spintronic platforms for biomedical applications. *Lab Chip* **2012**, *12*, 546–557. [CrossRef] [PubMed]
12. Gehanno, V.; Freitas, P.P.; Veloso, A.; Ferrira, J.; Almeida, B.; Soasa, J.B.; Kling, A.; Soares, J.C.; da Silva, M.F. Ion beam deposition of Mn-Ir spin valves. *IEEE Trans. Magn.* **1999**, *35*, 4361–4367. [CrossRef]

13. Freitas, P.P.; Ferreira, R.; Cardoso, S.; Cardoso, F. Magnetoresistive sensors. *J. Phys. Condens. Matter.* **2007**, *19*, 1–21. [CrossRef]
14. Walstra, P.; Wouters, J.; Geurts, T. *Dairy Science and Technology*, 2nd ed.; Taylor & Francis Group: New York, NY, USA, 2006.
15. Costa, T.; Piedade, M.S.; Germano, J.; Amaral, J.; Freitas, P.P. A neuronal signal detector for biologically generated magnetic fields. *IEEE Trans. Instrum. Meas.* **2014**, *63*, 1171–1180. [CrossRef]
16. National Mastitis Council (NMC). Sample collection and handling. In *Laboratory Handbook of Bovine Mastitis*; National Mastitis Council: Madison, WI, USA, 1999.
17. Koskinen, M.T.; Holopainen, J.; Pyörälä, S.; Bredbacka, P.; Pitkälä, A.; Barkema, H.W.; Bexiga, R.; Roberson, J.; Sølverød, L.; Piccinini, R.; *et al.* Analytical specificity and sensitivity of a real-time polymerase chain reaction assay for identification of bovine mastitis pathogens. *J. Dairy Sci.* **2009**, *92*, 952–959. [CrossRef] [PubMed]
18. Matsushita, T.; Dinsmore, R.P.; Eberhart, R.J.; Jones, G.M.; McDonald, J.S.; Sears, P.M.; Adams, D.S. Performance studies of an enzyme-linked immunosorbent assay for detecting *Staphylococcus aureus* antibody in bovine milk. *J. Vet. Diagn. Investig.* **1990**, *2*, 163–166. [CrossRef]
19. Taponen, S.; Salmikivi, L.; Simojoki, H.; Koskinen, M.T.; Pyörälä, S. Real-time polymerase chain reaction-based identification of bacteria in milk samples from bovine clinical mastitis with no growth in conventional culturing. *J. Dairy Sci.* **2009**, *92*, 2610–2617. [CrossRef] [PubMed]
20. Hiitiö, H.; Riva, R.; Autio, T.; Pohjanvirta, T.; Holopainen, J.; Pyörälä, S.; Pelkonen, S. Performance of a real-time PCR assay in routine bovine mastitis diagnostics compared with in-depth conventional culture. *J. Dairy Res.* **2015**, *82*, 200–208. [CrossRef] [PubMed]
21. Hovinen, M.; Aisla, A.-M.; Pyörälä, S. Accuracy and reliability of mastitis detection with electrical conductivity and milk color measurement in automatic milking. *Acta Agric. Scand. A Anim. Sci.* **2006**, *56*, 121–127.
22. Henriksen, A.D.; Wang, S.X.; Hansen, M.F. On the importance of sensor height variation for detection of magnetic labels by magnetoresistive sensors. *Sci. Rep.* **2015**, *5*. [CrossRef] [PubMed]
23. Quinn, P.J.; Carter, M.E.; Markey, B.; Carter, G.R. *Veterinary Clinical Microbiology*; Elsevier: London, UK, 1994; pp. 127–136.
24. Van der Woude, M.W.; Baümler, A.J. Phase and antigenic variation in bacteria. *Clin. Microbiol. Rev.* **2004**, *17*, 581–611. [CrossRef] [PubMed]
25. Duarte, C.M.; Fernandes, A.C.; Cardoso, F.A.; Bexiga, R.; Cardoso, S.; Freitas, P.P. Magnetic Counter for Group B Streptococci Detection in Milk. *IEEE Trans. Magn.* **2015**, *51*, 5100304. [CrossRef]
26. Mortari, A.; Lorenzelli, L. Recent sensing technologies for pathogen detection in milk: A review. *Biosens. Bioelectron.* **2014**, *60*, 8–21. [CrossRef] [PubMed]

4

Sensing of Salivary Glucose Using Nano-Structured Biosensors

Yunqing Du [1,*], Wenjun Zhang [1] and Ming L. Wang [1,2]

1 Interdisciplinary Engineering Program, College of Engineering, Northeastern University, 360 Huntington Ave, 400 SN, Boston, MA 02115, USA; zhang.wenj@husky.neu.edu (W.Z.); mi.wang@neu.edu (M.L.W.)
2 Civil and Environmental Engineering, and Bioengineering Department, Northeastern University, 360 Huntington Ave, 429 SN, Boston, MA 02115, USA
* Correspondence: du.yu@husky.neu.edu

Academic Editor: Domenico Caputo

Abstract: The anxiety and pain associated with frequent finger pricking has always been troublesome for diabetics measuring blood glucose (BG) in their daily lives. For this reason, a reliable glucose monitoring system that allows noninvasive measurements is highly desirable. Our main objective is to develop a biosensor that can detect low-level glucose in saliva (physiological range 0.5–20 mg/dL). Salivary glucose (SG) sensors were built using a layer-by-layer self-assembly of single-walled carbon nanotubes, chitosan, gold nanoparticles, and glucose oxidase onto a screen-printed platinum electrode. An electrochemical method was utilized for the quantitative detection of glucose in both buffer solution and saliva samples. A standard spectrophotometric technique was used as a reference method to validate the glucose content of each sample. The disposable glucose sensors have a detection limit of 0.41 mg/dL, a sensitivity of 0.24 $\mu A \cdot s \cdot dL \cdot mg^{-1}$, a linear range of 0.5–20 mg/dL in buffer solution, and a response time of 30 s. A study of 10 healthy subjects was conducted, and SG levels between 1.1 to 10.1 mg/dL were successfully detected. The results revealed that the noninvasive SG monitoring could be an alternative for diabetes self-management at home. This paper is not intended to replace regular BG tests, but to study SG itself as an indicator for the quality of diabetes care. It can potentially help patients control and monitor their health conditions, enabling them to comply with prescribed treatments for diabetes.

Keywords: saliva diagnostics; noninvasive; diabetes; glucose monitoring; biosensor; layer-by-layer assembly

1. Introduction

Diabetes mellitus is considered to be the most rapidly growing chronic disease of this century. It is a disease in which a person suffers from high blood sugar, either because the pancreas does not produce enough insulin (Type I), or because cells do not respond to the insulin that is produced (Type II). In 2014, 29.1 million Americans, about 9.3% of the total US population, were diagnosed with diabetes [1]. Besides inducing negative impacts on the life quality of patients, the epidemic of diabetes is resulting in more costs to the government health care budget each year. For the self-management of diabetes, most patients need to test their blood glucose (BG) levels periodically, actively dosing with insulin, or taking an oral drug in combination with controlling their diet. Typically, a blood sample for analysis is obtained through a finger prick, which often causes physical and mental stress to patients. Therefore, there is a great need for a point-of-care glucose monitoring system that allows for noninvasive, rapid and painless measurements. Saliva has been studied as a better indicator of disorders and diseases than blood [2]. Specifically, the salivary glucose (SG) level is considered an indicator of diabetes. According to preliminary studies, a good correlation between the BG level and the SG level has been verified [3–6]. Thus, the tracking of BG through the continuous monitoring of SG levels is very promising. Saliva offers great advantages as a diagnostic fluid over other body fluids such as blood, tears, sweat, urine and so forth. First, it is easily tested by individuals with modest training; second, it is noninvasive, so the risk of infection or cross-contamination caused by frequent finger pricks is eliminated; third, it is convenient for people who face difficulty extracting blood samples such as infants, the elderly and haemophiliacs; and, last but not the least, saliva contains numerous disease-related biomarkers, including those typically found in blood [7]. Taking these into account, this study developed a noninvasive SG sensing system which can be transformed into a saliva-based multiplex biomarkers detection system for the management of diabetes.

Various technologies, including infrared spectroscopy, fluorescence spectroscopy, raman spectroscopy, liquid chromatography–mass spectrometry (LC-MS) and gas chromatography–mass spectrometry (GC-MS), were proved capable of detecting glucose in clinical specimens [8–12]. However, the requirements of expensive equipment and complicated operation prohibited them from being applied to home-based care. Hence, SG sensors introduced in this study were developed based on electrochemical sensing technology, which has attracted more and more attention due to its high selectivity, repeatability, accuracy, strong biocompatibility, and low cost [13]. A typical sensor consists of a bioreceptor and transducers. The bioreceptor recognizes a target analyte and specifically reacts with it. Transducers are then used to convert the recognition event into a measurable electrical signal. For the purpose of glucose detection, the most commonly used bioreceptor is glucose oxidase (GOx) enzyme. In 1978 the first BG biosensor was designed relying on catalytic enzyme reactions [14]. It detected the hydrogen peroxide (H_2O_2) product that was generated from the glucose and GOx reaction when oxygen (O_2) was present. However, the measurement of H_2O_2 was easily altered by the product (H_2O_2) accumulation and also limited by the concentration of O_2 [15]. Due to these concerns, the second-generation glucose sensor was rendered by replacing O_2 with a synthetic electron acceptor (mediator), which was capable of shuttling electrons from the redox center of the enzyme to the surface of the electrode [13]. Measuring the electron transfer carried by mediators instead of products has successfully eliminated the drawbacks of the first generation. Nevertheless, there were still unsolved problems such as the potential leaching, low stability, and toxicity of mediators. That was when the third-generation glucose sensor came along, with the promise of a mediator-free glucose detection system based on direct electron transfer (DET). It is crucial to have a short distance or efficient electron-transfer pathway between the electrode and the reaction site which allows DET to happen. The third generation eliminated the interferences caused by O_2 concentration, H_2O_2 accumulation, and mediators leaching during the reaction, so more stable and precise electron transfer was captured [16]. Because of these advantages, we developed a third-generation glucose sensor using screen-printed sensor chips as bases.

Screen printing technology was widely used to mass produce disposable sensor chips. This technology was favored since it had flexible choices of cheap bulk materials, a mature process development, a fast production line, and high manufacturing capability and capacity. Table 1 displays a list of screen-printed glucose biosensors: here, it is evident that the third-generation glucose sensors achieved a lower limit of detection (LOD) with a faster response time compared to the first- and second-generation. Some sensors in this table display a broader range of detection or a faster response time when compared to our sensors. However, none of them have ever successfully detected glucose from real saliva samples. Unlike the other similar electrochemical biosensors reported in literature, developed sensors in this study demonstrate the capability of a real time SG measurement within 2 min (including saliva collection and testing). In addition, sensors presented in this paper provide a sufficient glucose detection range of 1.1–45 mg/dL, pinpointing the biological range of human SG (0.5–20 mg/dL), permitting them to be applicable for diabetic control and health surveillance [17]. Extremely low SG levels (<1.1 mg/dL) and high SG levels (>10.1 mg/dL) have not been examined yet since saliva samples of diabetic patients are excluded from this study. Here, an accurate, rapid, and portable SG measurement method is introduced to improve its clinical practicability and reduce pain for real-time diabetes management. Moving forward, our future goal is to measure extremely low/high SG levels in patients with diabetes as part of SG clinical validation study.

Table 1. Overview of screen-printed glucose biosensors.

Substrate	Electrode	Immobilization Method	Detection Range (mg/dL)	Reponse Time (Second)	Specimen	Generation	Reference
PET	RuO_2	GOx /Nafion	100–400	100	buffer	1st	[18]
PPy	Pt	PPD/GOx	9–540	N/A	buffer	1st	[19]
Paper	Graphite	ferricyanide/GOx	up to 500	60	buffer blood	2nd	[20]
PC	Graphite	HRP/PEGDGE/GOx /glutaraldehyde/BSA	9–540	N/A	buffer	2nd	[21]
PET	Carbon	pyocyanin/GOx	18–360	120	buffer soft drinks	2nd	[22]
Ceramic	Carbon	Tin(IV) oxide/GOx/Nafion	up to 200	N/A	blood	2nd	[23]
Unknown	Carbon	Rucoplex /$Ru(NH_3)_6Cl_3$ or $K_3Fe(CN)_6$ /FADGDH/GOx	100–800	2	blood	2nd	[24]
Ceramic	Carbon	Rhodium dioxide/				2nd	[25]
		m-phenylenediamine/GOx	10–500	25	honey		
		GDH/GOx/Nafion	10–200	120			
		glutaraldehyde/BSA/GOx	10–200	30	syrup		
		cellulose acetate/Nafion/GOx	10–200	240			
		pyrrole/GOx	50–250	35			
Unknown	SEC	CTC/GOx/gel	18–720	N/A	buffer	3rd	[26]
Ceramic	Pt	PPy-polystyrensulfonate /PA/GOx	up to 180	11	serum	3rd	[27]
Aluminum	Carbon	CNT/GOx/Nafion	1.8–16.2	20	buffer	3rd	[28]
Ceramic	**Pt**	**SWNT/(chitosan/gold nanoparticles/GOx)$_3$**	**0.5–20** **1.1–45**	**30**	**buffer** **saliva**	**3rd**	**Current study**

Abbreviations of Table 1: N/A, not applicable because glucose is measured from continuous flow; SWNT, single-walled carbon nanotubes; PET, polyethylene terephthalate; PC, polycarbonate; PPy, polypyrrole; PPD, poly(o-phenylenediamine); HRP, horseradish peroxidase; PEGDGE, polyethylene glycol diglycidyl ether; BSA, bovine serum albumin; $Ru(NH_3)_6Cl_3$, hexaammineruthenium (III) chloride; $K_3Fe(CN)_6$, potassium ferricyanide; FAD, flavin adenine dinucleotide; FADGDH, FAD-dependent glucose dehydrogenase; GDH, glucose dehydrogenase; SEC, shapable electroconductive film, a polyanion-doped polypyrrole film; CTC, stable charge transfer complex, tetrathiafulvalene-tet-racyanoquinodimethane; PA, polyacrylamide; RuO_2, ruthenium dioxide; GOx, glucose oxidase; Pt, platinum; CNT, carbon nanotubes.

2. Experimental Section

In this study, the developed glucose-sensing system can accurately measure the SG levels of healthy subjects. Sensors were fabricated through a layer-by-layer (LBL) self-assembly process on screen-printed electrodes. They were designed to help diabetics manage their health conditions and treatment results by monitoring SG levels. However, this study is not intended to replace BG tests. We believe that SG itself could potentially be considered as means for diabetes monitoring. The clinical applicability of SG sensors will be clearer especially when the next steps of clinical studies are finished.

2.1. Sensor Fabrication

DS550 platinum (Pt) screen-printed sensor chips were purchased from DropSens (Metrohm USA Incorporated). The three metallic electrodes were a Pt working electrode (WE), a silver (Ag) reference electrode (RE), and a Pt counter electrode (CE) (Figure 1). Phosphate buffered saline (PBS, pH 7.4,

Sigma-Aldrich Co. LLC.) was dissolved in deionized (DI) water to yield 0.1 M PBS aqueous buffer solution. Carboxyl groups functionalized single-walled carbon nanotubes (SWNT–COOH, diameter: 1~2 nm; length: 2~5 μm, 4000 mg/L in DI water with 5~7 wt% COOH groups at the ends) were obtained from Brewer Science Company. Chitosan (CS, low molecular weight), spherical gold nanoparticles (GNp, colloid gold, 20 nm diameter stabilized suspension), GOx (type II lyophilized powder with at least 17,300 units/g solid, enzyme commission (EC) 1.1.3.4 enzyme from Aspergillus niger), and acetate buffer solution (pH 4.65) were purchased from Sigma-Aldrich Co. LLC. Before use, 400 μL of the SWNT suspension was dispersed in 10 mL DI water with the aid of ultrasonication for 2 h to obtain stable black stock suspension; 10 mg CS was dissolved thoroughly into 5 mL acetate buffer solution to yield 2 mg/mL CS suspension; 5 mg GOx was dissolved into 5 mL 0.1 M PBS to produce 1 mg/mL GOx suspension. Experiments were performed at room temperature at approximately 23 °C.

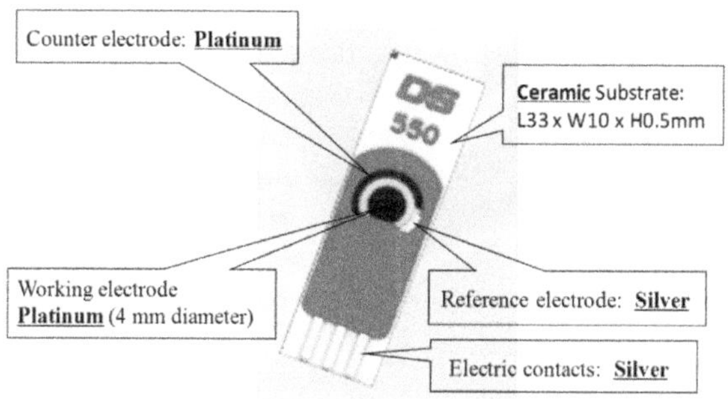

Figure 1. Schematic of screen-printed three-electrode sensor chips.

For sensor fabrication, all sensors were first rinsed with DI water and left to air dry. Only working electrodes were exposed while the other two electrodes were covered with dielectric tape (MSC industrial supply Co.). Then, 10 μL of SWNT suspension was cast onto each sensor and allowed to dry in desiccator (Terra Universal) under 10% relative humidity (RH). After 25 min, sensors were washed with 0.1 M PBS and dried up. The washing step was applied after the deposition of each layer (unless otherwise stated). Then, 10 μL of 2 mg/mL CS, 10 μL of GNp, and 10 μL of 1mg/mL GOx were cast onto the exposed electrode sequentially to form the first (CS/GNp/GOx) multi-layer film: each layer took 20 min to complete. Subsequently, two more multi-layer films were cast, and sensors were dried in the desiccator for 1 h without a washing step. After removing the dielectric tape, all resulting sensors were packed in gel-boxes (Gel-Pak) and then sealed in vacuum bags using a vacuum packaging machine (VACmaster pro110). Sensors were stored at 4 °C when not in use.

2.2. *Micro-Fabrication Imaging*

All micro-fabrication images were produced using a Supra 25 scanning electron microscope (SEM) from Gorge J. Kostas Nanoscale Technology and Manufacturing Research Center located at Northeastern University.

2.3. *Sensor Measurement*

Electrochemical measurements were carried out using a potentiostat (DY2100 mini, Digi-ivy), which was connected to a laptop with pre-installed post data processing software. A boxed adaptor for solid connection between single-use three-electrode sensors and potentiostat was purchased from DropSens. First, cyclic voltammetry (CV) electro-analytical tests were conducted and a suitable voltage to be applied between the WE and the RE was determined, under which the output current between the WE and the CE corresponded to the change of glucose concentrations. During the test, the applied voltage was sweeping from −0.2 V to 0.4 V at a scan rate of 50 mV/s. Current and voltage profiles of the third cycle were analyzed to determine a proper working potential. Then under a fixed working potential, amperometric tests were conducted to measure the glucose level, which is proportional to the output current signal. A 100 μL sample was dropped to cover all three electrodes before the selected voltage was applied between the WE and the RE constantly for 30 s. As glucose-GOx redox reactions happened on the WE, the output current between the WE and the CE illustrated how much charge passed along, quantitatively indicating the amount of glucose. In short, glucose concentrations were determined as a function of output current densities. As the reactions reached a steady state within 30 s, the output current in a time window of 27~30 s was integrated and used as the analytical signal. At the end of this 30 s test, a matlab script ran automatically to analyze the data and display results on a laptop.

2.4. Glucose Analysis with Reference Method

Spectrophotometric analysis based on enzymatic reactions by using ultraviolet-visible (UV-vis) spectroscopy was considered as a standard reference method for quantitative detection of glucose. Glucose assay kits (K606-100, Biovision incorporated) were used along with an ultraviolet (UV) spectrophotometer (mini1240, Shimadzu) and ultra-micro UV cuvettes (Brandtech scientific incorporated). This method detects 0.018–180 mg/dL glucose samples with a resolution of 7.2×10^{-5} mg/dL [29]. For each batch of measurements, a set of six standard glucose solutions were prepared following the manufacturer's protocol to provide a calibration curve. Samples were incubated in a water bath at 37 °C for 30–40 min and tested at a 570 nm wavelength. Absorbance readings were then converted into glucose concentrations using the calibration curve. All glucose concentrations in saliva/buffer samples were validated with standard UV tests.

2.5. Blood Glucose and Salivary Glucose Monitoring Test

Ten healthy volunteers in an age group of 20–60 years participated in an anonymous human subjects study. Diabetic and pre-diabetic subjects were excluded from this study. This project protocol was approved by Institutional Review Board of Northeastern University Human Subject Research Protection in February 2013 and was identified as #12-11-31. Each subject signed consent forms after fully understanding the purpose, procedure, and risks of the study, and were offered $12 compensation to purchase a lunch box at the completion of each session. Subjects were required to fast overnight without drinking/eating anything (except water) after 10 p.m. prior to the test date. In the morning, both blood and saliva samples of each subject in their fasted state were taken for analysis. Blood samples were measured by finger prick method using FreeStyle Lite BG monitoring systems (Abbott). Saliva samples for sensor tests were collected within 1–2 min following the saliva collection protocol as described in Section 2.6. The pH and viscosity of saliva samples were also recorded using pH test papers (6.0–8.0 range, FisherBrand) and a portable viscometer (Core-Parmer). The remaining saliva samples were prepared for spectrophotometric analysis. The preparation procedures included boiling samples at 100 °C for 30 to 60 min, and centrifuging them at 12,000× g for 6 min. The supernatant was then collected and analyzed for glucose concentrations as a reference method.

2.6. Saliva Collection Protocol

(a) Wait for 5 min after rinsing mouth with water;
(b) Minimize swallowing and hold saliva in mouth;
(c) Place sterilized dental cotton sponge in mouth and chew until it is soaked with saliva (typically < 1 min);
(d) Deposit sponge into syringe directly from the mouth without touching it to avoid contamination;
(e) Insert plunger into syringe;
(f) Squeeze saliva through pre-installed Westran S 0.2 μm polyvinylidene fluoride (PVDF) membrane (Sigma-Aldrich Co. LLC.) at the bottom of syringe and into sterilized tubes. Usually 1 ml of saliva samples is obtained through this process;

(g) Use pipette to drop 100 μL saliva onto a sensor to cover all three electrodes;
(h) Record measurement;
(i) Dispose of sensor after washing out residual salivary specimen.

The saliva collection method provides a reliable filtering performance to remove large biomolecules such as mucins from saliva samples. The collected saliva's viscosity usually ranges from 1.05 to 1.15 mPa· s, which is close to the viscosity of buffer solutions [30]. This is because the 0.2 μm pore size filter that comes pre-installed in collection devices is comprised of a fine PVDF material, which is widely used for protein blotting due to its high protein binding capability (over 200 $\mu g/cm^2$) [31]. Its high efficiency in mucins removal eliminates the matrix effects for saliva tests.

3. Results and Discussion

3.1. Layer-by-Layer Bio-Layer Construction

A variety of methods including physical adsorption, cross-linking, sol-gel matrix entrapment, covalent binding, membrane entrapment, and LBL self-assembly are widely used to fabricate glucose sensors. Among them, LBL self-assembly offers better uniformity, stability, sensitivity; it is also cost effective and has an easier operation processes [32]. This is due to the following: first, there are multiple interaction forces such as electrostatics forces, hydrogen bonds, covalent bonds, Van der Waals' interactions and hydrophobic interactions that we can choose from to build the most appropriate layer composition [33]; second, the LBL films often demonstrate close identical properties after deposition, no matter what substrate they are sitting on [34]; and, third, there is no complicated operation process involved, other than simply dipping the WE into different coating reagents. Thus, the LBL self-assembly method was selected for sensor fabrication.

Distinguished from biosensors that are fabricated for BG testing, SG sensors are developed using nano-materials to achieve better sensitivity, a lower detection limit, and a sufficient detection range for SG measurements. The bioreceptor GOx was used as a catalyst in the oxidation of glucose. During this reaction, electrons were transferred from the coenzyme flavin adenine dinucleotie (FAD) moieties to electrodes through the assembled transducers. Three transducers, SWNT-COOH, CS, and GNp, were selected and optimized in composition. Recent studies demonstrated that carbon nanotubes (CNT) promoted electron transfer reactions and enhanced the electrochemical reactivity of enzymes such as GOx [35]. SWNT was selected over multi-walled CNT due to its higher field emission current, conductivity and specific surface area [36]. The hydrophobic nature of SWNT also permitted it to easily bind onto Pt electrodes through a hydrophobic attraction. With its highly specific surface area and molecule capture capability, SWNT was well confined as a base layer. Wang's group [35] proved that CNT disturbed the secondary structure of GOx and forced its redox centers to move close to electrodes' surface, causing electrons to pass directly without mediators. By applying SWNT, DET from the enzyme to the electrode was realized via a series of "wired" relay centers to achieve lower glucose detection limit. CS was selected due to its outstanding biocompatibility, nontoxicity, stability, and low cost. It contains large numbers of protonated amino groups ($-NH^{3+}$) and hydroxyl groups (–OH) functional groups and is widely used as a bio-linker for enzyme immobilization. GNp has been commonly used in the design of electro-chemical sensors. As an electrocatalyst, GNp can promote electron transfer reactions and dramatically increase the specific surface area to capture a large amount of enzymes so that sensors' sensitivity is enhanced accordingly [37].

The stepwise modification process is described in Figure 2 with detailed information on composition layers [38–40]. The washing step between each layer was to remove un-bound chemicals. SWNT was first entrapped onto the porous Pt WE surface through physical adsorption, hydrophobic attraction, and electrostatic forces. As reported by the manufacturer, their carboxylation process yielded SWNT–COOH with a strong negative charge, while CS carried positive charges which were contributed by protonated amine groups. Thus, the first CS layer was deposited and linked to the SWNT film through electrostatics forces due to their opposite electric charges. Likewise, bonds between

GNp and CS were built through electrostatics forces relying on their opposite electric charges. After this, GOx with negatively charged FAD moieties were assembled onto the GNp layer through physical and covalent adsorption [41]. Some un-adsorbed GOx was also entrapped into underlayer matrices through physical adsorption as well as electrostatics interactions. After fabricating the first (CS/GNp/GOx) multi-layer film, the number of films was optimized based on the sensors' performance. The isoelectric point of GOx is reported as 4.2 by Sigma-Aldrich Co. LLC [42]. So under the enzyme immobilization process when the pH was 7.4, the overall net charge on GOx was negative. When the second multi-layer film was applied, GOx and CS bonds were formed through electrostatic interactions. The rest of the process was repeated as more layers were added.

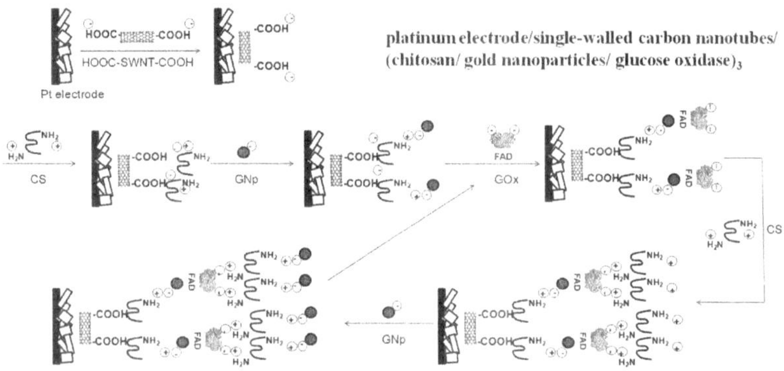

Figure 2. Schematic illustration of the layer-by-layer self-assembly procedure.

A surface imaging technique, SEM was used to obtain information about sensor surface topography and composition. The selected screen-printed sensor chips chose Pt as WE for two reasons: first, its coarse surface morphology with gaps and pinholes permits its large surface areas to entrap many biomolecules (Figure 3A); second, as a noble metal, Pt is chemically inert and tends to provide a stable working potential. Another noble metal, Ag, was chosen as RE because it did not participate in reactions and, as a result, prevented electrode fouling.

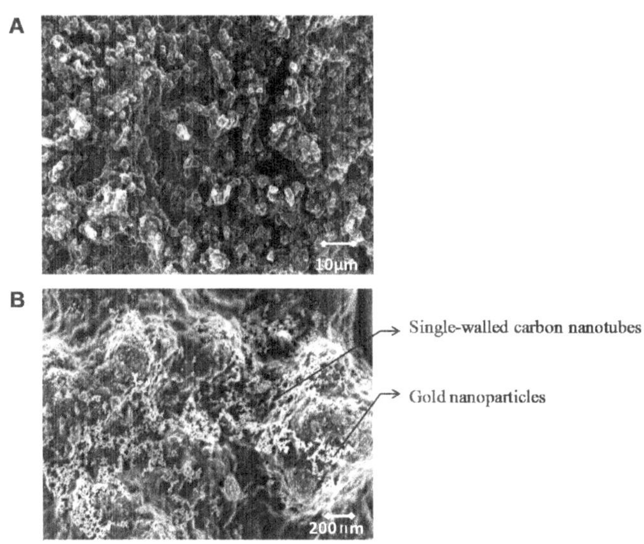

Figure 3. (**A**) Scanning electron microscope (SEM) image of platinum (Pt) electrode surface. (**B**) SEM image of one layer Pt/single-walled carbon nanotubes/chitosan/gold nanoparticles film on Pt electrode surface.

In the SEM image in Figure 3B, a single layer of GNp (white dots) was well dispersed on the SWNT (white short bars) formed matrix layer. GNp's comparable size to GOx provided GOx with more active binding sites and, as a result, immobilized more enzymes through physical adsorption and electrostatics force [43]. Although the covalent attachment method is also widely used to immobilize GOx with high stability, it normally leads to moderate or severe inactivation of enzymes due to conformational changes induced by the strong bonds [43]. Therefore, higher enzyme reactivity is retained through this LBL method since the applied adsorption method does not change the secondary structure of GOx. Here, the SEM image illustrates that multi-layers films are well distributed and provided large surface areas for GOx immobilization.

3.2. Number of Bio-Layers

The working potential was determined to be as low as 0.05 V for three layers, and 0.2 V for six layers, through CV tests. Saliva samples were treated through filtration, boiling and centrifuging processes, and then spiked with glucose to attain different glucose concentrations. Glucose was spiked as concentrated solution by adding 1 part solution to 40 parts treated saliva. The saliva matrix effect was eliminated because the viscosity of spiked saliva samples was close to the viscosity of the buffer solution (about 1.1 mPa· s). By comparing the amperometric results of three and six layers of multi-layer film fabricated sensors, the three-layered film demonstrated a better sensing linearity, intra-repeatability, and lower detection limit (Figure 4A,B). Both tests demonstrated that the absolute values of current density were proportional to glucose concentrations under a fixed working potential. However, the direction of current flow was different with these two type of sensors. This is because, when conducting CV tests, the working potential was picked in a region where anodic current dominated (forward sweep) with three layers of sensors, while with six layers sensors it dropped in a region where cathodic current dominated (backward sweep). With a $(CS/GNp/GOx)_3$ layer composition, sensors achieved a linear glucose detection range up to 45 mg/dL, and the linear regression was with 99% confidence limits. Theoretically, although films with more layers can immobilize larger amounts of GOx, films become thicker and so conductivity is reduced. Moreover, the extended distance between GOx and electrodes may eliminate DET and cause major interferences to glucose detection. As a result, three-layers composition was applied to achieve better sensor performance with less cost of materials and a faster fabrication process.

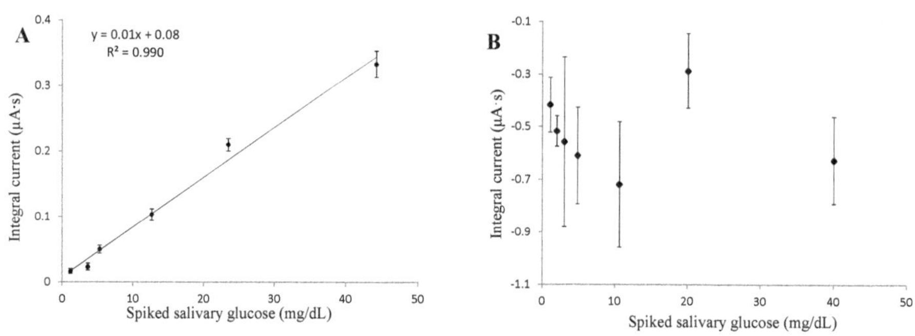

Figure 4. Amperometric tests with effect of different number of (chitosan/gold nanoparticles/glucose oxidase) multi-layer films on electrode (**A**) three multi-layer films; (**B**) six multi-layer films. Error bars = ±standard deviation and $n = 3$.

3.3. Glucose Sensing

With fixed three-layer composition, an appropriate working potential as low as 0.05 V was determined for amperometric tests. A high voltage may include many other redox reactions and cause interferences to glucose detection; thus, a consistent minimum voltage is required to capture all electron transfers for the glucose-GOx reactions alone. Through CV analysis, only the third cycles were analyzed because the signal tended to be more stable after two cycles (48 s). An extremely low working potential was selected with the use of elevated glucose concentrations in PBS, and the calibration curve at steady-state was plotted in Figure 5. This low applied potential further confirmed the DET between enzyme's active sites and the electrode surface [44].

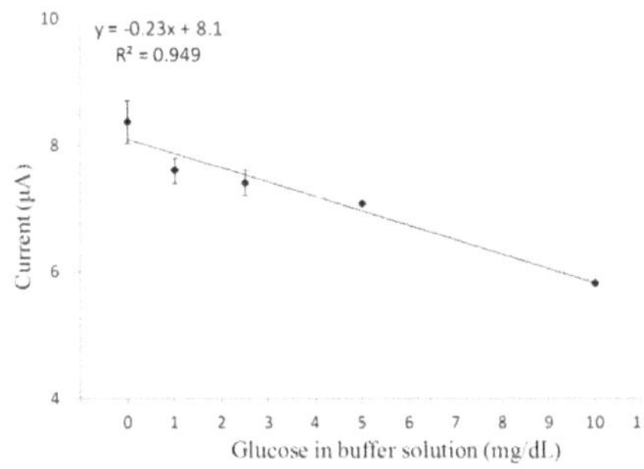

Figure 5. Cyclic voltammetry tests determined steady-state calibration curve of the single-walled carbon nanotubes/(chitosan/gold nanoparticles/glucose oxidase)$_3$ functionalized platinum electrode. Error bars = ±standard deviation and n = 3.

Amperometric tests of Pt/SWNT/(CS/GNp/GOx)$_3$ functionalized sensors were conducted under a selected working potential by using elevated glucose in PBS. It demonstrated a linear detection range of 0.5–20 mg/dL and the linear regression was with 98% confidence limits (Figure 6A). In order to study the SWNT's effect on layer composition and sensing efficiency, the same tests with Pt/(CS/GNp/GOx)$_3$ functionalized sensors were conducted under optimized working potential of −0.05 V. The results showed less repeatable readings with weaker linearity within this glucose range (Figure 6B). The comparison of sensor performances in Table 2 demonstrated sensors with SWNT had higher intra-repeatability, linearity, and lower LOD. Through this study, the high repeatability benefited from a uniformly confined SWNT matrix and well stabilized LBL multi-layer films on electrodes [45]. Concurrently, a lower glucose level was detectable in favor of the better conductivity and signal-to-noise ratio with the aid of SWNT [46]. The good linearity revealed that the immobilized GOx amount was sufficient for glucose detection up to 20 mg/dL, and that benefited from the large specific surface area provided by SWNT. As a result, this study concluded that SWNT played an essential role in promoting more repeatable measurements (coefficient of variance <10%), lower LOD (0.41 mg/dL), and a sufficient linear detection range (0.5–20 mg/dL with R^2 = 0.98). With optimized sensor layer composition, a human subjects study was conducted to evaluate the sensors' performance in SG measurements.

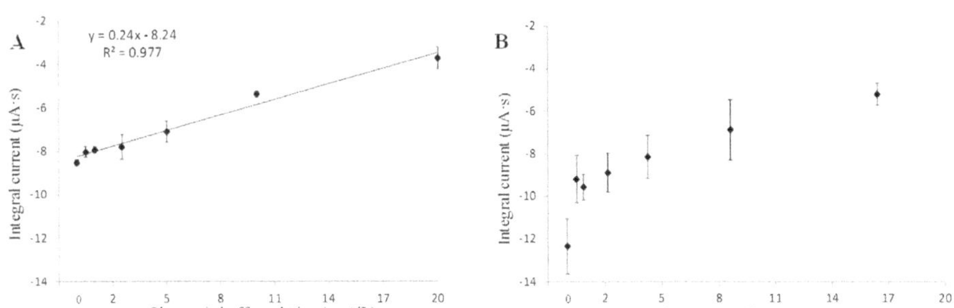

Figure 6. Amperometric tests with the effect of SWNT in support of sensor functionalization (**A**) single-walled carbon nanotubes/(chitosan/gold nanoparticles/glucose oxidase)$_3$ functional layers; (**B**) (chitosan/gold nanoparticles/glucose oxidase)$_3$ functional layers without single-walled carbon nanotubes. Error bars = ±standard deviation and n = 3.

Table 2. A comparison between sensors immobilized with and without single-walled carbon nanotubes.

Amperometric Test	$Pt/SWNT/(CS/GNp/GOx)_3$	$Pt/(CS/GNp/GOx)_3$
Detection range (glucose in PBS)	0–20 mg/dL	0–20 mg/dL
[a] Repeatability	<10%	<20%
[b] Limit of detection (LOD)	0.41 mg/dL	4.94 mg/dL
[c] linearity	0.98	0.78

[a] Repeatability was presented by the coefficient of variation produced from at least four single-use sensors; [b] LOD was calculated by dividing the sum of an average blank signal (x) plus three times the standard deviation of x by the slope of regression line; [c] The linearity was evaluated by the R-squared (R^2), which was a statistical measure of how close the data were to the fitted regression line. SWNT, single-walled carbon nanotubes; PBS, phosphate buffered saline; Pt, platinum; CS, chitosan; GNp, gold nanoparticles; GOx, glucose oxidase.

3.4. *Glucose in Saliva*

Two major objectives of the human subjects studies were as follows: (1) to understand the relationship between BG and SG of healthy people at a fasting state; (2) to screen for diabetes by measuring SG at fasting. Saliva samples were collected through the saliva collection protocol and tested immediately using glucose sensors. A linear correlation between the sensor's signal and the reference method (UV method) that measured SG concentrations was found in a range of 1.1 to 10.1 mg/dL ($R^2 = 0.931$), including 287 individual sensors' measurement (Figure 7A). A conversion formula SG = (Signal + 0.249)/0.0653 mg/dL was derived from the linear regression curve (Figure 7A), and applied to convert sensors' signal into SG levels. The intra-repeatability of SG levels measurements by at least three single-use glucose sensors achieved a variance <15%. Technically, BG levels at fasting are considered as a crucial index to evaluate peoples' health conditions and, more importantly, as a tool to screen for diabetes. Normal BG levels are typically less than 100 mg/dL, while diabetes is diagnosed if the fasting BG is 126 mg/dL or higher [47,48]. In this study, subjects A and B demonstrated that their fasting BG levels were lower than 100 mg/dL. Correspondingly, their SG levels were monitored over a year and plotted in Figure 7B. The normal range of fasting SG was 1.4 to 1.6 mg/dL for subject A, and 1.1 to 1.4 mg/dL for subject B, respectively. There were a couple of data points (circled) when subjects were not in good health conditions, either having a cold/fever or were in menstruation. That was when an elevated SG level was recorded. In conclusion, the healthy individual fasting SG was relatively consistent over time as long as the subjects' health conditions were unchanged.

Similar tests were further performed by eight healthy subjects. An interesting finding that was the BG (mg/dL)/SG (mg/dL) ratio of each subject at fasting was unique and the value was individually dependent (Table 3). For instance, subject B's fasting BG/SG ratio was 69.8 with a variance of 7.1% based on a 39-day study; for subject A, the fasting BG/SG ratio was 64.8 with a variance of 10.8% based on an 11-day study. Thus, with the aid of an initial calibration to determine the individual's BG/SG ratio at fasting, BG levels are predictable by measuring fasting SG levels on a daily basis. Thus, we propose an alternative method by measuring SG levels at fasting to evaluate glycemic levels and monitor health conditions. The findings indicate that SG levels at fasting can potentially be used to screen for diabetes. In the future, complete clinical validation including diabetic patients are crucial to apply the same concept obtained from this study for appropriate self-management of diabetes.

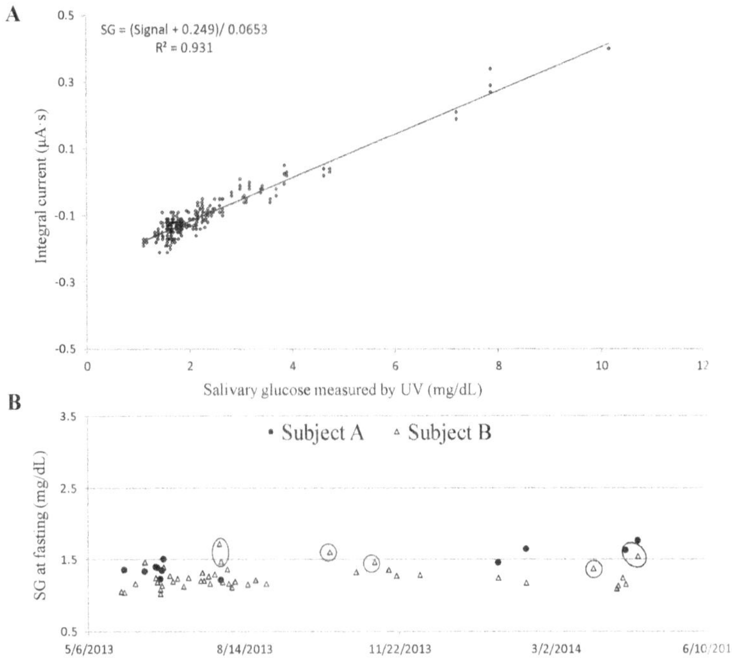

Figure 7. (**A**) Linear correlation between sensor and ultra-violet visible (UV) measured salivary glucose (SG) with obtained conversion formula; (**B**) Fasting SG monitoring history of two healthy females.

Table 3. Ten healthy subjects' blood glucose (BG)/salivary glucose (SG) ratios at fasting.

Subjects	Gender	Age	BG (mg/dL)	SG (mg/dL)	BG/SG Ratio
A	female	20s	92.7	1.43	64.8
B	female	20s	85.2	1.22	69.8
C	male	40s	96.5	1.39	69.6
D	male	50s	114.6	1.99	57.6
E	male	50s	108	2.4	45
F	male	50s	101	1.46	69.2
G	male	50s	99.7	1.43	69.7
H	male	20s	91.6	1.55	59.1
I	male	20s	100.3	1.73	58
J	female	20s	91.6	1.05	87.2

4. Conclusions

A disposable electrochemical sensor which could detect trace glucose levels down to 0.41 mg/dL has been developed. With a linear glucose detection range of 1.1–45 mg/dL, the sensors demonstrate good accuracy in SG measurements with the detection of variances of less than 15%. The human subjects studies, which included ten healthy subjects, have successfully accomplished a SG detection range of 1.1–10.1 mg/dL. Validation through the use of a reference UV method proves that the SG sensors are capable of accurate and reliable detection of glucose in real saliva. Also, the individual SG levels at fasting are found to be unique and relatively consistent over time if subjects' health conditions are unchanged. This discovery reveals that fasting SG levels are a crucial indicator of health conditions and can potentially be used for diabetes management. In the near future, it will be important to extend clinical trials that include diabetics to verify: (1) the efficiency of using SG levels to predict BG levels in real time; (2) whether sensors can detect extremely low/high SG levels as indications of dangerous hypoglycemia/hyperglycemia conditions. In conclusion, noninvasive SG glucose sensors have successfully been applied to measure a person's glucose level. The two-minute saliva test, including the preparation of samples, has great potential to be a viable alternative to BG measurement at fasting, and can even be applied for national screening programs for undiagnosed diabetes.

Acknowledgments: Part of our research work was conducted at the Gorge J. Kostas Nanoscale Technology and Manufacturing Research Center at Northeastern University. We would like to acknowledge a partial funding from Keyghobad Ventures LLC under Grant No. 0731102. We are grateful for the volunteers who participated in clinical studies.

Author Contributions: Yunqing Du, Wenjun Zhang, and Ming L. Wang conceived and designed the experimental protocols. Yunqing Du designed and performed the experiments, analyzed the data, and wrote the paper. All authors contributed to the writing of the manuscript.

Conflicts of Interest: The authors declare no conflict of interest.

References

1. National Diabetes Statistics Report. 2014. Available online: http://www.cdc.gov/diabetes/pubs/statsreport14/national-diabetes-report-web.pdf (accessed on 30 December 2015).
2. Kaufman, E.; Lamster, I.B. The diagnostic application of saliva—A review. *Crit. Rev. Oral Biol. Med.* **2002**, *13*, 197–212. [CrossRef] [PubMed]
3. Agrawal, R.P.; Sharma, N.; Rathore, M.S.; Gupta, V.B.; Jain, S.; Agarwal, V.; Goyal, S. Noninvasive method for glucose level estimation by saliva. *J. Diabetes Metab.* **2013**, *4*. [CrossRef]
4. Mirzaii-Dizgah, I.; Mirzaii-Dizgah, M.R.; Mirzaii-Dizgah, M.H. Stimulated saliva glucose as a diagnostic specimen for diabetes mellitus. *J. Arch. Mil. Med.* **2013**, *1*, 24–27. [CrossRef]
5. Mitsumori, M.; Yamaguchi, M.; Kano, Y. A new approach to noninvasive measurement of blood glucose using saliva analyzing systems. In Proceedings of the 20th Annual International Conference of the Engineering in Medicine and Biology Society, Hong Kong, China, 29 October–1 Noverber 1998; pp. 1767–1770.
6. Yamaguchi, M.; Mitsumori, M.; Kano, Y. Development of noninvasive procedure for monitoring blood glucose levels using saliva. In Proceedings of the 20th Annual International Conference of the Engineering in Medicine and Biology Society, Hong Kong, China, 29 October–1 Noverber 1998; pp. 1763–1766.
7. Yeh, C.K.; Christodoulides, N.J.; Floriano, P.N.; Miller, C.S.; Ebersole, J.L.; Weigum, S.E.; Floriano, P.N.; Miller, C.S.; Ebersole, J.L.; Weigum, S.E.; *et al.* Current development of saliva/oral fluid-based diagnostics. *Tex. Dent. J.* **2010**, *127*, 651–661. [PubMed]
8. Zeller, H.; Novak, P.; Landgraf, R. Blood glucose measurement by infrared spectroscopy. *Int. J. Artif. Organs* **1989**, *12*, 129–135. [PubMed]
9. D'Auria, S.; Lakowicz, J.R. Enzyme fluorescence as a sensing tool: New perspectives in biotechnology. *Curr. Opin. Biotechnol.* **2001**, *12*, 99–104. [CrossRef]
10. Shao, J.; Lin, M.; Li, Y.; Li, X.; Liu, J.; Liang, J.; Yao, H. *In vivo* blood glucose quantification using raman spectroscopy. *PLoS ONE* **2012**, *7*. [CrossRef] [PubMed]
11. Mclntosh, T.S.; Davis, H.M.; Matthews, D.E. A liquid chromatography-mass spectrometry method to measure stable isotopic tracer enrichments of glycerol and glucose in human serum. *Anal. Biochem.* **2002**, *300*, 163–169. [CrossRef] [PubMed]
12. Vahjudi, P.N.; Patterson, M.E.; Lim, S.; Yee, J.K.; Mao, C.S.; Lee, W.N. Measurement of glucose and fructose in clinical samples using gas chromatography/mass spectrometry. *Clin. Biochem.* **2010**, *43*, 198–207.
13. Wang, J. Electrochemical Glucose Biosensors. In *Sensors, Biosensors and Their Biomedical Applications*, 1st ed.; Zhang, X., Ju, H., Wang, J., Eds.; Academic Press: Burlington, MA, USA, 2008; Volume 3, pp. 57–69.
14. Lubrano, G.J.; Guilbault, G.G. Glucose and l-amino acid electrodes based on enzyme membranes. *Anal. Chim. Acta* **1978**, *97*, 229–236. [CrossRef]
15. Yoo, E.H.; Lee, S.Y. Glucose biosensors: An overview of use in clinical practice. *Sensors* **2010**, *10*, 4558–4576. [CrossRef] [PubMed]
16. Ghindilis, L.A.; Atanasov, P.; Wilkins, E. Enzyme-catalyzed direct electron transfer: Fundamentals and analytical applications. *Electroanalysis* **1997**, *9*, 661–674. [CrossRef]
17. De Almeida Pdel, V.; Grégio, A.M.; Machado, M.A.; de Lima, A.A.; Azevedo, L.R. Saliva composition and functions: A comprehensive review. *J. Contemp. Dent. Pract.* **2008**, *9*, 72–80. [PubMed]
18. Chou, J.; Tsai, Y.; Cheng, T.; Liao, Y.; Ye, G.; Yang, S. Fabrication of arrayed flexible screen-printed glucose biosensor based on microfluidic framework. *IEEE Sens. J.* **2014**, *14*, 178–183. [CrossRef]

19. Jing, J.; Hong, Y. Amperometric glucose sensor based on coimmobilization of glucose oxidase and poly(p-phenylenediamine) at a platinum microdisk electrode. *Anal. Biochem.* **2000**, *280*, 221–226. [CrossRef] [PubMed]
20. Nie, Z.; Deiss, F.; Liu, X.; Akbulut, O.; Whitesides, G.M. Integration of paper-based microfluidic devices with commercial electrochemical readers. *Lab Chip* **2010**, *10*, 3169–3169. [CrossRef] [PubMed]
21. Liu, J.; Sun, S.; Liu, C.; Wei, S. An amperometric glucose biosensor based on a screen-printed electrode and os-complex mediator for flow injection analysis. *Measurement* **2011**, *44*, 1878–1883. [CrossRef]
22. Ohfuji, K.; Sato, N.; Hamada-sato, N.; Kobayashi, T.; Imada, C.; Okuma, H.; Watanabe, E. Construction of a glucose sensor based on a screen-printed electrode and a novel mediator pyocyanin from pseudomonas aeruginosa. *Biosens. Bioelectron.* **2004**, *19*, 1237–1244. [CrossRef] [PubMed]
23. Berisha, L.; Kalcher, K.; Hajrizi, A.; Arbneshi, T. A new biosensor for glucose based on screen-printed carbon electrodes modified with Tin (IV)-oxide. *Am. J. Anal. Chem.* **2013**, *4*, 27–35. [CrossRef]
24. Yamaoka, H.; Sode, K. A disposable electrochemical glucose sensor using catalytic subunit of novel thermostable glucose dehydrogenase. *Open Biotechnol. J.* **2007**, *1*, 26–30. [CrossRef]
25. Polan, V.; Soukup, J.; Vytřas, K. Screen-printed carbon electrodes modified by rhodium dioxide and glucose dehydrogenase. *Enzyme Res.* **2010**, *2010*. [CrossRef] [PubMed]
26. Khan, G.F.; Ohwa, M.; Wernet, W. Design of a stable charge transfer complex electrode for a third-generation amperometric glucose sensor. *Anal. Chem.* **1996**, *68*, 2939–2945. [CrossRef] [PubMed]
27. Retama, J.R.; Cabarcos, E.L.; Mecerreyes, D.; López-ruiz, B. Design of an amperometric biosensor using polypyrrole-microgel composites containing glucose oxidase. *Biosens. Bioelectron.* **2004**, *20*, 1111–1117. [CrossRef] [PubMed]
28. Yang, T.; Hung, C.; Ke, J.; Zen, J. An electrochemically preanodized screen-printed carbon electrode for achieving direct electron transfer to glucose oxidase. *Electrochem. Commun.* **2008**, *10*, 1094–1097. [CrossRef]
29. Glucose Colorimetric/Fluorometric Assay Kit. 2014. Available online: http://www.biovision.com/manuals/K606.pdf (accessed on 22 January 2016).
30. Du, Y.; Zhang, W.; Wang, M.L. An on-chip disposable salivary glucose sensor for diabetes control. *J. Diabetes Sci. Technol.* **2016**. in press.
31. Whatman Westran PVDF Membranes. 2016. Available online: http://www.sigmaaldrich.com/catalog/product/aldrich/z671010?lang=en®=US (accessed on 22 January 2016).
32. Costa, R.R.; Mano, J.F. Layer-by-layer self-assembly techniques for nanostructured devices in tissue engineering. In *Nanomaterials in Tissue Engineering: Characterization, Fabrication and Applications*, 1st ed.; Gaharwar, A.K., Sant, S., Hancock, M.J., Hacking, S.A., Eds.; Woodhead Pulishing Ltd: Cambridge, UK, 2013; Volume 4, pp. 88–118.
33. Kumara, M.T.; Tripp, B.C.; Muralidharan, S. Layer-by-layer assembly of bioengineered flagella protein nanotubes. *Biomacromolecules* **2007**, *8*, 2718–2722. [CrossRef] [PubMed]
34. Rubner, M.F.; Cohen, R.E. Layer-by-layer processed multilayers: Challenges and opportunities. In *Multilayer Thin Films: Sequential Assembly of Nanocomposite Materials*, 2nd ed.; Decher, G., Schlenoff, J.B., Eds.; Wiley-VCH Verlag & Co. KGaA: Weinheim, Germany, 2012; Volume 1, pp. 23–41.
35. Wang, Y.; Yao, Y. Direct electron transfer of glucose oxidase promoted by carbon nanotubes is without value in certain mediator-free applications. *Microchim. Acta* **2012**, *176*, 271–277. [CrossRef]
36. Andzane, J.; Tobin, J.M.; Li, Z.; Prikulis, J.; Baxendale, M.; Olin, H.; Holmes, J.D.; Erts, D. Selection of application specific single and multi walled carbon nanotubes by *in situ* characterization of conductive and field emission properties. *AZojono-J. Nanotechnol. Online* **2007**, *3*. [CrossRef]
37. Tang, J.L.; Wang, J.N. Chemical sensing sensitivity of long-period grating sensor enhanced by colloidal gold nanoparticles. *Sensors* **2008**, *8*, 171–184. [CrossRef]
38. Zhang, W.; Wang, M.L. Saliva Glucose Monitoring System. U.S. Patent US 14/153.647, 17 July 2014.
39. Zhang, W.; Du, Y.; Wang, M.L. Noninvasive glucose monitoring using saliva nano-biosensor. *Sens. Biosens. Res.* **2015**, *4*, 23–29. [CrossRef]
40. Zhang, W.; Du, Y.; Wang, M.L. On-chip ultra-sensitive glucose sensing using multilayer films composed of single-walled carbon nanotubes-gold nanoparticles-and glucose oxidase. *Sens. Biosens. Res.* **2015**, *4*, 96–102.
41. Petkova, G.A.; Záruba, C.K.; Zvátora, P.; Král, V. Gold and silver nanoparticles for biomolecule immobilization and enzymatic analysis. *Nanoscale Res. Lett.* **2012**, *7*. [CrossRef] [PubMed]

42. Product Information. 2002. Available online: http://www.sigmaaldrich.com/content/dam/sigma-aldrich/docs/Sigma/Product_Information_Sheet/2/g6125pis.pdf (accessed on 22 January 2016).
43. Ma, S.; Mu, J.; Qu, Y.; Jiang, L. Effect of refluxed sliver nanoparticles on inhibition and enhancement of enzymatic activity of glucose oxidase. *Colloids Surf. A Physicochem. Eng. Asp.* **2009**, *345*, 101–105. [CrossRef]
44. Ruzgas, T.; Csöregi, E.; Emnéus, J.; Gorton, L.; Marko-Varga, G. Peroxidase-modified electrodes: Fundamentals and application. *Anal. Chim. Acta* **1996**, *330*, 123–138. [CrossRef]
45. Paloma, Y.; Jordi, R.; Jose, M.P.; Xavier, R. Electrochemical sensing based on carbon nanotubes. *Trends Anal. Chem.* **2010**, *29*, 939–953.
46. Dai, M.; Maxwell, S.; Vogt, B.D.; La-Belle, J.T. Mesoporous carbon amperometric glucose sensors using inexpensive, commercial methacrylate-based binders. *Anal. Chim. Acta* **2012**, *738*, 27–34. [CrossRef] [PubMed]
47. Diagnosing Diabetes and Learning about Prediabetes. 2014. Available online: http://www.diabetes.org/diabetes-basics/diagnosis/ (accessed on 2 March 2016).
48. Bower, B.F.; Moore, R.E. The interpretation of laboratory tests 97 György Abel and Michael Laposata. In *Clinical Laboratory Medicine*, 2nd ed.; McClatchey, K.D., Ed.; Lippincott Williams & Wilkins: Maywood, IL, USA, 2002; p. 339.

5

Computational Assessment of Neural Probe and Brain Tissue Interface under Transient Motion

Michael Polanco [1], Sebastian Bawab [1] and Hargsoon Yoon [2,*]

[1] Department of Mechanical and Aerospace Engineering, Old Dominion University, Norfolk, VA 23529, USA; mpola002@odu.edu (M.P.); sbawab@odu.edu (S.B.)
[2] Department of Engineering, Center for Materials Research, Norfolk State University, Norfolk, VA 23504, USA
* Correspondence: hyoon@nsu.edu

Academic Editor: Jeff D. Newman

Abstract: The functional longevity of a neural probe is dependent upon its ability to minimize injury risk during the insertion and recording period *in vivo*, which could be related to motion-related strain between the probe and surrounding tissue. A series of finite element analyses was conducted to study the extent of the strain induced within the brain in an area around a neural probe. This study focuses on the transient behavior of neural probe and brain tissue interface with a viscoelastic model. Different stages of the interface from initial insertion of neural probe to full bonding of the probe by astro-glial sheath formation are simulated utilizing analytical tools to investigate the effects of relative motion between the neural probe and the brain while friction coefficients and kinematic frequencies are varied. The analyses can provide an in-depth look at the quantitative benefits behind using soft materials for neural probes.

Keywords: neural electrodes; brain; finite element analysis; viscoelasticity

---

1. Introduction

Various neural probes have been developed for neuro-chemical and electrical signal sensing inside the brain [1–9]. By using chronically implanted probing devices, single neural cell and/or multi-neural ensemble recording could be available over a long period of time. Efforts continue to enhance the yield and longevity of chronic neural recordings in laboratory animals. Even with successful implementation of neural sensing devices in the brain, it is important to address longevity issues in chronic neural recording. The recording capabilities of microelectrodes have been mostly limited to a few months; they then degrade over time due in part to neuronal cell degeneration and cell layer formation on the electrodes from the inflammatory immune response caused by the chronic implantation and operation [10,11]. It is reported that the inflammatory response to mechanical impact also gives rise to Interleukin-1β, a proinflammatory cytokine derived from the caspase-1 enzyme [12,13]. Recent studies have shown a promising result for pharmacologic intervention that proves that the recording capabilities of electrodes can be improved by blocking caspase-1 activity [14].

To mitigate cellular and molecular response to the implanted probe, various materials and designs of neural probes and the local delivery of anti-inflammatory drug have been investigated to enhance electrode longevity [15–19]. Some other approaches such as nerve growth factor application or rejuvenation process using electrical pulses may be another useful strategy to prolong the lifetime of chronically implanted microelectrodes [20–22]. Many researchers have focused on using soft materials to mediate tissue and cell damage from mechanical motion in the brain [18,19].

While silicon and metal probes have traditionally been utilized for neural sensing applications, soft polymer materials may have an advantage due to their greater flexibility and biocompatibility [18,23,24].

One major problem that occurs when interfacing neural probes and brain tissue is related to the large difference in Young's Modulus (10^5–10^7 Pa) between them [25]. During chronic recording, the brain is subjected to movement brought upon by external motion of the body due to cardiac pulse, breathing, rapid head movement or impact collision. The difference in material stiffness between the brain and the probe makes the brain microvasculature and neural cells more susceptible to mechanical damage such as glial scarring. To mitigate these damage mechanisms, it is advantageous to design a probe that will minimize damage to the brain by limiting relative motion between the embedded neural probe and brain tissue, and ultimately enhance the quality of neural sensing and functional lifetime of the probe.

There have been several research efforts to implement materials with stiffness values close to that of brain tissue [26–31]. In Kim's research, hydrogel coatings were applied to surface of neural electrodes for better integration and mechanical buffering between the electrodes and neural tissue. Kipke's group tested Polydimethylsiloxane (PDMS) probes in an agarose *in vitro* brain model using stiff silicon insertion shuttles that can resolve a conflicting issue of precise implantations and mechanical softness. A composite neural probe with Parylene-C and polyethylene glycol (PEG) with integrated microfluidic channels was investigated. In this approach, PEG inside the microchannels makes the probe stiff and allows for precise positioning of the probe into a cortex. The PEG dissolves upon insertion into the brain resulting in a mechanically soft structure. Work continues in this area to quantify the mechanical compliance of softer probes for coupling with the brain.

To aid in increasing longevity of neural probes, previous research using finite element analysis has addressed the effects that micromotion can have on the brain when an embedded neural probe is present using different coatings and probe material properties [12,32–35]. Studies have also been conducted examining the brain tissue over a period of weeks using embedded probes of varying stiffnesses [36]. However, the analyses have been largely limited to static deformation, and limited research has been performed to understand the effect of transient motion, or frequency, on the brain. The effects of transient motion have been studied by Zhang [37], who only looked at the brain's response to a silicon probe during the motion. Time history displacement test data was acquired from Differential Variable Reluctance Transducers (DVRT) that were placed on the surface of anesthetized rat brains [38,39]. The displacements recorded in the brain due to respiration can range between 2 and 25 μm while the frequencies corresponding to those displacements are approximately 1–2 Hz [38,39]. Likewise, the displacements corresponding to cardiac pulse are slightly lower at 1–4 μm [38,39] with frequencies reaching up to 5 Hz. These measurements were taken with the brain exposed and a portion of the skull removed.

The major interest of this study is to investigate the transient motion of the brain with frequencies between 1 and 40 Hz applying mechanically-compliant materials for a neural probe and illustrate the post-insertion behavior of the probes during head movements that are likely to produce significant micromotion between the probes and surrounding brain tissue. While rat physiology will be employed in the studies, the frequencies are chosen such that practical applicability to humans can be extrapolated. For example, the frequencies in humans that can be generated within the head during walking can reach approximately 24 Hz at resonance [40]. Previously, transient frequencies at 1 and 5 Hz and Young's Moduli ranging from 165 GPa (silicon) to 6 MPa were considered [41]. The latter was driven by a finding shown in Lee [33] showing silicon microelectrodes to be capable of producing strains up to approximately 25% within the brain under a 1 μm longitudinal static displacement during initial insertion, or no coupling between the probe and the brain. The present study, using Finite Element Analysis techniques, covers a full range of friction coefficients to simulate different events in the probe implantation period from initial insertion to bonding, as represented by the formation of microglia/microphages around the implant site.

The intention of this study is to capture the interaction of the probe onto the brain due to relative micromotion. The configuration assumes that the probe being fixed to the skull complies with conventional animal experimental conditions using depth probes. It is expected that the relative motion between the probe and the brain still occurs [42] despite being enclosed in the skull where micromotion may be more inhibited. The outcome of this configuration can be applied and useful for future analysis of floating electrodes on the cortical surface including the cerebrospinal fluid within a hydrostatically sealed cranial structure. Since the state-of-the-art is gravitating towards manufacturing mechanically compliant neural probes to increase its longevity, a low modulus value of 200 kPa resembling hydrogel-type materials is studied and compared with a traditionally used silicon probe in the assessment of mechanical mismatch reduction between the probe and the brain.

2. Materials and Methods

The same quarter-symmetry finite element model (FEM) and boundary conditions described in [41] were utilized for this study. Quarter-symmetry boundary conditions assume that, in a full-scale representation, all kinematic motion and behavior from the interaction between the probe and the brain is mirrored along all symmetry planes, and has been utilized in previous studies [33,34,36,37]. The probe dimensions for the Michigan electrode were taken for our study and are described in [33], which represents a typical geometric representation of a silicon microelectrode. The probe was assumed to be placed in the center of a full brain model. Accordingly, the dimensions of the probe for the quarter-symmetry model were 7.5 μm thick, 60 μm wide, and 3000 μm long (note that both the half thickness and half widths were modeled in accordance with quarter-symmetry dimensions). Since microelectrodes can record from neurons within a radius of approximately 140 μm radius from the implant site [43], and damage due to micromotion could occur in cells within a 60 μm radius [25], the dimensions were chosen to be much greater than 140 μm to sufficiently capture deformation patterns within the brain. Thus, the dimensions of the brain model are 750 μm wide, 750 μm thick and 5000 μm long. The model contained a total of 11,860 elements and 14,794 nodes. A mesh bias was applied to concentrate the higher element density towards the interface between the brain and the probe, where the maximum deformation was expected to occur.

The nonlinear transient finite element code LS-DYNA [44] Version 971 R6.0 was utilized since the nature of the micromotion profiles was transient. A reduced integration formulation for solid elements [45] in LS-DYNA was utilized to characterize elements in both the probe and the brain. Using traditional contact definitions [46] within the software, three coefficients of friction were chosen for the simulations: 0.3, 0.6, and 1. The coefficients were chosen to simulate different periods of time for the probe to brain interface. A coefficient of friction of 0.3 signifies a period of initial insertion, or no coupling, a coefficient of 0.6 simulates increased, yet loose, bonding of the probe to the brain due to microglia formation, while a coefficient of 1 represents full bonding denoted by the microglia formation.

An elastic formulation on the probe was employed for the 200 kPa Young's Modulus similar to the property of some hydrogels ($v = 0.33$), while a rigid formulation was employed for the silicon probe to prevent allow for quicker run times in LS-DYNA ($E = 165$ GPa, $v = 0.22$). These property values for silicon were the same values utilized in Lee [33]. A literature survey on properties conducted by Yang [47] highlights the various methods researchers have used to characterize the brain, including hyperelastic [48], elastic, and viscoelastic [49–52] formulations, sometimes with user-defined material models [52,53]. For our application, a linear viscoelastic material model with properties acquired from [54] for head impact studies was used to characterize the brain since small displacements on the order of tens of micrometers were included in our modeling. The material properties utilized for the brain can be found in Table 1. The shear behavior for a linear viscoelastic model is characterized using the following constitutive equation as a function of time: $G(t) = G_\infty + (G_o - G_\infty)e^{-\beta t}$, where β is the decay constant, while being elastic in compression. The bulk modulus utilized here has been derived from testing [55] and has been commonly used for brain injury research. The shear properties utilized for this study account for the stiffness in the brain due to ventricles, and, as stated by [56], the ratio between bulk and shear moduli is approximately 10^5, to define the incompressible nature of the brain and its low stiffness in shear. As the intent of this study is to capture the interaction of the probe onto the brain solely due to relative micromotion, cerebrospinal fluid was absent from the analyses at this time for simplicity and comparative analysis with previous studies.

Table 1. Brain viscoelastic material properties.

	Density (kg/mm^3)	Bulk Modulus (GPa)	Short-term Shear Modulus, G_o (kPa)	Long-term Shear Modulus, G_∞ (kPa)	Decay constant, β ($m \cdot s^{-1}$)
Brain	1.05×10^{-6}	2.1	10	2	0.08

The top surface of the probe was fixed to represent an attachment of the neural probe to the skull. All input pulses were applied to the bottom surface of the brain in accordance with micromotion propagation onto the probe. The frequencies chosen and applied in the analyses, ranging from 1 Hz to 40 Hz, are most pertinent to the transient motion brought upon by rigorous motion that has the neural probe embedded in their brain. For this study, a low magnitude displacement of 4 μm was chosen to cover the 1–40 Hz frequency range being considered for the transient analyses. Only longitudinal motion was considered for the analyses since it has been shown to inflict greater injury by the probe during mechanical motion [33,34,37]. To assess the behavior of the brain at higher frequencies over time, the cases were run for three cycles using the 4 μm magnitude using a less stiff probe (200 kPa) over the 1–40 Hz frequency range. Due to long run times as a result of higher moduli associated with the probe, analyses using the silicon probe were relegated to only one cycle of motion. The intent was to capture the deformation of the brain at peak displacement after the probe has been inserted into the brain, as maximum strain was expected to take place at the initial period of displacement such as the onset of head impact.

3. Results

Both Von Mises stress and strain were examined in the analyses to take into account the combined compression-extension and shearing that takes place along the probe interface during brain motion. Stress and strain values were acquired for FEM elements that are adjacent to the interface, expecting that the deformation would be greatest in this region of the brain. Tables 2 and 3 show the side stresses and strains at the tip of the probe-brain interface at maximum displacement of the brain for the first motion cycle using various friction coefficients for both probes. The stresses increase monotonically with the applied displacement frequency by over 1000 Pa. Values in the tables show two things: differences in stress and strain values over various degrees of probe/brain coupling, and peak deformation values converge as bonding increases along the interface. In addition, the stress level is kept relatively steady and small compared to silicon when Young's Modulus is reduced to 200 kPa over the frequency range of 1 to 40 Hz. Over lower frequencies, the softer probe exhibits high stress and strain levels compared to the characteristics at higher frequencies due to a conversion of brain kinetic energy to strain energy in the probe. Around 20–30 Hz, however, a slight increase is seen due to an increase in impulsive effects between the probe and the brain, though the levels never reach as high as those seen around 1–5 Hz. The relative reduction in stress and strain compared to silicon does not go below approximately 95% over the 1–40 Hz frequency range compared to silicon.

Table 2. Maximum stress side interface values for 165 GPa (silicon)/0.0002 GPa probe at the tip.

Frequency	Interface Stress (Pa) with 0.3 COF	Interface Stress (Pa) with 0.6 COF	Interface Stress (Pa) with 1 COF
1 Hz	325/14.7	304/6.62	291/3.92
5 Hz	607/12.9	570/5.27	545/2.92
10 Hz	857.5/11.6	813/3.7	764/2.96
15 Hz	1010/10	955/3.38	906/3.46
20 Hz	1149/9.3	1080/4.02	1011/3.67
30 Hz	1310/10	1230/5.06	1146/4.79
40 Hz	1400/10.8	1350/6.2	1260/5.53

Table 3. Maximum strain side interface values for 165 GPa (silicon)/0.0002 GPa probe at the tip.

Frequency	Side Interface Strain with 0.3 COF	Side Interface Strain with 0.6 COF	Side Interface Strain with 1 COF
1 Hz	0.0503/2.14e−3	0.0474/1.03e−3	0.0448/5.67e−4
5 Hz	0.052/1.45e−3	0.049/6e−4	0.0463/3.29e−4
10 Hz	0.0529/9.38e−4	0.0497/3.27e−4	0.0472/2.3e−4
15 Hz	0.0535/7.11e−4	0.05/2.58e−4	0.0478/2.08e−4
20 Hz	0.0539/5.91e−4	0.0511/2.42e−4	0.0487/1.94e−4
30 Hz	0.054/5.24e−4	0.0514/2.42e−4	0.0487/2.06e−4
40 Hz	0.0583/5.05e−4	0.0552/2.74e−4	0.0515/2.33e−4

The effect of frequency change and adhesion on stress and strain can be found in Figures 1 and 2, all shown for the first cycle of motion for the 200 kPa probe. The hysteresis loop, shown for a friction coefficient of 0.6, encompasses a wider range of stress and strain at lower frequencies due to a longer time of contact between the probe and the brain during the first cycle and returning close to its original state. As the frequency increases to 20 Hz, the stress levels decrease compared with 5 Hz, possibly due to strain energy being absorbed by the soft probe as a result of the kinetic energy increase. Sinusoidal effects are present due to the increased presence of friction along the probe-brain interface. However, when the frequency reaches 40 Hz, the stress levels increase again, possibly due to inertial effects being present, leading to increased indentation with larger kinetic energies present. The strain levels also end at the same values before undergoing another cycle of motion. A low friction coefficient (COF = 0.3) unsurprisingly exhibits high stresses and strains before settling at a strain value during the first cycle. However, once the friction coefficient reaches 0.6, the stress and strain behavior is nearly similar to that with a friction coefficient of 1, or total bonding. This behavior suggests similarity with other degrees of bonding once it has been achieved. The strain, or deformation, energy in the 200 kPa probe is shown in Figure 3. The energy increases directly both with friction, or the degree of interface bonding, and frequency in the brain as work done by friction acts to resist the motion in the brain in creating increased deformation. The silicon probe is not shown as the strain energy was shown to be negligible due to its relatively high stiffness.

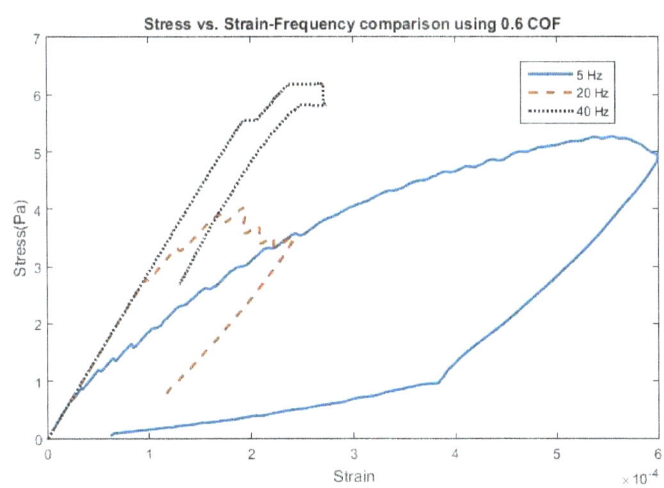

Figure 1. Stress *vs.* Strain for a 4-micron amplitude at various applied frequencies using a coefficient of friction (COF) of 0.6.

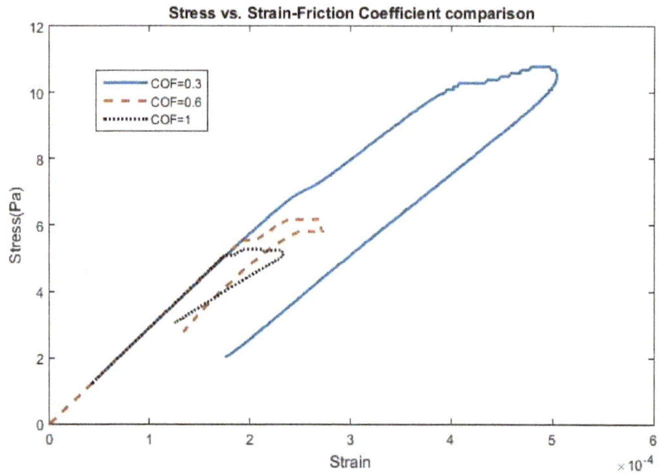

Figure 2. Stress *vs.* Strain for a 4-micron amplitude at 40 Hz using various COFs.

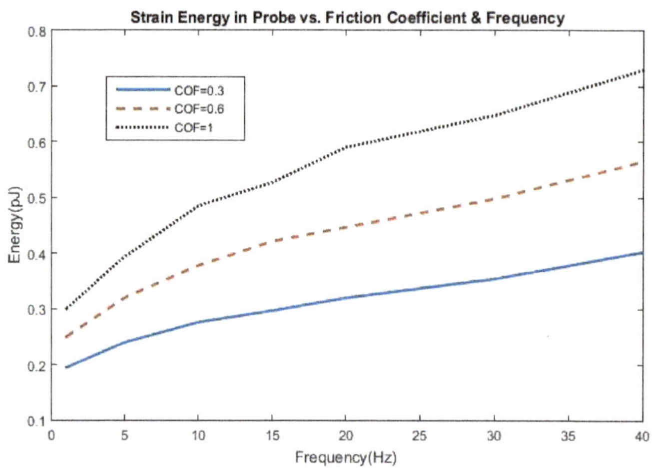

Figure 3. Strain Energy in the 200 kPa probe as a function of friction coefficient and frequency.

Fringe plots for the brain at peak strain levels can be found in Figure 4 for the 20 Hz applied displacement frequency. The strain levels scale goes to 0.001 while the stress levels scale goes to 1×10^{-7} Pa. This is not a reflection of the peak stresses and strains that occur during the duration of the displacement cycle, but was chosen to show how the distributions are distributed at peak displacement. The deformation profiles when the Young's Moduli of silicon and 200 kPa are employed are shown. As the Young's Modulus of the probe decreases, the deformations of the brain also decrease around the tip region and do not spread out as far from the interface, eventually showing negligible deformation around the tip when Young's Modulus is 200 kPa. It is noted also that the stresses and strains exhibit linear behavior until reaching the taper at position 2.3 mm, where both compression and shear deformations occur and exhibit their highest values. Sinusoidal effects are present in the traces due to the coupled role of friction and probe strain energy during motion of the brain.

A time history of strain element response in the tip region, as far away as approximately 73 microns from the interface and 164 microns from the actual tip of the probe, can be found in Figures 5 and 6 for both silicon and the probe with 200 kPa Young's Modulus at 5 Hz and 4 microns to depict the brain response, or deformation levels from the probe, during vascular pulsation. Each output is compared with the input micromotion profile. The elements graphed are highlighted in Figure 7. The graphs show that the highest strain level occurs near the interface where the probe tip is located (denoted in red as x = 0 and y = 0) and decreases the farther away one gets from the interface. The locations plotted in Figures 4 and 5 are denoted by numbers 1–4 in Figure 6. The strain level is highest at approximately 50 ms, when the pulse reaches its amplitude before decreasing. A discontinuity is shown at approximately 90 ms within the simulation for a silicon probe in Figure 4, which signifies that the probe is still in contact with the brain for a short duration as it changes direction in motion. The discontinuity is not seen in the graphs; however, for the softer probe (200 kPa), indicating that the probe is soft enough to absorb the energy from brain micromotion and would not result in contact with the tip for extended periods of time. Compared with use of the silicon probe, the brain experiences a time lag in peak deformation using a softer probe due to energy absorption within the probe during motion. As the silicon probe deformation is negligible, peak deformations in the brain do not lag with respect to time.

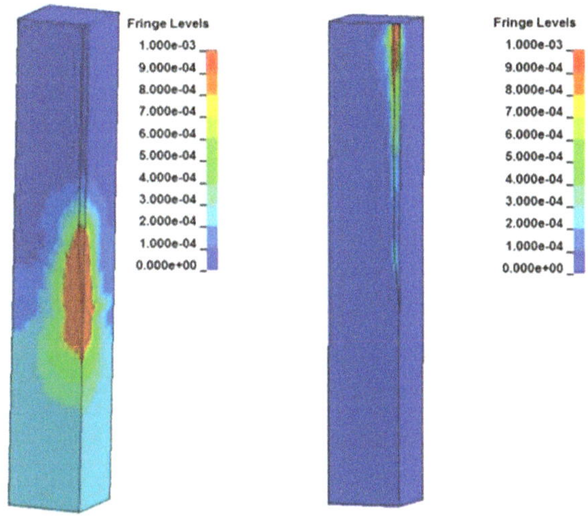

(a) (b)

Figure 4. Strain distribution of the brain using a micromotion displacement of 4 μm and interfaced with a (**a**) silicon probe and (**b**) 200 kPa stiff probe.

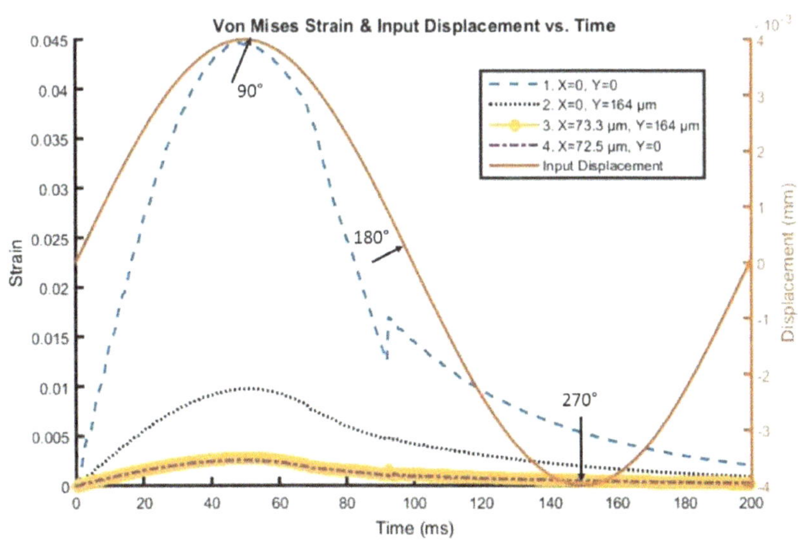

Figure 5. Von Mises Strain *versus* time along the interface of the Silicon probe with the brain.

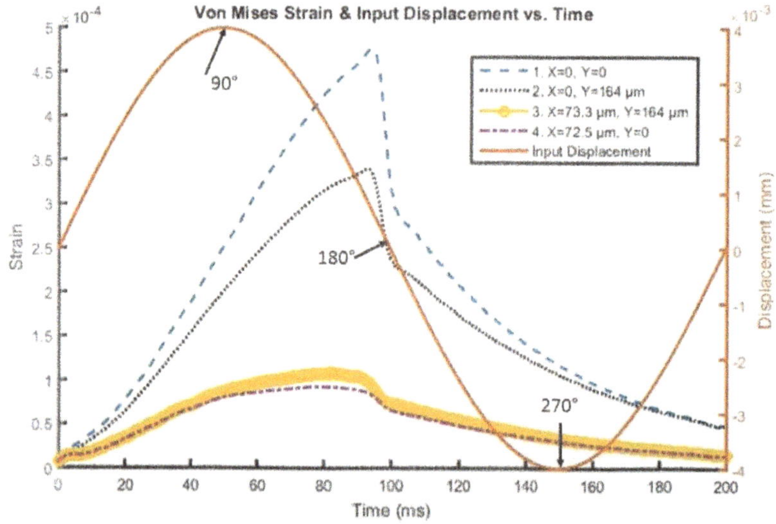

Figure 6. Von Mises Strain *versus* time along the interface of the 200 kPa stiff probe with the brain.

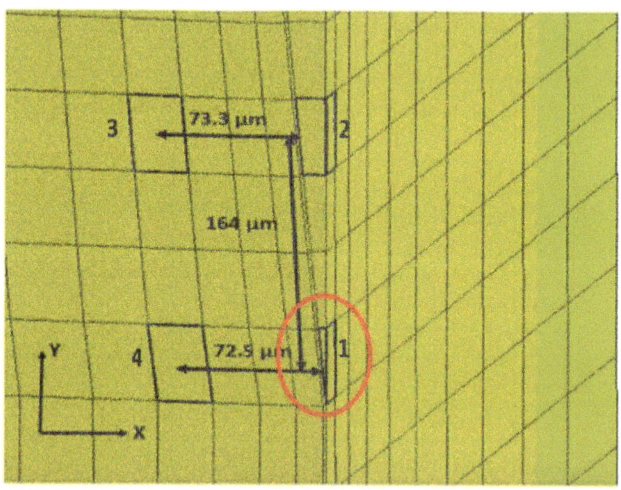

Figure 7. Element locations along interface tip for time history traces corresponding to graphs in Figures 5 and 6.

Finally, examples of stress and strain behavior over multiple cycles of motion can be seen for a 200 kPa probe in Figure 8 for a 4 μm displacement pulse at both 5 Hz and 40 Hz for a COF of 0.6. At 5 Hz, the stress and strain behavior is almost identical between the initial and third cycles, indicating that the kinetic energy from the brain is not sufficient to produce deformations higher than its initial value. At 40 Hz, the stress levels are higher, but also the strains are not as high as they are at lower frequencies due to the strain energy of the probe becoming more prevalent with the increase of the brain's kinetic energy. The traces also indicate the role that strain relaxation time plays between indentation cycles and their contribution to the strain experienced within the brain.

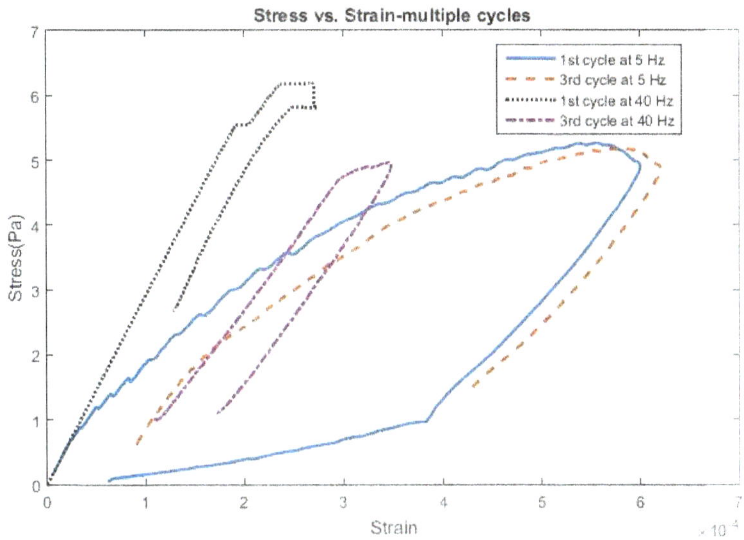

Figure 8. Stress *vs.* Strain for 4 microns comparing first 3 cycles of motion using 200 kPa Young's Modulus.

4. Discussion

Using state-of-the-art tools in Finite Element Analysis, an examination of the behavior of structures under various loading conditions can be performed, providing insight on what parameters are important when designing neural probes. For this problem, researchers have been looking at ways to reduce the strains seen at the tip of the probe along the brain tissue interface as a result of mechanical mismatch between the neural probe and brain tissue. The results presented attempt to provide guidance on what is needed to avoid injury to the brain around the probe tip resulting from mechanical motion of the brain. To the authors' knowledge, the transient aspects of motion within the brain utilizing materials for the probe compatible to the brain had not yet been addressed, and, in conjunction, the benefit probes with lower Young's Moduli play in providing strain relief under different motion profiles was investigated in this study. Through incorporation of frequency, the study offers a more realistic approach to examining the probe to brain interface over time due to micromotion.

The aim of the analysis was to show the motion in the first few moments after the onset of mechanical impact during various stages of probe insertion. The brain tissue was presumed to be more vulnerable to the mechanical damage during the initial period of interface. By utilizing probes closely resembling mechanical characteristics of the brain, the deformation levels can be reduced as highlighted by the scenarios in this study. A Young's Modulus of 200 kPa was examined as it was hypothesized that strain levels at the tip region of the brain could be alleviated. These values for the probe were tried in several research efforts by implementing hydrogel materials [27,28]. Over time, while the strain levels may continuously build up, in any micromotion profile, they are considered miniscule enough using softer probes that they likely would not cause any injury to surrounding tissue, as evidenced by the hysteresis plots presented. A limitation of the study included run times that ranged between eight hours to over a day depending on the frequency employed to run the models on four CPUs. In addition, while some of the micromotion profiles applied were based on previously conducted rat experiments [34,35,38,39], overall the analyses provide an approximation on the implications movement from pulsation, breathing, and walking can have on a human patient.

Introducing different friction coefficients to simulate bonding between the probe and the brain also provides insight as to how the brain is affected over the period of implantation with respect to frequency and Young's Modulus. In the event that the brain undergoes rigorous motion due to walking or head movement, more energy can be absorbed by the probe as the degree of bonding increases over time due to better material compatibility. In addition, the simulations suggest that once bonding is introduced, the strain levels, or potential for scarring, decrease significantly compared with scenarios where the probe has initially been implanted into the brain and the damage to tissue is more imminent. However, as astro-glial sheath formation can occur as early as approximately 2 to 4 weeks after initial insertion into the brain [57], the probe's ability to record neuronal activity can diminish from separation between neural spike sources and sensing electrodes on the probe [58,59]. To facilitate bonding to the brain during implantation, a coating around the probe can help in alleviating deformation levels as suggested in Lee and Subbaroyan [33,34].

It should be noted that a linear viscoelastic formulation was utilized to characterize the brain in this study. Previous research investigated the effects of micromotion [33,34] using small displacements (1–4 μm) in the static regime, accordingly characterizing the brain using an elastic formulation. However, when dealing with variable strain rates and transient, or impact, motion, it is most appropriate to characterize the brain using either a viscoelastic or hyperelastic formulation to effectively capture brain deformation under different micromotion profiles primarily due to shearing from the probe.

The analyses presented provide an initial step in validating the interfacial effects between the probe and the brain in accordance with physics due to relative brain motion. More in-depth examinations on the effects of cerebrospinal fluid on interaction between the probe and the brain can be conducted in the future as it is expected to dampen motion when the fluid fills the voids within the brain. Moreover, application of a lower probe Young's Modulus in the analyses serves as a precursor to wider applications in neural probe design. Future studies can be extended to include transient models incorporating stiffer probes integrated with softer materials such as Silk, PEG, or Polydimethylsiloxane (PDMS), as a surface coating layer of probe or a bioresorbable backing structure. Using a viscoelastic model for the brain and exploring material alternatives for neural probes provides insight for a next generation of neural interface technology. In the future, boundary conditions can be modified to model an untethered probe in the cerebral cortex for chronic recordings in human and large animal applications in an air-tight seal skull condition, which incorporates a dominant tangential component of deformation, or an electrode tethered to the skull by way of a flexible cable [42].

5. Conclusions

A series of transient brain motion profiles were employed and the assessment of mechanically compliant neural probes examined at the interface between the probe and brain tissue was completed. The frequency was varied between 1 and 40 Hz to determine the behavior of the rat brain under mechanical motion as a result of various motor functions such as vascular pulsation, respiration, and walking. The cases were run to three cycles of motion using a probe Young's Modulus of 200 kPa as running multiple cycles resulted in negligible change in stress and strain. Deformation levels in the brain start converging when bonding becomes more present along the interface, as simulated with higher friction coefficients. The stress-strain profiles also differed vastly between motion cycles as frequencies increased while low deformation levels were maintained. By applying transient pulses, the interaction between the probe and the brain as the kinetic energy varies was examined, and revealed the importance of strain relaxation within the brain on deformation levels between indentation cycles. Furthermore, at least a 95% reduction in stress and strain was present at the tip when a 200 kPa Young's Modulus was utilized for the probe, highlighting the importance of using probes mechanically similar to that of the brain to reduce long-term injury to surrounding tissue.

Acknowledgments: Special thanks are expressed to Douglas McCreery for his sincere comments on this work. This work is partially supported by the NSF-CREST Grant (HRD 1036494) and the NSF-RISE Grant (HRD 1345215).

Author Contributions: Both Michael Polanco and Sebastian Bawab conducted the transient analyses of the neural probe to brain tissue interface and analytical data acquisition. Hargsoon Yoon is the primary designer of the neural probes. All three authors revised and wrote different sections of the manuscript.

Conflicts of Interest: No conflicts of interest exist among all authors.

References

1. Wise, K.D.; Angell, J.B.; Starr, A. An integrated-circuit approach to extra cellular microelectrodes. *IEEE Trans. Biomed. Eng.* **1970**, *17*, 238–247. [CrossRef] [PubMed]
2. Campbell, P.K.; Jones, K.E.; Huber, R.J.; Horch, K.W.; Normann, R.A. A silicon-based, three-dimensional neural interface: Manufacturing processes for an intercortical electrode array. *IEEE Trans. Biomed. Eng.* **1991**, *38*, 758–768. [CrossRef] [PubMed]
3. Donoghue, J.P. Connecting cortex to machines: Recent advances in brain interfaces. *Nat. Neuroscience.* **2002**, *5*, 1085–1088. [CrossRef] [PubMed]
4. Lebedev, M.A.; Nicolelis, M.A.L. Brain-machine interfaces: Past, present and future. *Trends Neurosci.* **2006**, *29*, 536–546. [CrossRef] [PubMed]
5. Zhang, J.; Atay, T.; Nurmikko, A.V. Optical detection of brain cell activity using plasmonic gold nanoparticles. *Nano Lett.* **2009**, *9*, 519–524. [CrossRef] [PubMed]
6. Kneipp, K.; Moskovits, M.; Kneipp, H. Surface-enhanced Raman scattering: Physics and applications. In *Topics in Applied Physics*; Springer: Berlin, Germany, 2006; pp. 47–66.
7. Wang, J.; Wagner, F.; Borton, D.A.; Zhang, J.; Ozden, I.; Burwell, R.D.; Nurmikko, A.; van Wagenen, R.; Diester, I.; Deisseroth, K. Integrated device for combined optical neuromodulation and electrical recording for chronic *in vivo* applications. *J. Neural Eng.* **2012**, *9*, 16001–16014. [CrossRef] [PubMed]
8. Tidswell, T.; Gibson, A.; Bayford, R.H.; Holder, D.S. Three-dimensional electrical impedance tomography of human brain activity. *Neuroimage* **2001**, *13*, 283–294. [CrossRef] [PubMed]
9. Yoon, H.; Hankins, P.; Oh, S.; Haubaugh, R.E.; Varadan, V.K. Heterostructured IrO_2/Au nanowire electrodes and unit recordings from hippocampal rat brain. *J. Nanotech. Eng. Med.* **2010**, *1*. [CrossRef]
10. Polikov, V.S.; Tresco, P.A.; Reichert, W.M. Response of brain tissue to chronically implanted neural electrodes. *J. Neurosci. Meth.* **2005**, *148*, 1–18. [CrossRef] [PubMed]
11. Xie, Y.; Martini, N.; Hassler, C.; Kirch, R.K.; Stieglitz, T.; Seifert, A.; Hofmann, U.G. *In vivo* monitoring of glial scar proliferation on chronically implanted neural electrodes by fiber optical coherence tomography. *Front. Neuroeng.* **2014**, *7*. [CrossRef] [PubMed]
12. Kozai, T.D.; Catt, K.; Li, X.; Gugel, Z.V.; Olafsson, V.T.; Vasquez, A.L.; Cui, X.T. Mechanical failure modes of chronically implanted planar silicon-based neural probes for laminar recording. *Biomaterials* **2015**, *37*, 25–39. [CrossRef] [PubMed]
13. Rosenzweig, J.M.; Lei, J.; Burd, I. Interleukin-1 receptor blockade in perinatal brain injury. *Front. Pediatr.* **2014**, *2*. [CrossRef] [PubMed]
14. Kozai, T.D.; Li, X.; Bodily, L.M.; Caparosa, E.M.; Zenonos, G.A.; Carlisle, D.L.; Friedlander, R.M.; Cui, X.T. Effects of caspase-1 knockout on chronic neural recording quality and longetivity: Insight into cellular and molecular mechanisms of the reactive tissue response. *Biomaterials* **2014**, *35*, 9620–9624. [CrossRef] [PubMed]
15. Misra, A.; Kondaveeti, P.; Nissanov, J.; Barbee, K.; Shewokis, P.; Rioux, L.; Moxon, K.A. Preventing neuronal damage and inflammation *in vivo* during cortical microelectrode implantation through the use of poloxamer P-188. *J. Neural Eng.* **2013**, *10*. [CrossRef] [PubMed]
16. Gutowski, S.M.; Shoemaker, J.T.; Templeman, K.L.; Wei, Y.; Latour, R.A.; Bellamkonda, R.V.; LaPlaca, M.C.; Garcia, A.J. Protese-degradable PEG-maleimide coating with on-demand release of IL-1Ra to improve tissue response to neural electrodes. *Biomaterials* **2015**, *44*, 55–70. [CrossRef] [PubMed]
17. Lee, H.J.; Son, Y.; Kim, J.; Lee, C.J.; Yoon, E.-S.; Cho, I.-J. A multichannel neural probe with embedded microfluidic channels for simultaneous *in vivo* neural recording and drug delivery. *Lab Chip* **2015**, *15*, 1590–1597. [CrossRef] [PubMed]
18. Altuna, A.; Berzango, J.; Fernandez, L.J. Polymer SU-8-based microprobes for neural recording and drug delivery. *Front. Mater.* **2015**, *2*, 2. [CrossRef]
19. Jeong, J.W.; McCall, J.G.; Zhang, Y.; Huang, Y. Soft microfluidic neural probes for wireless drug delivery in freely behaving mice. In Proceedings of the 18th International Conference on Solid State Sensors, Actuators, and Microsystems, Anchorage, AK, USA, 21–25 June 2015; pp. 2264–2267.
20. HajjHassan, M.; Chodavarapu, V.; Musallam, S. NeuroMEMS: Neural probe microtechnologies. *Sensors* **2008**, *8*, 6704–6726. [CrossRef]
21. Motta, P.S.; Judy, J.W. Multielectrode microprobes for deep-brain stimulation fabricated with a customizable 3-D electroplating process. *IEEE Trans. Biomed. Eng.* **2005**, *52*, 923–933. [CrossRef] [PubMed]

22. Mercanzini, A.; Cheung, K.; Buhl, D.; Boers, M.; Maillard, A.; Colin, P.; Bensadoun, J.; Bertsch, A.; Carleton, A.; Renaud, P. Demonstration of cortical recording and reduced inflammatory response using flexible polymer neural probes. In Proceedings of the IEEE MEMS Conference, Kobe, Japan, 21–25 January 2007; pp. 573–576.
23. Rousche, P.J.; Pellinen, D.S.; Pivin, D.P., Jr.; Williams, J.C.; Kipke, D.R. Flexible polyimide-based intracortical electrode arrays with bioactive capability. *IEEE Trans. Biomed. Eng.* **2001**, *48*, 361–371. [CrossRef] [PubMed]
24. Cheung, K.C.; Renaud, P.; Tanila, H.; Djupsund, K. Flexible polyimide microelectrode array for *in vivo* recordings and current source density analysis. *Biosens. Bioelectron.* **2007**, *22*, 1783–1790. [CrossRef] [PubMed]
25. Edell, D.J.; Toi, V.V.; McNeil, V.M.; Clark, L.D. Factors influencing the biocompatibility of insertable silicon microshafts in cerebral cortex. *IEEE Trans. Biomed. Eng.* **1992**, *39*, 635–643. [CrossRef] [PubMed]
26. Kim, D.H.; Abidian, M.; Martin, D.C. Conducting polymers grown in hydrogel scaffolds coated on neural prosthetic devices. *J. Biomed. Mater. Res. A* **2004**, *71*, 577–585. [CrossRef] [PubMed]
27. Kozai, T.D.; Kipke, D.R. Insertion shuttle with carboxyl terminated self-assembled monolayer coatings for implanting flexible polymer neural probes in the brain. *J. Neurosci. Methods* **2009**, *184*, 199–205. [CrossRef] [PubMed]
28. Felix, S.H.; Shah, K.G.; Tolosa, V.M.; Sheth, H.J.; Tooker, A.C.; Delima, T.L.; Jadhay, S.P.; Frank, L.M.; Pannu, S.S. Insertion of flexible neural probes using rigid stiffeners attached with biodissolvable adhesive. *J. Vis. Exp.* **2013**, *79*. [CrossRef] [PubMed]
29. Sridharan, A.; Nguyen, J.K.; Capadona, J.R.; Muthuswamy, J. Compliant intracortical implants reduce strains and strain rates in brain tissue *in vivo*. *J. Neural Eng.* **2015**, *12*. [CrossRef] [PubMed]
30. Arreaga-Salas, D.E.; Avendaño-Bolivar, A.; Simon, D.; Reit, R.; Garcia-Sandoval, A.; Rennaker, R.L.; Voit, W. Integration of high-charge-injection-capacity electrodes onto polymer softening neural interfaces. *ACS Appl. Mater. Interfaces* **2015**, *7*, 26614–26623. [CrossRef] [PubMed]
31. Ware, T.; Simon, D.; Hearon, K.; Kang, T.H.; Maitland, D.J.; Voit, W. Thiol-click chemistries for responsive neural interfaces. *Macromol. Biosci.* **2013**, *13*, 1640–1647. [CrossRef] [PubMed]
32. Zhu, R.; Huang, G.L.; Yoon, H.; Smith, C.S.; Varadan, V.K. Biomechanical strain analysis at the interface of brain and nanowire electrodes on a neural probe. *J. Nanotechnol. Eng. Med.* **2011**, *2*. [CrossRef]
33. Lee, H.; Bellamkonda, R.V.; Sun, W.; Levenston, M.E. Biomechanical analysis of silicon microelectrode-induced strain in the brain. *J. Neural Eng.* **2005**, *2*, 81–89. [CrossRef] [PubMed]
34. Subbaroyan, J.; Martin, D.C.; Kipke, D.R. A finite-element model of the mechanical effects of implantable microelectrodes in the cerebral cortex. *J. Neural Eng.* **2005**, *2*, 103–113. [CrossRef] [PubMed]
35. Muthuswamy, J.; Saha, R.; Gilletti, A. Tissue micromotion induced stress around brain implants. In Proceedings of the 3rd Annual International IEEE EMBS Special Topic Conference on Microtechnologies in Medicine and Biology, Kahuku, Oahu, HI, USA, 12–15 May 2005; pp. 102–103.
36. Nguyen, J.K.; Park, D.J.; Skousen, J.L.; Hess-Dunning, A.E.; Tyler, D.J.; Rowan, S.J.; Weder, C.; Capadona, J.R. Mechanically-compliant intracortical implants reduce the neuroinflammatory response. *J. Neural Eng.* **2014**, *11*. [CrossRef] [PubMed]
37. Zhang, W.; Li, Z.; Gilles, M.; Wu, D. Mechanical simulation of neural electrode-brain tissue interface under various micromotion conditions. *J. Med. Biol. Eng.* **2013**, *34*, 386–392. [CrossRef]
38. Muthuswamy, J.; Gilletti, A.; Jain, T.; Okandan, M. Microactuated neural probes to compensate for brain micromotion. In Proceedings of the 25th Annual International Conference of IEEE EMBS 2, Cancun, Mexico, 17–21 September 2003; pp. 1941–1943.
39. Gilletti, A.; Muthuswamy, J. Brain micromotion around implants in the rodent somatosensory cortex. *J. Neural Eng.* **2006**, *3*, 189–195. [CrossRef] [PubMed]
40. Rao, B.K.N.; Jones, B. Some studies on the measurement of head and shoulder vibration during walking. *J. Ergonomics* **1975**, *18*, 555–566. [CrossRef]
41. Polanco, M.; Yoon, H.; Bawab, S. Micromotion-induced dynamic effects from a neural probe and brain tissue interface. *J. Micro Nanolithogr. MEMS MOEMS* **2014**, *13*. [CrossRef]
42. Sankar, V.; Sanchez, J.C.; McCumiskey, E.; Brown, N.; Taylor, C.R.; Ehlert, G.J.; Sodano, H.A.; Nishida, T. A highly compliant serpentine shaped polimide interconnect for front-end strain relief in chronic neural implants. *Front. Neurol.* **2013**, *4*. [CrossRef] [PubMed]
43. Buzsaki, G. Large-scale recording of neuronal ensembles. *Nat. Neurosci.* **2004**, *7*, 446–451. [CrossRef] [PubMed]

44. Hallquist, J.Q. *LS-DYNA Keyword User's Manual I and II, 971*; Livermore Software Technology Corporation: Livermore, CA, USA, 2008.
45. Erhart, T. Review of solid element formulations in LS-DYNA: Properties, limits, advantages, disadvantages. In Proceedings of the LS-DYNA Developers' Forum, Stuttgart, Germany, 12–13 October 2011.
46. Tabiei, A. *Contact in LS-DYNA*; Livermore Software Technology Corporation: Livermore, CA, USA, 2007.
47. Yang, K.H.; Hu, J.; White, N.A.; King, A.I.; Chou, C.C.; Prasad, P. Development of numerical models for injury biomechanics research: A review of 50 years of publications in the Stapp car crash conference. *Stapp Car Crash J.* **2006**, *50*, 429–490. [PubMed]
48. Seshaiyer, P.; Humphrey, J. A sub-domain inverse finite element characterization of hyper elastic membranes including soft tissues. *J. Biomed. Eng.* **2003**, *125*, 363–371.
49. Hrapko, M.; Van Dommelen, J.A.W.; Peters, G.W.M.; Wismans, J.S.H.M. The mechanical behavior of brain tissue: Large strain response and constitutive modeling. *J. Biorhel.* **2006**, *43*, 623–636.
50. Miller, K.; Chinzei, K. Constitutive modeling of brain tissue: Experiment and theory. *J. Biomech.* **1997**, *30*, 1115–1121. [CrossRef]
51. Bischoff, J.; Arruda, E.; Grosh, K. A rheological network model for the continuum anisotropic and viscoelastic behavior of soft tissue. *J. Biomech. Model. Mechanobiol.* **2004**, *3*, 56–65. [CrossRef] [PubMed]
52. Prevost, T.; Balakrishnan, A.; Suresh, S.; Socrate, S. Biomechanics of brain tissue. *J. ActaBiomater.* **2011**, *7*, 83–95. [CrossRef] [PubMed]
53. Miller, K. Constitutive model of brain tissue suitable for finite element analysis of surgical procedures. *J. Biomech.* **1999**, *32*, 531–537. [CrossRef]
54. Zhang, L.; Yang, K.H.; Dwarampudi, R.; Omori, K.; Li, T.; Chang, K.; Hardy, W.N.; Khalil, T.B.; King, A.I. Recent development in brain injury research: A new human head model development and validation. *Stapp Car Crash J.* **2001**, *45*, 369–394. [PubMed]
55. Stalnaker, R. Mechanical Properties of the Head. Ph.D. Thesis, West Virginia University, Morgantown, WV, USA, 1969.
56. Donnelly, B.R.; Medige, J. Shear properties of human brain tissue. *J. Biomed. Eng.* **1997**, *119*, 423–432.
57. Turner, J.N.; Shain, W.; Szarowski, D.H.; Anderson, M.; Martins, S.; Isaacson, M.; Craighead, H.G. Cerebral astrolyte response to micromachined silicon implants. *J. Exp. Neurol.* **1999**, *156*, 33–49. [CrossRef] [PubMed]
58. Szarowski, D.H.; Andersen, M.D.; Retterer, S.; Spence, A.J.; Isaacson, M.; Craighead, H.G.; Turner, J.N.; Shain, W. Brain responses to micro-machined silicon devices. *J. Brain Res.* **2003**, *983*, 23–35. [CrossRef]
59. McConnell, G.C.; Schneider, T.M.; Owens, D.J.; Bellamkonda, R.V. Extraction force and cortical tissue reaction of silicon microelectrode arrays implanted in the rat brain. *IEEE Trans. Biomed. Eng.* **2007**, *54*, 1097–1107. [CrossRef] [PubMed]

6

Optimal Magnetic Field for Crossing Super-Para-Magnetic Nanoparticles through the Brain Blood Barrier: A Computational Approach

Maysam Z. Pedram [1], Amir Shamloo [1,*], Aria Alasty [1] and Ebrahim Ghafar-Zadeh [2,*]

[1] Department of Mechanical Engineering, Sharif University of Technology, Tehran, PO Box: 11365-11155, Iran; maysam.pedram@gmail.com (M.Z.P.); aalasti@sharif.edu (A.A.)
[2] Department of Electrical Engineering, York University, Toronto, ON M3J1P3, Canada
* Correspondence: shamloo@sharif.edu (A.S.); egz@cse.yorku.ca (E.G.-Z.)

Academic Editor: Jeff D. Newman

Abstract: This paper scrutinizes the magnetic field effect to deliver the superparamagnetic nanoparticles (SPMNs) through the Blood Brain Barrier (BBB). Herein we study the interaction between the nanoparticle (NP) and BBB membrane using Molecular Dynamic (MD) techniques. The MD model is used to enhance our understanding of the dynamic behavior of SPMNs crossing the endothelial cells in the presence of a gradient magnetic field. Actuation of NPs under weak magnetic field offers the great advantage of a non-invasive drug delivery without the risk of causing injury to the brain. Furthermore, a weak magnetic portable stimulator can be developed using low complexity prototyping techniques. Based on MD simulation results in this paper, SPMNs can cross the cell membrane while experiencing very weak mechanical forces in the range of pN. This study also derives guidelines for the design of the SPMNs dedicated to crossing the BBB using external magnetic fields.

Keywords: Molecular Dynamics simulation; force steering; Blood Brain Barrier; superparamagnetic nanoparticles

1. Introduction

Recent advances in micro- and nanotechnologies have greatly attracted the attentions of researchers for the development of magnetic nanoparticles (MNPs). MNPs offer great advantages for the diagnostics of various diseases, such as glioblastoma, Alzheimer, and Epilepsy [1–3]. MNPs have also demonstrated great advantages as contrast agents for Magnetic Resonance Imaging (MRI). Naturally occurring, the endothelium patterning around the cerebral micro vessels with strong tight junctions accurately controls the transportation of biomolecules necessary for neural signaling. However, the Blood-Brain Barrier (BBB) prevents the delivery of large drug molecules or NPs into the brain [4]. To overcome this problem, many papers have reported non-invasive chemical techniques to increase the permeability of the BBB [5–7]. Based on these papers, the improper surface chemistry hinders crossing through the BBB when the recognition of these NPs takes place along with receptors on the surface of the endothelial cells. Figure 1a shows the selectivity of these non-invasive chemical techniques that enable specific molecules to cross the BBB. As seen in Figure 1(a-i), there are many lipid-soluble molecules, or so-called *Passive partitioners*, that can cross the BBB and enter the Central Nervous System (CNS). The relation between the translocation rate and the degree of solubility of molecules in lipids has been elucidated in [5]. There are various methods for computing the permeability of the BBB for lipid-soluble non-polar molecules under the effect of passive diffusion.

Diffusion parameters could then be evaluated based on experimental results. A rigorous formulation is provided for *in vivo* purposes. In addition to passive partitioners, there are many solutes and drugs called *ATP-Binding Cassette (ABC) transporters* that have much lower CNS entry rates than expected. These substances are actively transported through the capillary endothelium by means of the ABC transporter family (Figure 1(a-ii)). As mentioned above, the chemical techniques for crossing the BBB are selective and they allow the translocation of nutrients that are necessary for metabolisms, such as glucose and amino acids. Therefore, for transporting these essential nutrients to the brain, endothelium cells must contain a number of specific *Solute Carriers (SLCs)* which can play the role of transporters of those substances essential for brain activity and homeostasis. In addition, endothelial cells can use transport proteins for a wide variety of solutes and nutrients. Some of these transport proteins are polarized in their expression and are inserted into either the luminal or abluminal membrane only; others are inserted into both membranes of endothelial cells. The direction of the molecular transportation (e.g., Glucose, amino acids, nucleosides, monocarboxylates, small peptides, FFAs, organic anions, and organic cations) is from the blood to the brain and *vice versa* (Figure 1(a-iii)).

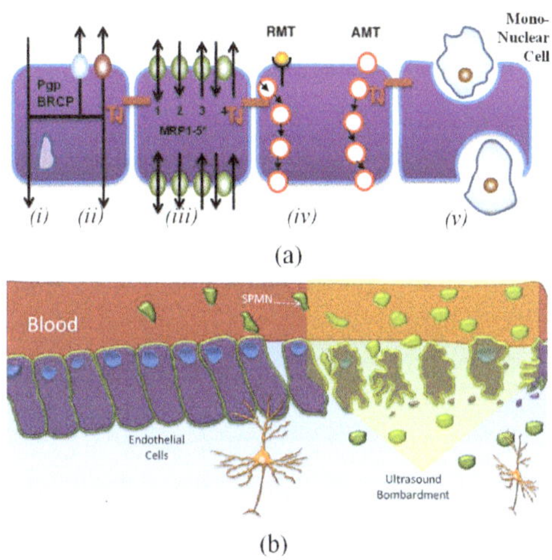

Figure 1. Methods of crossing the blood-brain barrier: (**a**) chemical methods and (**b**) a physical method (e.g., ultrasound). The chemical methods are separated into five different groups RMT (receptor-mediated transcytosis), AMT (adsorptive-mediated transcytosis), BRCP (bovine retinal capillary pericytes), and MRP (multidrug resistance protein). The physical methods rely on the effect of solid particles or electromagnetic/mechanical waves on endothelial cells.

The transportation of macromolecules through the BBB via endocytotic mechanisms is another important method for crossing the BBB. Although large molecular-weight solutes, such as proteins and peptides, are prevented from entering the CNS, there are a few transcytotic mechanisms capable of transporting large molecules. Figure 1(a-iv) illustrates such a mechanism. Transferin, melanotransferrin, lipoproteins, Amyloid β, clycosylated proteins, IgG, Insulin, Leptin, TNFα, and EGF (Epidermal Growth Factor) translocate to CNS via this mechanism. Furthermore, Figure 1(a-v) shows that cells from the bone-marrow derived monocyte lineage enter the brain during embryonic development and form colonies of residents and immunologically competent micro-glia. Moreover, mononuclear leukocytes, monocytes, and macrophages are able to be recruited by the CNS in pathological conditions, and play a complementary role to those of the resident micro-glia; in some cases they may transform into a microglial phenotype. Cationised albumin, histone, avidin, TAT, and synB are used in this method for facilitating the tansport.

Additionally, high-frequency electromagnetic field radiation and ultrasonic techniques have enabled the delivery of NPs or large biomolecules into the brain by creating nanoscale openings in the endothelium, as observed in Figure 1b [8–16]. Despite these advances, the development of a non-invasive or minimally invasive technique to deliver drugs or NPs into the brain is a key challenge. In this paper, we address this challenge by proposing a low complexity technique to deliver SPMNs in the brain.

As the result of this minimally invasive technique, these energized SPMNs penetrate through the membrane. Hence, we analyze the complexity of this technique using the molecular dynamic computational tool. This computational study deals with the molecular-level simulations to fathom the interaction between the energetic SPMNs and the endothelial cells membranes. Furthermore, this MD approach is crucial to obtain the optimal magnetic field energizing the SPMNs in order to cross the BBB. In other words, it is crucial to obtain the minimum gradient and/or amplitude of applied magnetic field for this purpose. Based on the literature, an MRI system can be practiced as a viable technique to energize such SPMNs [17,18]. As seen in Figure 2a, a handheld magnetic stimulator can also be used to generate the magnetic forces. Figure 2b reveals the structure of a capillary blood vessel. This figure also depicts how SPMNs translocate from the blood stream to the parenchymal tissue of the brain. An anisotropic transportation of SPMNs can be observed in this figure. In the remainder of this paper, the mathematical and MD models are described in Sections 2 and 3. Section 4 demonstrates and discusses the results, and is followed by a conclusion in Section 5.

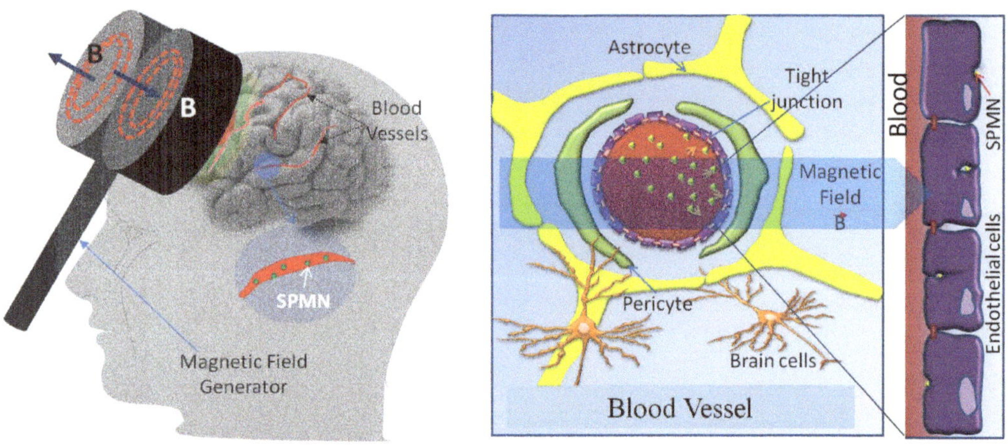

(a) (b)

Figure 2. Magnetic superparamagnetic nanoparticles (SPMN) delivery into the brain: (**a**) Portable magnetic stimulator, and (**b**) Mechanism of crossing the blood brain barrier (BBB) based on the applied magnetic field. In this method, regarding the magnetic field applied to the magnetic nanoparticle, magnetic force created nanoparticles are crossing through the BBB.

2. Mathematical Models

In this section, we present the simplified mathematical models of the required magnetic field for applying magnetic forces on SPMNs. In Section 4, we demonstrate and discuss the simulation results and practical guidelines using MATLAB and MD computational tools based on these models.

Magnetic Force

The relationship between the magnetic force subjected on a magnetic dipole $\vec{m}$, in an applied magnetic field $\vec{B}$, is obtained from Equation (1):

$$\vec{F} = \left(\vec{m}.\nabla\right)\vec{B} \tag{1}$$

By substituting $\vec{m} = \chi_{bead} V \vec{B}/\mu_0$ into Equation (1) [19], the following equation is obtained.

$$\vec{F} = \frac{V\chi_{bead}}{\mu_0}(\vec{B}.\nabla)\vec{B} \tag{2}$$

where the magnetic susceptibility χ_{bead} and volume of the bead is expressed by χ_{bead} and V. μ_0 is the permeability constant.

By assuming $\vec{B} = b_z \vec{a}_z$, the magnetic force is obtained from the following equation.

$$\vec{F} = \frac{V\chi_{bead}}{\mu_0}(b_z \frac{\partial b_z}{\partial z})\vec{a}_z \tag{3}$$

By assuming that b_z is a function of time and z or $Y(z,t) = b_z$ and $\vec{F} = F_z(t)\hat{e}_z$, U(t) can be defined as follows.

$$U(t) = \frac{F_z(t)\mu_0}{V\chi_{bead}} \tag{4}$$

$U(t)$ is proportional to magnetic force $F_z(t)$, therefore, by substituting Equation (4) into Equation (3), and by assuming that $Y(z,t) = b_z$, Equation (5) is achieved.

$$Y(z,t)\frac{\partial Y(z,t)}{\partial z} = U(t) \tag{5}$$

Let us assume that the magnetic generator (e.g., MRI system) is linear $\partial Y(z,t)/\partial z = 1/k$ where k is a constant value. Conclusively, the following equation is obtained.

$$Y(z,t) = kU(t) \tag{6}$$

The magnetic field profile is obtained through extracting $U(t)$ from the MD simulation results, based on Equation (6). The guidelines for designing the magnetic field will be discussed in Section 3.

3. Molecular Dynamic Models

In this section, we discuss the MD model of each component, including the BBB membrane and SPMNs. Then, we present the MD specifications.

3.1. MD Modeling

BBB Structure: The brain microvasculature is composed of three cellular elements including the BBB endothelial cells, astrocyte endfeet, and pericytes, as depicted in Figure 2. Tight junctions (TJs) present in the gap between the cerebral endothelial cells create a diffusive barrier, which selectively prevents the entrance of most blood-borne substances to the brain. The BBB endothelial cells differ from endothelial cells in the rest of the body by the absence of fenestrations, more extensively tight junctions (TJs), and sparse pinocytic vesicular transport [20]. In this study, only the cell membrane is modeled because the latter manifests no significant resistance to nano-particles when crossing the cytoplasm. It is noteworthy that this assumption is valid where the nanoparticle is crossing the cell membrane. In the case of crossing through tight junctions, a more complicated interaction should be modeled [21]. Selection of the correct size of NP would help to increase the rate of penetration. It has been experimentally observed that the tight junction can be opened for a NP with a size less than 20 nm, and this size of NPs can select this pathway for crossing the BBB [22]. A membrane is a lipid bilayer. In the literature, DMPC (DiMyristoyl PhosphoCholine) and POPC (Palmitoyl Oleyl Phosphatidyl Choline) are widely used to simulate BBB endothelial cell membranes. The membrane is a POPC lipid bilayer modeled by the VMD (Visual Molecular Dynamics) plugin Membrane Builder and merged by NP using a TCL (Tool Command Language) code [23,24].

SPMNs Model: In this model, Iron Oxide (Fe_3O_4) is used as a core and gold (Au) is applied as a shell of the SPMNs. Au plays an important role in this approach. Au is a biocompatible material [25]. Moreover, Au has proven its advantage for crossing BBB in a non-invasive manner based on the experimental results reported in [22]. Additionally, the uniform distribution of Au in the brain after crossing the BBB has been also proved from the experimental point of view. However, the role of Au remains unknown in the above mechanisms [22]. Furthermore, it is also assumed that the magnetic saturation curve of the SPMNs is linear in this computational study [26]. Figure 3 illustrates the magnetization curve used in MD simulations. Based on this curve, $\chi_{bead} = 0.17$ and the maximum magnetic field should be less than 2.5 T. In the literature, the rigidity of SPMNs is also argued [27] since the atomic bonds between the nano-particles of metallic atoms are much stronger than the chemical connections between (e.g., van der Walls interactions) the nano-particle atoms and the atoms of organic compounds are used in this study.

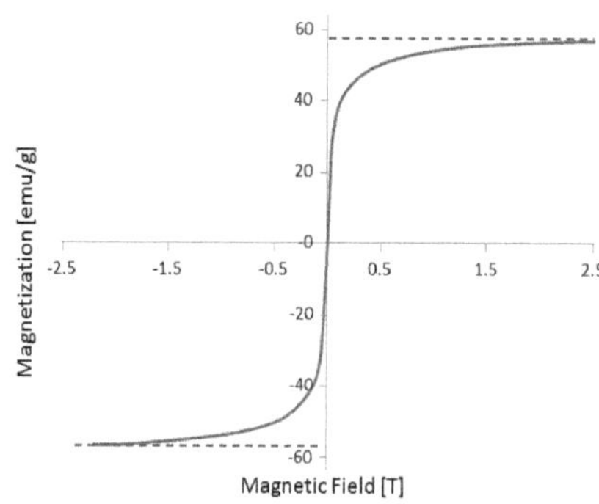

Figure 3. Magnetization curve for Fe_3O_4 magnetic suspension. In this figure, the threshold of saturation is demonstrated.

Figure 3 shows the estimated strength of the magnetic field that can be applied on a NP. In regards to [28], coated and uncoated gold/magnetic NPs' saturation values are similar, but coated NPs with gold saturation are a little higher, as reported in this paper. The maximum permitted magnetic field is defined, and it can be considered as the maximum value of the magnetic field. Although a higher magnetic field can be applied, due to the saturation effect, the effective magnetic force is the same. Figure 4 displays the 2 nm NP above the POPC membrane after 100 ps relaxation time. This figure indicates the structure of the NP. This NP forms a single rigid body with Au coating. Despite the fact that SPMNs can be considered as rigid particles, they are still deformable to some extent. Since Fe_3O_4 SPMNs are coated with Au, their structure can be considered as FFC (Face-Centered Cubic). In this MD modeling process, FCC is created using VMD plugin Inorganic builder. Then, a sphere with the desired radius is extracted from the FCC by a TCL code. Thus, the PDB (Protein Data Bank) and PSF (Protein Structure File) files were written. The van der Waals interactions are considered for all types of atoms (truncated at 12 A). This step runs for the second time using a Fe_3O_4 NP coated with gold. Thus, the material under the gold surface is considered in the interaction potential due to its cut-off distance [29]. It is noteworthy that in this computational study, the spheral-shape NPs are used. Therefore, the rotation of nanoparticles is not considered as a key factor. Due to the symmetrical shape of NPs, only the magnetic force in the defined direction is crucial. In [30], the direction of the magnetic field was taken into account; however, in this study, a magnetic field in a certain single direction is applied. It is noteworthy that, in the stability mode, the buoyancy force is canceled with the gravity force. The fluid resulting in the drag force is important, but in this study the NPs are located on the surface of enthotleial cells, and, in fact, we are supposed to calculate the force needed to cross through the BBB. The goal of this paper is to derive the minimum force required for crossing the BBB. Furthermore, it is well understood that Brownian motion is a function of temperature. In this study the Browning motion should also be taken into account. However, the average of Brownian motion is negligible due to the fact that the direction of the NPs' motion is aligned with the direction of the magnetic field.

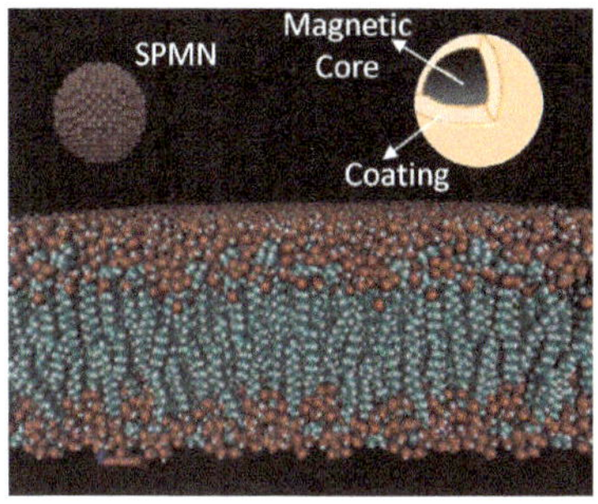

Figure 4. 100 × 100 membrane and core/shell magnetic nanoparticle (NP).

3.2. Molecular Dynamics Criteria

The MD simulation was performed with the Nanoscale Molecular Dynamics Package NAMD, and visualizations and analysis were performed using the Molecular Graphics Viewer VMD. The CHARMM27 All-Atoms (AA) force field was employed to model atomic interactions in the model. Based on the Langevin dynamics, all simulations were performed at a constant temperature equal to 310 K using a Langevin thermostat. In fact, the Langevin piston Nos'e–Hoover method was used to maintain a pressure at 101.3 kPa. The cutoff distance for the pairwise Lennard-Jones non-bonded interactions was set at 12 Å with a pair list distance extended to 14 Å.

Figure 4 reveals that the magnetic NP consists of two materia—Fe_3O_4 and gold. To date, many researchers, including León *et al.* [31], have reported the development of submicron hollow Fe_3O_4 that can be coated with Au; however, in this paper we want to put forward the manufacturing process not the magnetic properties of Fe_3O_4 coated with gold. The gold coating is needed for its biocompatibility, and also core-shell Au/Fe_3O_4 nanoparticles for drug delivery. As described in [32,33], the role of the gold shell functionalized with many functional groups is to increase the permeability of NPs crossing the BBB.

As already mentioned, all simulations consist of a cell membrane and a NP. The cell membrane is a POPC lipid bilayer with dimensions of 100 × 100 Å^2, consisting of 50,318 atoms. Periodic boundary conditions are applied in all directions. The water molecules were modeled by the TIP3P method. Moreover, the time step is set to 2 fs. The initial energy of the system was minimized for 50 ps, thereafter the SMD (Steered Molecular Dynamics) simulation applied to the NP. This energy was used so that NPs cross the membrane at a constant velocity ranging from 0.0005 Å/Step to 0.1 Å/Step. During this process the exerted force on the nanoparticles was also recorded. The applied computational resources were necessary for the simulation. The simulation was performed on a personal workstation using a 2.67 GHz XEON processor for about seven days

4. Results and Discussion

In this paper, the MD modeling and simulation were carried out to investigate the non-invasive penetration of SPMNs into the brain through the BBB. Table 1 provides a summary of MD key parameters and results.

Table 1. Molecular dynamics key parameters.

Parameter	Quantity or Name
NP Type	$(Fe_2O_3)\ Au,\ \chi_{bead} = 0.17$
NP Size	Diameter = 2 nm
Gold Thickness	2 A
Temperature	310 K, Langevin thermostat
Velocity of NPs	0.0005–0.1 Å /Step
Processor	XEON
Time	7 days
Relaxation time	20 nS
Membrane molecular dynamic (MD) model	POPC (Palmitoyl Oleyl Phosphatidyl Choline)
Membrane simulation area	$100 \times 100\ Å^2$

4.1. *Magnetic Force*

After 50 ps relaxation time, the NPs crossed the membrane at constant velocities ranging from 0.0005 Å/step to 0.1 Å/step. The applied force on the single NP as the effect of the magnetic field was recorded is shown in Figure 5a. As already discussed, a similar force profile must be applied on the NP in order to cross the BBB at the range of 0.0005–0.1 Å/Step. Based on our study, this figure shows that we need an alternative magnetic field in order to generate an appropriate force. As seen in Figure 5a, it needs a sharp burst of force amplitude. This mechanical force signal reaches its steady state after 3~4 oscillations. The rise time of this profile is about 10 pS (=2000 time steps). Figure 5a signifies that an effective SPMN translocation can be performed in such an oscillatory mode of acceleration for which we can discern the negative and positive cycles. Since a dummy spring has been considered as a means to express the softness of tissue in MD simulations, the oscillations are expected from the related governing equation of dynamic system. Despite this fact, moving in two directions could help crossing more easily, however, it results in a complicated magnetic field generator. Therefore, time and force are two factors that should be taken into account in order to push NPs effectively in a specific direction. Furthermore, the maximum amplitude of force when NPs pass the cell membrane plays a crucial role. Consequently, we omitted the negative oscillation and only the positive force in the effective direction was considered. For further simplicity, we can consider the minimum and maximum forces for crossing the BBB corresponding to two ranges of velocities. Figure 5b presents these minimum and maximum force values. It expresses that any force magnitude chosen from the interval between these two boundaries will assure crossing the BBB. In another simulation, different sizes of NPs have been examined. The applied forces on SPMNs with different sizes between 5 nm and 45 nm are obtained for crossing the BBB. Figure 5c shows that the SPMNs with various diameter sizes require different forces for crossing the membrane, however, these particles can move almost with the same force inside the cells.

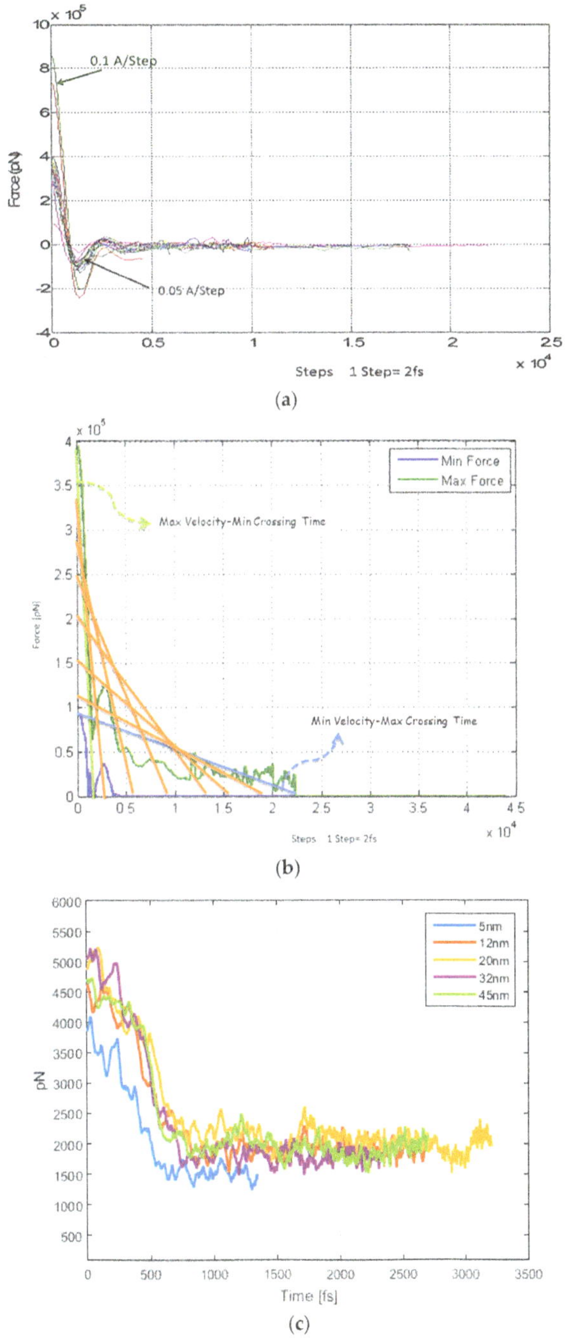

Figure 5. (**a**) Force Profile. Colored lines are related to different velocities of NPs. In this figure, the force profile needed for crossing nanoparticles is illustrated; (**b**) Diagram of minimum and maximum forces which are needed for crossing the BBB. Colored lines are related to different velocities of NPs; (**c**) Magnetic force *versus* time for different sizes of NPs ranging from 5 to 45 nm.

4.2. Magnetic Field

In these MD simulations, a static magnetic field strength of 3[T] with a maximum spatial gradient magnetic field of 3.3[T/m] is singled out to achieve the required SPMN velocities. As already discussed, Figure 5a shows the magnetic force for energized SPMNs with different velocities. In other words, if the force applied on SPMNs is the same force applied to the membrane, the particles should move by a constant velocity. It is assumed that SPMNs can reach the assigned speed in this simulation in the presence of the aforementioned magnetic field's strength and gradient. On the other hand, the magnetic field $Y(z, t)$ can be obtained as shown and is discussed in Figure 5a based on the Equation (2). Since the maximum magnetic field value permitted for a nano-particle should not reach the saturation point, the effective magnetic field intensities simulated in this work should not have exceeded 2.5[T] for the core/shell (Fe_3O_4/Au). Based on the Equations (2) and (3), and using the constant values (μ_0, V, χ_{bead}) from Table 1, the applied magnetic field ($Y(z,t)$) should be $0.6 < Y(z,t) = b_z < 2.5$.

It is expected that the required time for crossing the membrane varies between 1.5 *min* to 7 *min* using various magnetic fields. The required time can be calculated through rescaling the travelling NPs in the upper velocity to lower velocities in the same distance and restricted magnetic field. Regarding these calculations, it is possible to exert alow magnetic field with higher duty cycle time and *vice versa*, while SPMNs can still cross the BBB. As described before, each endothelial cell features two barriers, one membrane when entering the endothelial cell and the other one when exiting the blood vessel. Inside the cells, the materials are softer than the membrane. As a result, the required force applied at a specific time is dedicated to pass the first barrier.

5. Non-Invasive BBB Crossing

Figure 6 features the successive simulation frames at different moments for a few specific velocities. The steps in this figure were captured from the video output frequency. In this simulation, the video output frequency was a frame per 10 computational steps. It means that this figure was generated after 6000 steps of the numerical simulation when the nanoparticle crossed the BBB. As demonstrated in these images, the SPMN opens a gap in the membrane in order to cross the membrane. The corresponding deformation or other changes of the membrane are reversible. This process is totally non-invasive. Based on these simulation results, the SPMNs can cross the membrane by applying a magnetic force while these NPs can move through the cells with a much lower magnetic force, as shown in Figure 7.

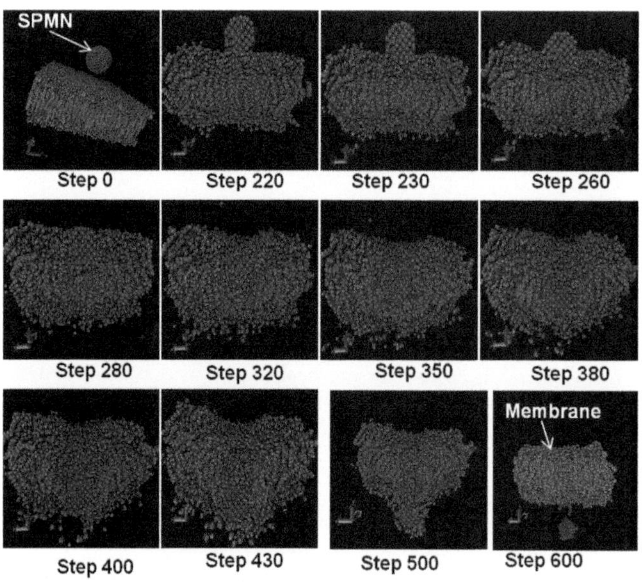

Figure 6. Several Steps of Crossing Through the BBB. These steps come from simulation, and the main goal is to show how the membrane is opened and how it can rehabilitate itself upon the completion of the crossing. In this figure, the receptor and insulin have been omitted in order to have a good view of the crossing.

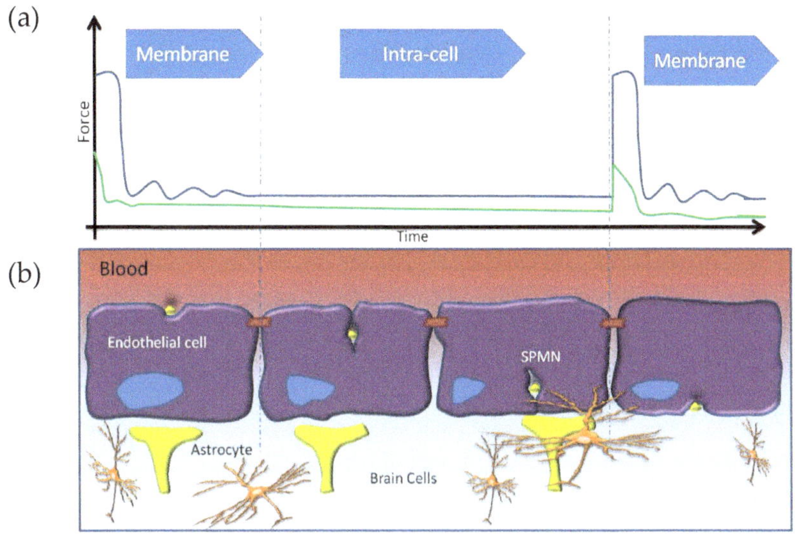

Figure 7. The process of NPs crossing through the BBB. The figure specifies how force should be exerted during the penetration of an endothelial cell and the penetration into the brain parenchyma. (**a**) force required for crossing through the cell vs Time. The blue line points to upper limit of the force and green line points to lower limit of the force. (**b**) status of nanoparticle inside the cell regarding the applied force during the time.

6. Conclusions

In this work, we studied the advantage of using SPMNs in the presence of a gradient magnetic field to cross the BBB for disease diagnostics and subsequent treatment purposes. The core/shell (Fe_2O_3)Au structure with 2 nm diameter was used as a biocompatible SPMN. The focus of this paper was placed on the modeling and simulation of SPMNs in the course of crossing the endothelial membrane under a magnetic field. In this paper, we demonstrated new results showing the required magnetic field which can be obtained by simulating the applied force on SPMNs that interacted with the membrane molecules. Based on the simulation results, the magnetic field should be in the range of 0.6 T to 2.5 T. Also, depending on the nanoparticle size, the maximum magnetic force would be changed from 4000 pN to 5000 pN for 5 nm to 45 nm nanoparticle sizes, respectively. In addition, the crossing time is extracted according to the force profile diagram, and it can be controlled by varying the magnetic pattern and magnetic field strength during the process. The simulation results as depicted in Figures 5 and 6 provide promising guidelines for the development of experimental protocols suitable for clinical applications.

Author Contributions: M.Z.P., A.S., A.A. and E.G.-Z. developed the concepts and wrote the paper; and M.Z.P. performed the simulations.

Conflicts of Interest: The authors declare no conflict of interest.

References

1. Pedram, M.Z.; Shamloo, A.; Alasty, A.; Ghafar-Zadeh, E. Toward Epileptic Brain Region Detection Based on Magnetic Nanoparticle Patterning. *Sensors* **2015**, *15*, 24409–24427. [CrossRef] [PubMed]
2. Akhtari, M.; Bragin, A.; Cohen, M.; Moats, R.; Brenker, F.; Lynch, M.D.; Vinters, H.V.; Engel, J., Jr. Functionalized magnetonanoparticles for MRI diagnosis and localization in epilepsy. *Epilepsia* **2008**, *49*, 1419–1430. [CrossRef] [PubMed]
3. Jordan, A.; Scholz, R.; Wust, P.; Fähling, H.; Felix, R. Magnetic fluid hyperthermia (MFH): Cancer treatment with AC magnetic field induced excitation of biocompatible superparamagnetic nanoparticles. *J. Magn. Magn. Mater.* **1999**, *201*, 413–419. [CrossRef]

4. Tang, J.; Xiong, L.; Zhou, G.; Wang, S.; Wang, J.; Liu, L.; Li, J.; Yuan, F.; Lu, S.; Wan, Z.; *et al.* Silver nanoparticles crossing through and distribution in the blood-brain barrier *in vitro*. *J. Nanosci. Nanotechnol.* **2010**, *10*, 6313–6317. [CrossRef] [PubMed]
5. Abbott, N.J.; Romero, I.A. Transporting therapeutics across the blood-brain barrier. *Mol. Med. Today* **1996**, *2*, 106–113. [CrossRef]
6. Begley, D.J. ABC transporters and the blood-brain barrier. *Curr. Pharm. Des.* **2004**, *10*, 1295–1312. [CrossRef] [PubMed]
7. Cima, M.J.; Lee, H.; Daniel, K.; Tanenbaum, L.M.; Mantzavinou, A.; Spencer, K.C.; Ong, Q.; Sy, J.C.; Santini, J.; Schoellhammer, C.M.; *et al.* Single compartment drug delivery. *J. Control. Release* **2014**, *190*, 157–171. [CrossRef] [PubMed]
8. Choi, J.J.; Feshitan, J.A.; Baseri, B.; Wang, S.; Tung, Y.S.; Borden, M.A.; Konofagou, E.E. Microbubble-size dependence of focused ultrasound-induced blood-brain barrier opening in mice *in vivo*. *IEEE Trans. Biomed. Eng.* **2010**, *57*, 145–154. [CrossRef] [PubMed]
9. Jolesz, F.A.; McDannold, N.J. *MRI-Guided Focused Ultrasound, in Intraoperative Imaging and Image-Guided Therapy*; Springer: New York, NY, USA, 2014; pp. 403–412.
10. Jolesz, F.A. Science to Practice: Opening the Blood-Brain Barrier with Focused Ultrasound—A Potential Treatment for Alzheimer Disease? *Radiology* **2014**, *273*, 631–633. [CrossRef] [PubMed]
11. Kinoshita, M.; McDannold, N.; Jolesz, F.A.; Hynynen, K. Noninvasive localized delivery of Herceptin to the mouse brain by MRI-guided focused ultrasound-induced blood-brain barrier disruption. *Proc. Natl. Acad. Sci. USA* **2006**, *103*, 11719–11723. [CrossRef] [PubMed]
12. McDannold, N.; Arvanitis, C.D.; Vykhodtseva, N.; Livingstone, M.S. Temporary disruption of the blood-brain barrier by use of ultrasound and microbubbles: Safety and efficacy evaluation in rhesus macaques. *Cancer Res.* **2012**, *72*, 3652–3663. [CrossRef] [PubMed]
13. Vykhodtseva, N.; McDannold, N.; Hynynen, K. Progress and problems in the application of focused ultrasound for blood-brain barrier disruption. *Ultrasonics* **2008**, *48*, 279–296. [CrossRef] [PubMed]
14. George, M.S. Stimulating the brain. *Sci. Am.* **2003**, *289*, 66–73. [CrossRef] [PubMed]
15. D'Andrea, J.A.; Chou, C.K.; Johnston, S.A.; Adair, E.R. Microwave effects on the nervous system. *Bioelectromagnetics* **2003**, *24*, S107–S147. [CrossRef] [PubMed]
16. Salford, L.G.; Brun, A.; Sturesson, K.; Eberhardt, J.L.; Persson, B.R. Permeability of the blood-brain barrier induced by 915 MHz electromagnetic radiation, continuous wave and modulated at 8, 16, 50, and 200 Hz. *Microsc. Res. Tech.* **1994**, *27*, 535–542. [CrossRef] [PubMed]
17. Weinberg, I.N.; Urdaneta, M.G.; Stepanov, P.Y.; Beylin, D.; Nacev, A.; Sarwar, A.; Shapiro, B.; Rodriguez, O.C.; Albanese, C.; Probst, R.; *et al.* Non-invasive image-guided brain access with gradient propulsion of magnetic nanoparticles. In Proceedings of the 2012 IEEE Nuclear Science Symposium and Medical Imaging Conference (NSS/MIC), Anaheim, CA, USA, 27 October–3 November 2012.
18. Lampropoulos, N.; Karvelas, E.; Sarris, I. Computational Modeling of an MRI Guided Drug Delivery System Based on Magnetic Nanoparticle Aggregations for the Navigation of Paramagnetic Nanocapsules. *Soft Condens. Matter* **2015**. arXiv preprint arXiv:1504.03490.
19. Teste, B.; Malloggi, F.; Gassner, A.; Georgelin, T.; Siaugue, J.; Varenne, A.; Girault, H.; Descroix, S. Magnetic core shell nanoparticles trapping in a microdevice generating high magnetic gradient. *Lab Chip* **2011**, *11*, 833–840. [CrossRef] [PubMed]
20. Abbott, N.J.; Patabendige, A.A.; Dolman, D.E.; Yusof, S.R.; Begley, D.J. Structure and function of the blood-brain barrier. *Neurobiol. Dis.* **2010**, *37*, 13–25. [CrossRef] [PubMed]
21. Ballabh, P.; Braun, A.; Nedergaard, M. The blood-brain barrier: An overview: Structure, regulation, and clinical implications. *Neurobiol. Dis.* **2004**, *16*, 1–13. [CrossRef] [PubMed]
22. Masserini, M. Nanoparticles for brain drug delivery. *ISRN Biochem.* **2013**, *2013*. [CrossRef] [PubMed]
23. Fiedler, S.L.; Violi, A. Simulation of nanoparticle permeation through a lipid membrane. *Biophys. J.* **2010**, *99*, 144–152. [CrossRef] [PubMed]
24. Lin, J.; Zhang, H.; Chen, Z.; Zheng, Y. Penetration of lipid membranes by gold nanoparticles: Insights into cellular uptake, cytotoxicity, and their relationship. *ACS Nano* **2010**, *4*, 5421–5429. [CrossRef] [PubMed]

25. Weinstein, J.S.; Varallyay, C.G.; Dosa, E.; Gahramanov, S.; Hamilton, B.; Rooney, W.D.; Muldoon, L.L.; Neuwelt, E.A. Superparamagnetic iron oxide nanoparticles: Diagnostic magnetic resonance imaging and potential therapeutic applications in neurooncology and central nervous system inflammatory pathologies, a review. *J. Cereb. Blood Flow Metab.* **2010**, *30*, 15–35. [CrossRef] [PubMed]
26. Mathieu, J.-B.; Martel, S. Aggregation of magnetic microparticles in the context of targeted therapies actuated by a magnetic resonance imaging system. *J. Appl. Phys.* **2009**, *106*. [CrossRef]
27. Bayraktar, E.; Robert, M.H.; Miskioglu, I.; Bayraktar, A.T. Mechanical and Tribological Performance of Aluminium Matrix Composite Reinforced with Nano Iron Oxide (Fe_3O_4). In *Composite, Hybrid and Multifunctional Materials*; Springer: Cham, Switzerland, 2015; Volume 4, pp. 185–192.
28. León-Félix, L.; Chaker, J.; Parise, M.; Coaquira, J.A.H.; Valladares, L.D.L.S.; Bustamante, A.; Garg, V.K.; Oliveira, A.C.; Morais, P.C. Synthesis and characterization of uncoated and gold-coated magnetite nanoparticles. In *LACAME 2012*; Springer: Medellín, Colombia, 2013; pp. 173–182.
29. Yaghoobpour, E.; Ahmadpour, A.; Farhadian, N.; Shariaty-Niassar, M. Molecular dynamics simulation of carbon molecular sieve preparation for air separation. *Korean J. Chem. Eng.* **2015**, *32*, 494–500. [CrossRef]
30. Llandro, J.; Lee, D.; Mitrelias, T.; Palfreyman, J.J.; Hayward, T.J.; Cooper, J.; Bland, J.A.C.; Barnes, C.H.; Lees, M. Magnetic measurements of suspended functionalised ferromagnetic beads under DC applied fields. *J. Magn. Magn. Mater.* **2009**, *321*, 2129–2134.
31. León, L.; Bustamante, A.; Osorio, A.; Olarte, G.S.; Valladares, L.D.L.S.; Barnes, C.H.; Majima, Y. Synthesis and characterization of hollow α-Fe_2O_3 sub-micron spheres prepared by sol-gel. *Hyperfine Interact.* **2011**, *202*, 131–137. [CrossRef]
32. Hinterwirth, H.; Kappel, S.; Waitz, T.; Prohaska, T.; Lindner, W.; Lämmerhofer, M. Quantifying thiol ligand density of self-assembled monolayers on gold nanoparticles by inductively coupled plasma–mass spectrometry. *ACS Nano* **2013**, *7*, 1129–1136. [CrossRef] [PubMed]
33. Ulman, A. Formation and structure of self-assembled monolayers. *Chem. Rev.* **1996**, *96*, 1533–1554. [CrossRef] [PubMed]

7

Broadband 120 MHz Impedance Quartz Crystal Microbalance (QCM) with Calibrated Resistance and Quantitative Dissipation for Biosensing Measurements at Higher Harmonic Frequencies

Manuel Kasper [1,†], Lukas Traxler [2,†], Jasmina Salopek [3], Herwig Grabmayr [2,4], Andreas Ebner [2] and Ferry Kienberger [1,*]

1. Keysight Technologies Austria GmbH, Keysight Labs Linz, Gruberstrasse 40, 4020 Linz, Austria; manuel.kasper@keysight.com
2. Johannes Kepler University Linz, Biophysics Institute, Gruberstrasse 40, 4020 Linz, Austria; Lukas.Traxler@jku.at (L.T.); herwigreinhard.grabmayr@students.fh-wels.at (H.G.); Andreas.Ebner@jku.at (A.E.)
3. Faculty of Science, Department of Chemistry, Division of Physical Chemistry University of Zagreb, Horvatovac 102a, 10000 Zagreb, Croatia; jsalopek@chem.pmf.hr
4. University of Applied Sciences Upper Austria, School of Engineering, Stelzhamerstrasse 23, 4600 Wels, Austria

* Correspondence: ferry_kienberger@keysight.com

† These authors contributed equally to this work.

Academic Editor: Torsten Frosch

Abstract: We developed an impedance quartz crystal microbalance (QCM) approach with the ability to simultaneously record mass changes and calibrated energy dissipation with high sensitivity using an impedance analyzer. This impedance QCM measures frequency shifts and resistance changes of sensing quartz crystals very stable, accurately, and calibrated, thus yielding quantitative information on mass changes and dissipation. Resistance changes below 0.3 Ω were measured with corresponding dissipation values of 0.01 μU (micro dissipation units). The broadband impedance capabilities allow measurements between 20 Hz and 120 MHz including higher harmonic modes of up to 11th order for a 10 MHz fundamental resonance frequency quartz crystal. We demonstrate the adsorbed mass, calibrated resistance, and quantitative dissipation measurements on two biological systems including the high affinity based avidin-biotin interaction and nano-assemblies of polyelectrolyte layers. The binding affinity of a protein-antibody interaction was determined. The impedance QCM is a versatile and simple method for accurate and calibrated resistance and dissipation measurements with broadband measurement capabilities for higher harmonics measurements.

Keywords: quartz crystal microbalance; impedance analysis; biosensing; dissipation; higher harmonics

---

1. Introduction

Quartz crystal microbalance (QCM) is an acoustic sensing technique which uses the inverse piezoelectric effect for measuring different properties of surrounding media, such as mass adsorption or fluid viscosity. The mass changes per area ($\Delta m/A$) due to thin films deposited on the surface of a periodically-oscillating quartz crystal are related to a change in resonance frequency according to Sauerbrey's equation [1], $\Delta f = -\frac{2 \cdot n \cdot f_0^2}{\sqrt{\rho_q \cdot \mu_q}} \cdot \frac{\Delta m}{A}$, where Δf is the change in resonance frequency, f_0 is the fundamental resonance frequency and ρ_q and μ_q are the density (2.947×10^{11} g$\cdot$cm$^{-1}\cdot$s^2) and shear modulus of quartz (2.648 g$\cdot$ cm^{-3}), respectively. Due to its extraordinary mass sensitivity (<0.4 ng/cm^2 for a 5 MHz quartz crystal), the technique was used originally for gravimetric measurements [2]. Due to the introduction of an empirical model to describe the influence of viscosity and density of liquids on the change in resonance frequency [3,4], the applications were extended including process control, environment engineering, as well as bio-medical diagnosis. Biochemical functionalization of the quartz crystal electrode allows a label-free detection of specific molecular interactions with high sensitivity and specificity and a real-time determination of kinetic rates and affinity constants. This makes QCM a versatile bioanalytic screening tool for various applications ranging from the detection of single molecular monolayers, polymer films, complex macromolecules, to whole cells [5–7]. While the QCM tracks changes in the resonant frequency due to different fluid properties or mass deposition on the quartz surface, it offers additional advantages over similar biosensing techniques such as surface plasmon resonance [8,9]. As additional mass on the quartz plate does not only affect its oscillation frequency but also changes the oscillation behavior (more specifically the motional resistance), these changes correlate with the energy loss per stored energy during one oscillation cycle (referred in the following as dissipation factor) and provide information about the mechanical properties of the deposited mass. Rigid materials which are coupled tightly to the quartz plate will not influence the motional resistance significantly as they follow the oscillations more or less directly. By contrast, elastic materials such as cells or lipid layers with entrapped water are not following the oscillations perfectly which leads to internal frictions and, therefore, energy dissipation. Thus, dissipation serves as an additional parameter characterizing the deposited mass layer. This additional information is critical for many biomolecular systems, including the investigation of conformational effects of ligand binding to a DNA complex [10], DNA hybridization, and DNA–protein interactions [11,12], or protein adsorption to biomaterials [13–16].

With respect to QCM measurement technology, various approaches exist to read out the resonance frequency of quartz crystals [17,18]. In the following we describe three approaches, including single frequency oscillators, time domain-based methods, and advanced impedance analysis. *Method 1*: In the single frequency oscillator method a harmonic oscillator is implemented around the quartz under test (QUT) involving an amplifying circuit and active amplitude control to maintain a pre-defined oscillation level. A second control loop acts on the phase lag and maintains a zero degree phase-shift between QUT current and voltage, as the QUT is an inherent part of the oscillator circuitry, its stability and noise performance directly affects the measurement result, and it is not easily possible to use advanced techniques, like calibration and averaging for improving the signal-to-noise ratio. Additionally, only a limited frequency band can be covered with this approach limiting broadband harmonic frequency operation. *Method 2*: Dissipation analysis is implemented in the time domain. The QUT is stimulated with short excitation bursts which have a frequency close to the relevant resonance. After the excitation is switched off, the QUT continues to oscillate at its natural resonance frequency with decaying amplitude due to energy dissipation [19]. This decaying oscillation is acquired in the time domain and the resulting data is processed in order to extract the resonance frequency and the dissipation coefficient. Similar to the impedance analysis method the excitation can be in a broad frequency range allowing harmonic operation up to, typically, 70 MHz. *Method 3*: In standard impedance analysis the QUT impedance is analyzed in a certain frequency range around the relevant resonance frequency. By sweeping the frequency, data from various frequencies is acquired and advanced averaging and curve fitting can be applied. An excitation voltage is put at the QUT terminals and both the voltage and the flowing current are measured while the impedance is calculated. There are several methods to implement this impedance analyzer approach [20], and in each of them the circuitry parts for signal generation and measurement are completely separated which allows to optimize each part individually, resulting in a better signal-to-noise ratio. Furthermore, sensitive input amplifiers and high quality connections enables low drive level operation thus reducing the mechanical stress and the power dissipation in the QUT.

In the following we present an advanced impedance based QCM workflow (*Method 3*) that works up to 120 MHz allowing for higher harmonics measurements as well as accurate calibration of resistance and dissipation. For an avidin-biotin test sample we compare the performance of the impedance QCM with the single frequency oscillator (*Method 1*) resulting in better signal-to-noise on the resistance. Metrological grade impedance calibration procedures are used to get calibration of the resistance and the dissipation with a sensitivity that is better compared to time domain based dissipation methods (*Method 2*). Additionally we show overtone higher harmonics measurements of up to 11th order using the impedance QCM.

2. Materials and Methods

2.1. Measurement Setup and Liquid Chamber

For all QCM measurements an in house developed liquid chamber (Johannes Kepler University Linz, Austria, http://www.jku.at/biophysics) consisting of two parts was used (Figure 1e). The lower part holds the quartz crystal and provides the electrical contacts, whereas the upper part contains the tube connections together with the inlet and outlet fluidic channels. By putting the two parts together, the quartz crystal gets clamped between the two x-rings. The liquid chamber is then mounted in the flow-cell holder and fixed by a screw. The electrodes are contacted by two corresponding counter-electrodes installed in the liquid cell. The wiring from these electrodes to the calibration plane where the actual impedance is measured is very short in order to avoid significant parasitic circuit elements, such as series inductance. For this reason, the electrical connection to the impedance analyzer is provided by a BNC socket directly at the liquid cell. To suck the liquid through the liquid chamber a constant liquid flow rate is provided by an automatic programmable syringe pump (NE-1000, New Era Pump Systems Inc., New York, NY, USA). In this study, the running buffer was either degased phosphate buffered saline (PBS, pH 7.3) or 0.5 M NaCl aqueous solution.

2.2. Biological Interaction Analysis and Polyelectrolyte Formation Measurements

For the avidin-biotin-IgG biochemical test measurement, AT-cut quartz crystals (ICM, Oklahoma City, OK, USA) with a diameter of 13.7 mm and a nominal fundamental resonance frequency of 9.995 MHz were used (surface area of working electrode was 20.47 mm^2). At the beginning of the experiment, phosphate-buffered saline (PBS, 150 mM NaCl, 15 mM NaH_2PO_4, pH adjusted to 7.4) solution was run through the liquid chamber to equilibrate the system. As a first step of the biochemical reaction, NeutrAvidin, a deglycosylated version of native avidin (concentration 1.67 μM, molecular weight 60 kDa) known to adhere to bare gold surfaces [21], was injected into the liquid chamber via an automatic programmable syringe pump for approximately 15 minutes at a constant flow rate of 50 μL/min until saturation was reached. In saturation, a dense layer of NeutrAvidin is established on the gold electrode of the quartz crystal. Subsequent flushing with PBS solution was done in order to wash away loosely adsorbed NeutrAvidin. In the second step of the biochemical reaction, biotinylated goat IgG-antibody (concentration 0.5 μM, molecular weight 150 kDa, ~2 biotins per IgG) was injected into the liquid chamber for 15 min at a flow rate of 50 μL/min. In control measurements we observed an almost full saturation (>95%) of the biotin-binding sites of NeutrAvidin at a biotin-IgG concentration of 0.5 μM. Due to the high affinity between NeutrAvidin and biotin ($K_d \approx 10^{-15}$ M), biotin-IgG forms a stable complex with the NeutrAvidin layer. Again, after saturation the liquid chamber was flushed with PBS.

For the determination of the binding affinity of goat-IgG to protein G a similar approach was used. After adsorbing a chicken-avidin mutant (1.67 μM, described in detail in [22]) to the gold electrode of the quartz crystal, biotinylated goat IgG-antibody (0.5 μM) was bound on top of the avidin mutant layer. Upon saturation, bacterial cell wall protein G from *Streptococcus* sp. was injected at increasing concentrations ranging from 1.37 nM to 1000 nM (solutions prepared by a serial dilution by a factor of three) until reaching equilibrium. Before the next injection, the flow-cell was rinsed with PBS after each injection step.

For the formation of polyelectrolyte monolayers, a SiO_2 coated 5 MHz quartz crystal was used (Q-Sense, Gothenburg, Sweden). Stock solutions of Poly(allylamine hydrochloride) (PAH,

M_W = 15,000 g· mol^{-1}, degree of amine functionalization f = 0.89) and Poly(sodium 4-styrenesulfonate) (PSS, M_W = 70,000 g· mol^{-1}, degree of styrenesulfonate functionalization f = 0.83) were prepared by dissolving polyelectrolytes and NaCl in the aqueous solution of hydrochloric acid (c(HCl) = 0.1 mM) in order to assure the complete protonation of the polycation. Polyelectrolyte solutions were prepared of 50 mM (in monomer units) stock solutions by diluting the stock solutions with 0.1 mM· HCl. The concentration of the injected polyelectrolyte solutions was 1 mM (in 0.5 M NaCl). After exposing the sensor chip to the respective polyelectrolyte solution for approx. 10 min, it was rinsed with 0.5 M NaCl for approx. 5 min.

2.3. *Impedance Analyzer, Impedance Probe, and Impedance Calibration*

For impedance measurements the Keysight E4990 impedance analyzer (Keysight Technologies, Santa Rosa, CA, USA) is used within the frequency range of 20 Hz to 120 MHz. Alternatively, the Keysight 4294A impedance analyzer (Keysight Technologies) can also be used for frequencies of up to 110 MHz. Both impedance analyzers apply the auto-balancing-bridge measurement method [20] and have a four-terminal port for connecting the quartz crystal in the liquid chamber. The Keysight 42941A impedance probe (Keysight Technologies) is used to connect the impedance analyzer to the liquid chamber. This probe effectively converts the four terminal connection into a single coaxial one and adds only little additional noise and drift. The probe is equipped with a SMA connector; therefore, the connection to the liquid chamber is done using a SMA-BNC adaptor (*cf.* Figure 1a).

For the QCM calibration a two-step procedure is applied. In the first step, calibration is done with the impedance probe by running a procedure including phase correction, open, short, and load measurements. The calibration measurements are done over the full frequency span (20 Hz–120 MHz). Short and load calibration standards are included in the impedance probe kit, while open is not an explicit standard. The calibration effectively shifts the measurement plane directly to the SMA connector of the impedance probe, thereby eliminating any effects of the probe connection cable. For this first step it is typically enough to recalibrate after several months. In a second calibration step the parasitic effects of the liquid chamber and the quartz crystal including stray inductance and electrode capacitance C_0 are removed. This is done by a built-in fixture compensation assuming an open circuit and ignoring resonances. Due to the strong dependency on the individual quartz crystals this procedure is typically done before every measurement. The absolute impedance accuracy of the calibrated system is well within 1% for fundamental measurements and 3% for overtone measurements and traceable to metrology standards. The frequency reference is provided by a temperature-controlled time base resulting in 1 ppm accuracy and 0.5 ppm drift over a one year period.

2.4. *QCM Models and Data Analysis*

Figure 1a shows the QCM setup and Figure 1b shows a lumped circuitry model for the QCM in the acoustic domain and in the electrical domain. In the acoustic domain the oscillation mode is a thickness shear wave modelled as a harmonic spring-mass-damper oscillator. Based on the piezoelectric effect the quartz crystal acts as transformer between the acoustical and the electrical domain, thereby converting forces and displacements into currents and voltages, respectively. By measuring the electrical impedance Z ($Z = \frac{V_q}{I_q}$) between the two connectors of the quartz, the mechanical elements are replaced by an electrical equivalent circuitry model. This leads to an L-C-R equivalent circuit which, is also called the motional leg. The LCR circuit is in parallel to a static shunt capacitance C_0 which represents the electrode capacitance of the quartz crystal. This capacitance is a purely electric effect which has no equivalent in the acoustic domain. The complete electrical equivalent circuit is known as Butterworth–Van Dyke model. Figure 1c shows a sketch of a single resonance curve obtained from an LCR circuit. Two characteristic resonances, the series resonance and the parallel resonance, can be obtained. The first one is the serial resonance where the magnitude of the impedance drops to a minimum value R representing the losses in the system. The series resonance is characterized by the resonance frequency f_R and the quality factor Q, with the former given by $f_R = \frac{1}{2\pi\sqrt{L \cdot C}}$. The quality factor represents the losses of the system at resonance and is the ratio of stored energy and dissipated energy. Thus, it is influenced by both, the reactive components L and C, as well as the dissipative element R. The quality factor Q is given by $Q = 2\pi \cdot f_R \frac{L}{R}$. The inverse of the quality factor is called dissipation coefficient d = 1/Q. Both quantities are dimensionless and without units. Typical Q-values for the used quartz crystals are in the range of 1000 to 3000 in liquid environment and up to 100,000 in air. The parallel electrode capacitance C_0 causes the subsequent parallel resonance at high impedance where the motional leg becomes inductive at frequencies above the series resonance. The parallel resonance is however not used in QCM. At off-resonance frequencies the total impedance is defined mostly by the electrode capacitance C_0. Figure 1d shows the quantitative equivalent circuit analysis that is included in the impedance analyzer. To determine the circuit element values L, C, R, and C_0, a frequency sweep is performed around the resonance frequency with the C_0 compensation switched off. For instance, to characterize a 10 MHz quartz crystal a sweep between 1 MHz and 15 MHz is applied.

2.5. *QCM Software Control*

A graphical user interface (GUI) that controls the E4990 impedance analyzer has been implemented in MATLAB. The GUI monitors the resonance frequency over time as well as the corresponding resistivity. The GUI allows to set up the measurement, start-and-stop the data record, and has a built-in conversion model to calculate the quantitative mass adsorption based on the frequency shift. Dissipation values are calculated based on the measured resistance values. Before the measurement is started a wide span frequency sweep is done in order to extract the required equivalent circuit parameters (L, C, R, and C_0) using the impedance analyzer built-in circuit analysis software. For the typically high Q (quality factor) value resonances the effect of C_0 is a slight offset of the absolute resonance frequency. Therefore, fixture compensation is applied eliminating the effect of C_0 and parasitic circuit elements arising from the liquid cell. Subsequently, a search algorithm is used to find the relevant resonance frequencies. The implementation is done using the interpolation capabilities and corresponding tracking search markers of the impedance analyzer. The actual frequency sweep is software triggered every 0.5 s corresponding to a refresh rate of 2 Hz. If a frequency shift larger than 200 Hz occurs (e.g., due to air bubbles in the liquid cell) the frequency tracking could be lost. This case is detected and the resonance search is redone automatically.

3. Results and Discussion

3.1. *Biological Interaction Analysis*

For testing the performance of the calibrated impedance QCM we performed biosensing on the well characterized receptor-ligand system avidin-biotin which is known to be stable, robust, and having a high affinity [23]. Figure 2a shows the results of an avidin-biotin measurement on a 10 MHz fundamental frequency quartz crystal monitored with the impedance QCM (solid line) and compared to a commercial test oscillator QCM (dashed lines; Maxtek RQCM, Inficon). The first step of the biochemical reaction was to inject NeutrAvidin into the liquid cell leading to adsorption to the gold surface with a corresponding frequency shift of 240 Hz. In the second step biotinylated goat IgG-antibody was injected that binds specifically to the NeutrAvidin layer via biotin resulting in frequency shift of 195 Hz (*cf.* Materials and Methods). The frequency shift for both steps was the same either measured with the impedance QCM or the test-oscillator QCM. However, the corresponding resistance changes are significantly better resolved with the impedance QCM (Figure 2a, right axis), and a resistance change of 2.5 Ohms and 1 Ohm was obtained for the first and second step, respectively. The impedance-QCM results in a more than two times larger resistance signal compared to the test oscillator QCM. An accurate impedance calibration using open, short, and load measurements was done prior to the QCM experiments (*cf.* Materials and Methods). For the impedance QCM the absolute impedance accuracy of the calibrated system is better than 1% for fundamental resonance frequencies.

Relative impedance measurements can be even done at higher sensitivity, for instance a 50 mΩ change can be easily detected on top of a 1 kΩ signal. Similarly, using the impedance QCM the absolute frequency is measured with 1 ppm accuracy while the sensitivity for frequency changes is below 0.05 ppm. As such, the highly accurate measurement capabilities of the impedance analyzer result in stable QCM frequency and resistance measurements. Additionally, due to the open, short, and load calibration routine using the impedance probe kit, the resistance values are also calibrated and traceable to metrology standards.

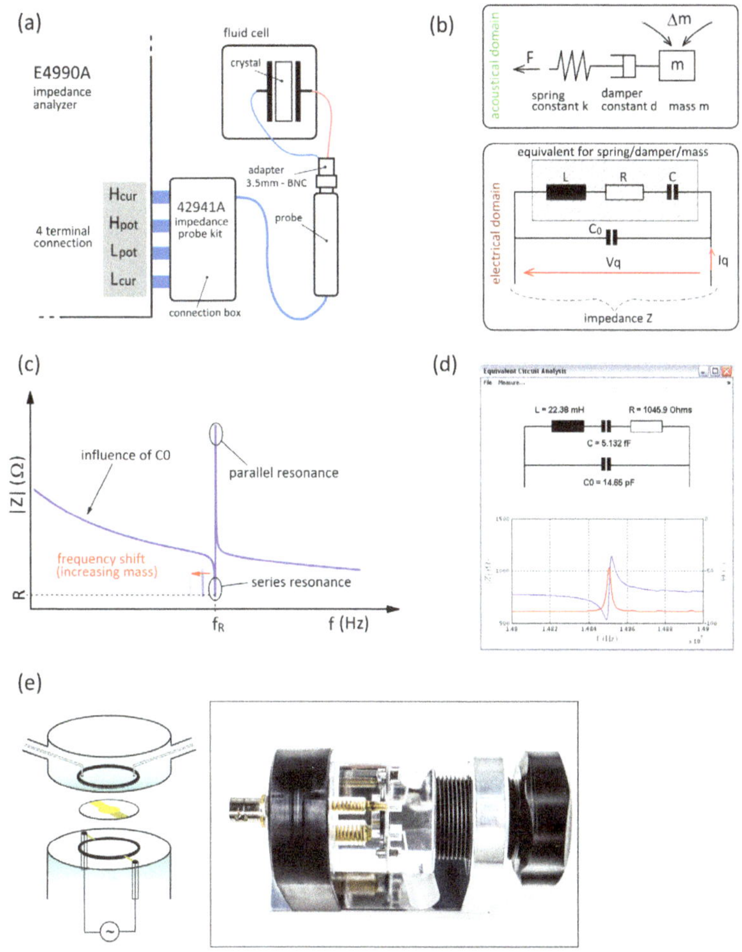

Figure 1. QCM setup and models. (**a**) Sketch of the impedance QCM setup. The impedance probe is used to connect the impedance analyzer with the liquid chamber; (**b**) mechanical (top) and electrical equivalent model (bottom) of the quartz resonator. V_q and I_q represent the voltage and the current applied to the quartz crystal, respectively. The impedance Z is equal to V_q/I_q; (**c**) sketch of a single resonance at f_R including the series and parallel resonance characteristics. For increasing mass adsorption the frequency is shifted to lower values (red arrow). The minimum impedance R represents the losses in the system. The electrode capacitance C_0 determines the impedance curve at off-resonance frequencies; (**d**) graphical user interface showing the equivalent circuit LCR analysis based on the impedance analyzer built in software functions. The measured impedance resonance is shown including the absolute impedance in blue (Ω) and the phase in red (degree); and (**e**) Left: sketch of the liquid cell and quartz crystal with the upper part providing the fluidic channels and the lower part the electrical contacts to the quartz electrodes. Right: The impedance analyzer is connected to the assembled liquid cell via a BNC-connector at the liquid cell holder.

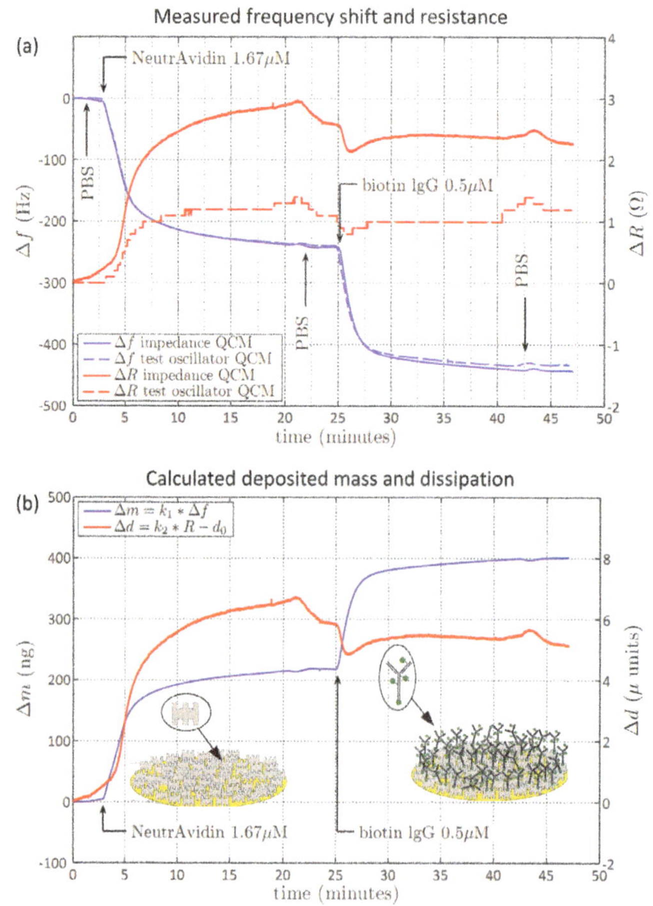

Figure 2. Impedance QCM measurement results of a simple bio-chemical test reaction. (a) The impedance QCM raw data (solid blue and red lines) is compared to the test oscillator QCM (dashed lines) (both with 9.995 MHz quartz crystals). Blue traces show frequency changes (Hz, left axis), and red traces show resistance changes (Ohm, right axis). After washing the liquid chamber with PBS (phosphate-buffered solution) the first step in this reaction is the adsorption of NeutrAvidin on gold (240 Hz shift) followed by the specific binding of biotin labeled antibodies (IgG, immunoglobulin G; 195 Hz shift); (b) based on the raw data the mass adsorption (ng; left axis) and the change in dissipation (micro-units; right axis) are calculated. The mass adsorption is inversely proportional to the frequency shift (k_1), while the dissipation is proportional (k_2) to the resistance. The sketches show the adsorption of avidin to the gold surface and the subsequent specific binding of biotin-IgG to the avidin layer.

Figure 2b shows the mass adsorption (left axis) and the dissipation changes (right axis) calculated from the raw frequency and resistance data. The mass uptake was calculated using Sauerbrey's equation which provides an inverse relationship to the frequency shift, given by $\Delta m = -\frac{A\cdot\sqrt{\rho_q\cdot\mu_q}}{2\cdot n\cdot f_0^2}\cdot\Delta f = -9.05\cdot 10^{-10}\cdot\Delta f$ (*cf.* Introduction). The first step of NeutrAvidin adsorption to the gold surface results in a mass uptake of 218 ng. Based on the NeutrAvidin molecular weight of 60 kDa this corresponds to 2.19×10^{12} NeutrAvidin molecules bound to the gold electrode, which is in good accordance to other studies [21]. The second step of biotin-IgG binding results in a mass uptake of 177 ng, corresponding to 7.11×10^{11} biotin-IgG molecules (molecular weight of 150 kDa). The factor of three lower number of biotin-IgG molecules, compared to NeutrAvidin, corresponds well to the theoretical number of biotin-IgG molecules that are bound to the NeutrAvidin monolayer, assuming a size of the antibody based on its 3D structure [24]. The red trace in Figure 2b represents the change in the dissipation calculated from the resistance data and the model parameters of the quartz equivalent circuit for the corresponding frequency (L, C, R, C_0). The equivalent circuit parameters were measured by acquiring an impedance sweep of sufficient bandwidth (*cf.* Materials and Methods). Based on the impedance sweep the equivalent circuit analysis software from the impedance analyzer automatically estimates the circuit parameters L, C, R, and C_0 (*cf.* Figure 1d). The dissipation (d) is proportional to the resistance according to $d=R/(\omega \times L)$, with R being the measured resistance, L the equivalent circuit inductance value and ω the circular frequency ($\omega = 2\pi f$). A change in dissipation of 6.5 μU (micro units) and 5.5 μU was obtained for the NeutrAvidin adsorption and the biotin-IgG binding, respectively. The dissipation values are mainly related to the layer viscoelasticity and layer softness and describe structural changes within the deposited mass. The dissipation values were compared to commercially available time domain-based dissipative QCM and similar values were obtained on the same biochemical reaction (data not shown). Based on the accurate resistance measurements and equivalent circuit parameters determination, very small dissipation coefficients below 0.05 μU can be detected without special efforts with the impedance QCM. Using averaging and curve fitting methods a minimum detection level of 0.01 μU is possible with the impedance analyzer which is better than time domain based dissipation methods that typically have a minimum detection level of 0.03 μU.

In Figure 3 we show the application of the impedance QCM for the quantitative determination of the binding affinity of goat-IgG to protein G based on the above described immobilization of biotinylated goat-IgG on top of a gold-adhered avidin mutant layer. Protein G, at seven different concentrations ranging from 1.37 nM to 1000 nM, was injected until reaching equilibrium. The respective decrease in resonance frequency per injection step was normalized, plotted against protein G concentration, and fitted with a logistic function (Figure 3 inset), yielding an equilibrium dissociation constant K_D of 129 ± 38 nM.

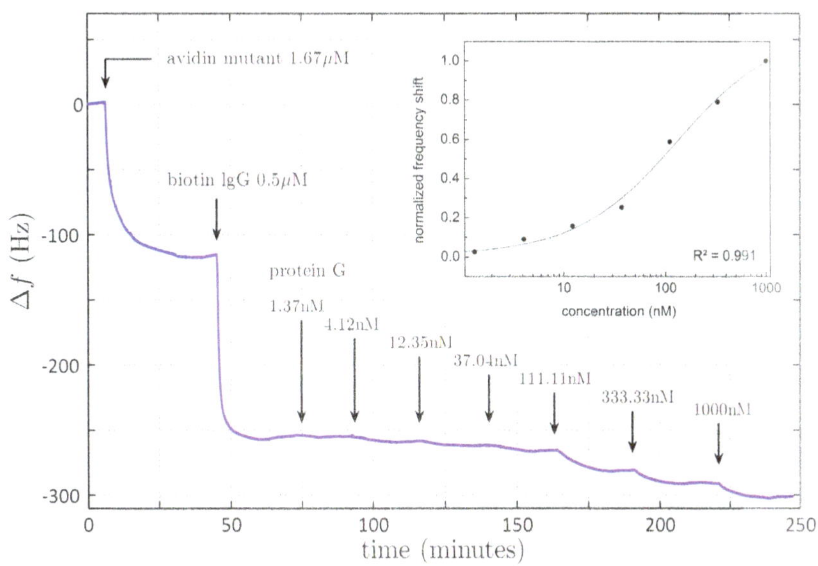

Figure 3. Impedance QCM measurement for the determination of the binding affinity of goat-IgG to protein G. Upon immobilization of biotinylated goat-IgG on a gold-adsorbed avidin-mutant layer, protein G was injected at different concentrations ranging from 1.37 nM to 1000 nM. For each step, the flow-cell was flushed with PBS after reaching equilibrium. Inset: Semi-logarithmic plot of normalized frequency shift per injection *versus* protein G-concentration, fitted with a logistic function.

3.2. Formation of Polyelectrolyte Multilayers

For investigating multi-layer formation with the impedance QCM we studied the resonance frequency and resistive dissipation of a polyelectrolyte multilayer (PEM) on a silicon dioxide

(SiO_2)-coated quartz crystal (Figure 4). For the PEM formation, solutions of poly(allylammonium hydrochloride) (PAH) and poly(sodium styrene sulfonate) (PSS) were injected subsequently into the liquid chamber in a multi-step process (Figure 4a). Each individual injection led to a mass deposition of the respective polymer on SiO_2 as indicated by the stepwise decrease in resonance frequency (Figure 4a, left axis). The corresponding dissipative changes of layer formation and trapping of water molecules are shown in the stepwise resistance data (Figure 4a, right axis). Figure 3b shows the calculated mass uptake per electrode area according to the Sauerbrey equation yielding, on average, 61 ng for PSS and 29 ng for PAH. One of the reasons for the larger mass adsorption of PSS compared to PAH is the higher mass per charge and monomer unit. The corresponding increase in dissipation during the multi-layer formation was 0.5 μU per polymer layer, followed by a decrease to the initial value during the rinsing with 0.5 M solution of NaCl. This indicates that the additional polymer layers do not have any significant viscoelastic impact and the layers behave like a homogenous rigid mass. However, due to the high sensitivity of our impedance based QCM, we were able to detect the difference in energy dissipation between tightly-assembled PEM layers and loosely-bound polyelectrolytes. Further QCM studies on the PEM will investigate layer thickness and nano-assembly with respect to different ionic strengths. It is expected that at higher ionic strengths the film thickness depends on the type of anion counterbalancing the polycation charge.

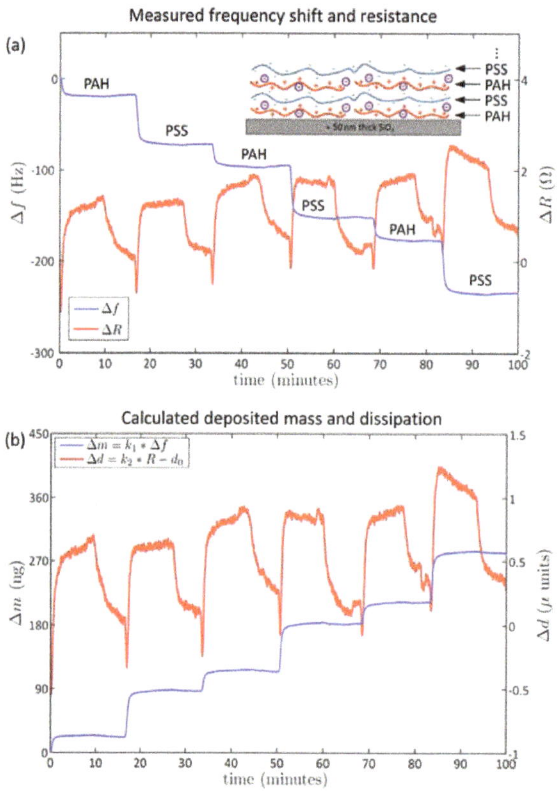

Figure 4. Impedance QCM measurement results of the formation of a polyelectrolyte multilayer (PEM) on top of a silicon dioxide coated quartz crystal (5 MHz resonance frequency). (**a**) Experimental data showing the stepwise decrease in resonance frequency (left axis, third harmonic, not normalized) and resistance (right axis) due to the sequential injection of solutions of poly(allylammonium hydrochloride) (PAH, 1 mM) and poly(sodium styrene sulfonate) (PSS, 1 mM) in the presence of NaCl (0.5 M). A 10 point moving average filter was applied to the raw data. The polymer was injected for 10 min at a flow rate of 50 μL/min followed by a 5 min injection of 0.5 M NaCl solution; and (**b**) calculated mass uptake (left axis) per electrode area and dissipation values (right axis) for the individual polymer layers.

3.3. *Higher Harmonic Impedance Measurements*

The impedance analyzer operates between 20 Hz and 120 MHz. Thus, higher harmonic resonances of the 10 MHz quartz crystal can also be investigated. Higher harmonics measurements have the advantage that the cheap, relatively thick, and easily-mountable 10 MHz crystal can be used at higher operating frequencies and it is not necessary to use a thinner and more expensive high-frequency quartz crystal. Figure 5a shows the measured broadband impedance spectrum of a pristine 10 MHz quartz crystal between 1 MHz and 120 MHz. The fundamental resonance at 10 MHz and the odd harmonics can be clearly identified up to the 11th harmonic at 110 MHz. For all quartz crystals and QCM setups, the even harmonic resonance numbers are not excited electrically. The overall impedance baseline falls with increasing frequency, which is caused by the parallel electrode capacitance C_0. The electrode capacitance C_0 is leading to a parallel resonance with a local impedance maximum that is following every series resonance with a local impedance minimum, resulting in the typical derivative resonance shape (*cf.* Figure 1). This resonance behavior can be obtained for all resonances and is shown as inset for the fundamental frequency, the 5th harmonics, and the 11th harmonics. The overall shape of the individual resonance curves is very similar. However, it can be observed that the quality factor decreases slightly at higher frequencies indicating increased losses. Additionally, spurious responses can be occasionally observed caused by additional resonant modes of the quartz crystal. Figure 5b shows a simulated impedance sweep in the same frequency range. The underlying circuitry model is shown in the inset and is composed of eleven parallel series resonant networks (only four LCR networks are shown in the sketch). A parallel shunt capacitance accounts thereby for the electrode capacitance C_0, and the resonant frequency is related to the inductance (L) and capacitance (C). It is required that the L and C values fulfil the relationship $L_n = L_1/n$ and $C_n = C_1/n$ for each harmonic number n, with L_n and C_n being the values for the harmonic resonator inductance and capacitance, and C_1 and L_1 being the corresponding values for the fundamental resonance. The applied circuitry model matches the experimental broadband impedance sweep very well for both the fundamental frequency and higher harmonic resonances.

Figure 5c shows higher harmonics measurements of the biochemical two-step reaction of NeutrAvidin adsorption to gold and subsequent biotin-IgG binding to avidin. The frequency shift is shown for the fundamental frequency (~10 MHz), the third harmonic (~30 MHz), the fifth harmonic (~50 MHz), and the seventh harmonic (~70 MHz). Both steps of NeutrAvidin adsorption and biotin-IgG binding can be properly seen in all resonances at the same center frequency. The absolute frequency change thereby increases with the resonance number and the highest frequency change is obtained at the highest harmonic resonance number. This is in line with the model where the frequency change is related to the fundamental frequency f_0 of the quartz crystal multiplied by the harmonic number n. Therefore, the expected frequency shift at higher harmonic oscillations is directly proportional to its order. Dividing each frequency shift by the harmonic number should, therefore, result in the same shift as measured at the fundamental resonance frequency. The inset of Figure 5c shows the normalized frequency shifts ($\Delta f/n$) for the harmonic and the fundamental frequency resonances. The curves are overlapping and the measured values are in good accordance to the expected behavior. This indicates that the assumptions of the Sauerbrey equation are fulfilled, including a thin, rigid, and uniformly distributed layer of NeutrAvidin and biotin-IgG. In addition to the 10 MHz quartz crystal we used a 25.4 mm diameter 5 MHz quartz crystal (Inficon, Inc., New York, NY, USA) and monitored the resonance frequency at the 23rd harmonic oscillation at 115 MHz over several hours in air (data not shown). For both quartz crystals the corresponding frequency curves are stable for several hours with a typical drift below 1 Hz/h, indicating the stability and high performance of the impedance analysis measurement.

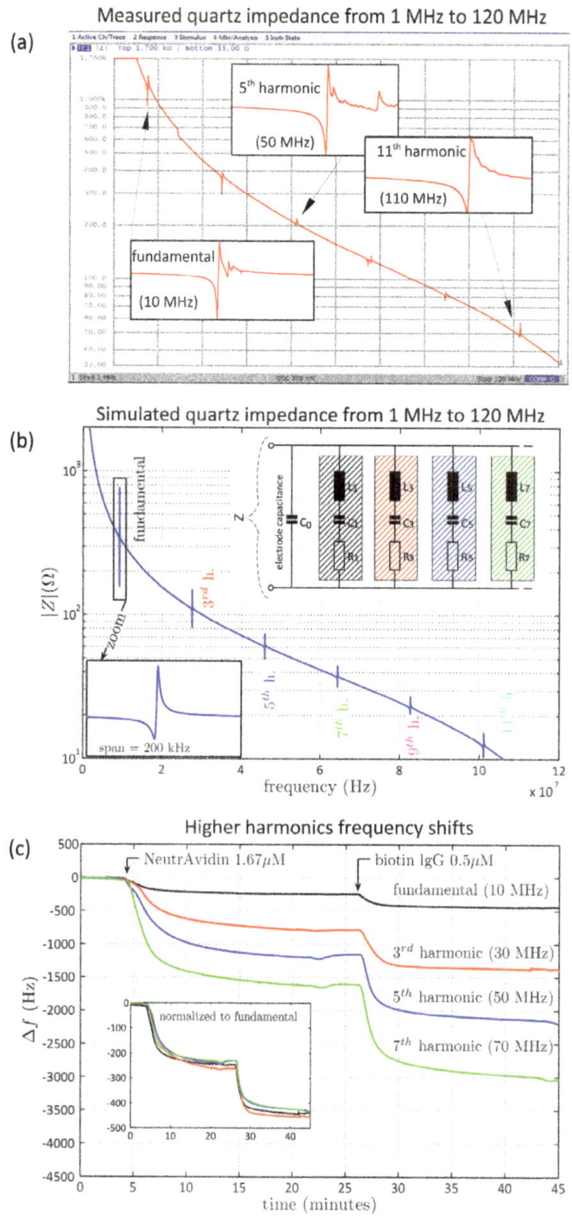

Figure 5. Harmonic measurements with the impedance QCM up to 120 MHz. (**a**) A broadband impedance sweep is done between 1 MHz and 120 MHz (1601 points). Based on the fundamental resonance frequency at 10 MHz, subsequent odd harmonic resonances are present up to 110 MHz corresponding to the 11th harmonics; (**b**) modeled impedance sweep using harmonic resonators. The individual resonances correspond to the multiple LCR circuits (sketches of LCR_1, LCR_3, LCR_5, and LCR_7 as inset) with the overall slope of the impedance curve mainly defined by the electrode capacitance C_0; and (**c**) experimental results of the higher harmonics impedance QCM. The two step bio-chemical reaction (first step is NeutrAvidin adsorption to gold; second step is biotin-IgG binding to the avidin layer) is measured at the fundamental frequency and at higher harmonics (third, fifth, and seventh harmonics). For the harmonic frequencies, both the absolute frequency and the frequency shifts are multiple integer values of the corresponding fundamental values. The normalized frequency shifts are shown in the inset.

4. Conclusions

An impedance QCM was used to measure the frequency shift and resistance for the multi-layer formation of polyelectrolytes and for specific avidin-biotin interaction. Furthermore, we applied this technique to determine and quantify the binding affinity between *Streptococcal* protein G and surface-bound goat-IgG. The broadband impedance measurement capabilities allow measurements between 20 Hz and 120 MHz including higher harmonic modes of up to 11th order for the 10 MHz fundamental resonance frequency quartz crystal. The Sauerbrey equation is used to convert the frequency shift into mass adsorption, while the dissipation is calculated from the measured resistance values. A full impedance calibration resulted in stable, quantitative and accurate resistance measurements with high sensitivity that is traceable to metrology standards. The calibration concept applied in this paper relies on traceable calibration standards (Short, Open, Load) which are consecutively connected to the impedance analyzer. By measuring the calibration standards first, all systematic errors due to different liquid cells, different cables, thermal drift and electrical connector degradation are corrected. This results in a significant accuracy improvement if small changes in impedance, respectively resistance and dissipation, are measured. We show this by measuring small resistance changes (0.3 Ω) at a high signal-to-noise ratio. The impedance calibrated QCM results in superior resistance signals compared to un-calibrated QCM systems, with respect to both the absolute accuracy and the relative signal-to-noise ratio. In un-calibrated systems where scale errors and offset errors are added to the real value of the physical resistance, the measurement of low absolute resistance values is not accurate. For instance, for the avidin adsorption on gold we measured a calibrated 2.5 Ω resistance change *versus* 1 Ω measured with an un-calibrated system. This corresponds to a relative error of 60% for un-calibrated systems. Comparing the performance of the method presented in this paper with traditional QCM methods, we can resolve smaller changes more robustly due to the advanced calibration and impedance measurement system. Additionally, quantitative measurements can be performed, and absolute dissipation values are comparable among different QCM machines. In summary, a high-performing impedance analyzer allows for fast and sensitive measurements in a broad frequency range, with the main advantage that calibrated and accurate resistance data can be acquired, which is important for robust dissipation analysis at higher modes. Future applications will focus on bio-medical detection of single virus particles in complex liquid environments where sensitivity, robustness and quantitative evaluation are of utmost importance.

Acknowledgments: We would like to thank Akihiko Oginuma and Hiroaki Ugawa from the Keysight impedance analyzer division (Kobe, Japan), Giovanni d'Amore from Keysight Europe, and WeiBeng Ng from Keysight Singapore for helpful technical discussions and hardware support; T. Vuletic (Institute of Physics, Zagreb, Croatia) for providing the QCM-D setup through support by UKF grant No. 17/13 "Confined DNA" and Vesa. P. Hytönen (BioMediTech, University of Tampere, Finland) for providing the avidin-mutant. For financial funding we thank the Austrian OEAD, Project WTZ HR 06/2014.

Author Contributions: M.K. and L.T. did the QCM experiments including hardware and software work, as well as data evaluation. J.S. worked on the polyelectrolyte multilayer chemistry, H.G. worked on the antibody QCM, A.E. and F.K. designed the study, planned the experiments and the overall implementation. All authors contributed to manuscript writing.

Conflicts of Interest: The authors declare no conflict of interest.

References

1. Sauerbrey, G. Verwendung von Schwingquarzen zur Wägung dünner Schichten und zur Mikrowägung. *Z. Phys.* **1959**, *155*, 206–222. (In German) [CrossRef]
2. Janshoff, A.; Galla, H.-F.; Steinem, C. Piezoelectric mass-sensing devices as biosensors—An alternative to optical biosensors? *Angew. Chem. Int. Ed.* **2000**, *39*, 4004–4032. [CrossRef]
3. Kanazawa, K.K.; Gordon, J.G. The oscillation frequency of a quartz resonator in contact with liquid. *Anal. Chim. Acta* **1985**, *175*, 99–105. [CrossRef]
4. Kanazawa, K.K.; Gordon, J.G. Frequency of a quartz microbalance in contact with liquid. *Anal. Chem.* **1985**, *57*, 1770–1771. [CrossRef]

5. Marx, K.A. Quartz crystal microbalance: A useful tool for studying thin polymer films and complex biomolecular systems at the solution-surface interface. *Biomacromolecules* **2003**, *4*, 1099–1120. [CrossRef] [PubMed]
6. Tang, D.; Li, Q.; Tang, J.; Su, B.; Chen, G. An enzyme-free quartz crystal microbalance biosensor for sensitive glucose detection in biological fluids based on glucose/dextran displacement approach. *Anal. Chim. Acta* **2011**, *686*, 144–149. [CrossRef] [PubMed]
7. Lin, T.Y.; Hu, C.H.; Chou, T.C. Determination of albumin concentration by MIP-QCM sensor. *Biosens. Bioelectron.* **2004**, *20*, 75–81. [CrossRef] [PubMed]
8. Vikinge, T.P.; Hansson, K.M.; Sandström, P.; Liedberg, B.; Lindahl, T.L.; Lundström, I.; Tengvall, P.; Höök, F. Comparison of surface plasmon resonance and quartz crystal microbalance in the study of whole blood and plasma coagulation. *Biosens. Bioelectron.* **2000**, *15*, 605–613. [CrossRef]
9. Su, X.; Wu, Y.-J.; Knoll, W. Comparison of surface plasmon resonance spectroscopy and quartz crystal microbalance techniques for studying DNA assembly and hybridization. *Biosens. Bioelectron.* **2005**, *5*, 719–726. [CrossRef] [PubMed]
10. Peh, W.Y.; Reimhult, E.; Teh, H.F.; Thomsen, J.S.; Su, X. Understanding ligand binding effects on the conformation of estrogen receptor alpha-DNA complexes: A combinational quartz crystal microbalance with dissipation and surface plasmon resonance study. *Biophys. J.* **2007**, *92*, 4415–4423. [CrossRef] [PubMed]
11. Nguyen, T.H.; Elimelech, M. Adsorption of plasmid DNA to a natural organic matter-coated silica surface: Kinetics, conformation, and reversibility. *Langmuir* **2007**, *23*, 3273–3279. [CrossRef] [PubMed]
12. Nguyen, T.H.; Elimelech, M. Plasmid DNA adsorption on silica: Kinetics and conformational changes in monovalent and divalent salts. *Biomacromolecules* **2007**, *8*, 24–32. [CrossRef] [PubMed]
13. Wittmer, C.R.; Phelps, J.A.; Saltzman, W.M.; van Tassel, P.R. Fibronectin terminated multilayer films: Protein adsorption and cell attachment studies. *Biomaterials* **2007**, *28*, 851–860. [CrossRef] [PubMed]
14. Scheideler, L.; Rupp, F.; Wendel, H.P.; Sathe, S.; Geis-Gerstorfer, J. Photocoupling of fibronectin to titanium surfaces influences keratinocyte adhesion, pellicle formation and thrombogenicity. *Dent. Mater.* **2007**, *23*, 469–478. [CrossRef] [PubMed]
15. Malmstrom, J.; Agheli, H.; Kingshott, P.; Sutherland, D.S. Viscoelastic modeling of highly hydrated laminin layers at homogeneous and nanostructured surfaces: Quantification of protein layer properties using QCM-D and SPR. *Langmuir* **2007**, *23*, 9760–9768. [CrossRef] [PubMed]
16. Atthoff, B.; Hilborn, J. Protein adsorption onto polyester surfaces: Is there a need for surface activation? *J. Biomed. Mat. Res. B Appl. Biomat.* **2007**, *80B*, 121–130. [CrossRef] [PubMed]
17. Arnau, A. A Review of Interface Electronic Systems for AT-cut Quartz Crystal Microbalance Applications in Liquids. *Sensors* **2008**, *8*, 370–411. [CrossRef]
18. Johannsmann, D. Viscoelastic, mechanical, and dielectric measurements on complex samples with the quartz crystal microbalance. *Phys. Chem. Chem. Phys.* **2008**, *10*, 4516–4534. [CrossRef] [PubMed]
19. Dixon, M.C. Quartz Crystal Microbalance with Dissipation Monitoring: Enabling Real-Time Characterization of Biological Materials and Their Interactions. *J. Biomol. Tech.* **2008**, *19*, 151–158. [PubMed]
20. Keysight Technologies. *Impedance Measurement Handbook: A Guide to Measurement Technology and Techniques*, 5th ed.; Agilent Technologies: Santa Clara, CA, USA, 2015.
21. Hianik, T.; Ostatná, V.; Sonlajtnerova, M.; Grman, I. Influence of ionic strength, pH and aptamer configuration for binding affinity to thrombin. *Bioelectrochemistry* **2007**, *70*, 127–133. [CrossRef] [PubMed]
22. Taskinen, B.; Zauner, D.; Lehtonen, S.I.; Koskinen, M.; Thomson, C.; Kähkönen, N.; Kukkurainen, S.; Määttä, J.A.E.; Ihalainen, T.O.; Kulomaa, M.S.; *et al.* Reversible Biofunctionalization of Surfaces with a Switchable Mutant of Avidin. *Bioconjug. Chem.* **2014**, *25*, 2233–2243.
23. Green, N.M. Avidin. *Adv. Protein. Chem.* **1975**, *29*, 85–113. [PubMed]
24. Kienberger, F.; Mueller, H.; Pastushenko, V.; Hinterdorfer, P. Following single antibody binding to purple membranes in real time. *EMBO Rep.* **2004**, *5*, 579–583. [CrossRef] [PubMed]

8

A Flow SPR Immunosensor Based on a Sandwich Direct Method

Mauro Tomassetti [1,*], Giorgia Conta [1], Luigi Campanella [1], Gabriele Favero [2], Gabriella Sanzò [2], Franco Mazzei [2] and Riccarda Antiochia [2]

[1] Department of Chemistry, Sapienza University of Rome, P.le Aldo Moro 5, 00185 Rome, Italy; giorgia.conta@libero.it (G.C.); luigi.campanella@uniroma1.it (L.C.)

[2] Department of Chemistry and Drug Technologies, Sapienza University of Rome, P.le Aldo Moro 5, 00185 Rome, Italy; gabriele.favero@uniroma1.it (G.F.); gabriella.sanzo@uniroma1.it (G.S.); franco.mazzei@uniroma1.it (F.M.); riccarda.antiochia@uniroma1.it (R.A.)

* Correspondence: Mauro.tomassetti@uniroma1.it

Academic Editor: Nicole Jaffrezic-Renault

Abstract: In this study, we report the development of an SPR (Surface Plasmon Resonance) immunosensor for the detection of ampicillin, operating under flow conditions. SPR sensors based on both direct (with the immobilization of the antibody) and competitive (with the immobilization of the antigen) methods did not allow the detection of ampicillin. Therefore, a sandwich-based sensor was developed which showed a good linear response towards ampicillin between 10^{-3} and 10^{-1} M, a measurement time of $\leqslant$20 min and a high selectivity both towards β-lactam antibiotics and antibiotics of different classes.

Keywords: ampicillin; flow immunosensor SPR; sandwich method

---

1. Introduction

β-lactams antibiotics are a class of antibiotics with a structure containing a β-lactam ring, *i.e.*, a four-term cyclic amide. The action mechanisms of most of these antibiotics interfere with the synthesis of the cell wall of the bacteria foreign to the human body [1]. Therefore, the β-lactam antibiotics generally act as bactericides. However, some bacteria are capable of producing particular enzymes, called β-lactamases, that are able to inactivate the same antibiotics, making them completely ineffective [1]. Among the antibiotics of the penicillin group, ampicillin shows a broader spectrum of activity than penicillin G. The cephalosporins, such as ceftriaxone (which will also be considered in this study), do not belong to the group of penicillins, but they belong to the same class of β-lactam antibiotics. Therefore, they have the same action mechanism of penicillins, although they show a wider antibacterial spectrum and a greater resistance to β-lactamase.

Of course, several strategies have been developed for the analytical determination of these antibiotics, for example chromatographic [2–5], mass-spectrometry [6–9], or microbial screening methods [10,11], but also methods based on sensors, biosensors and immunosensors [12–19]. Our research group developed different sensors for β-lactam antibiotics detection, initially ISES (Ion Selective Electrodes) [20] and most recently amperometric immunosensors [21].

Recent research carried out in our laboratories have been aimed at developing a traditional highly sensitive amperometric immunosensor [21] for penicillin G and other β-lactam antibiotics based on the competitive method, obtaining results that support the validity of this approach [21]. The LOD (low detection limit) was of the order of 10^{-10} M, but the analysis time was very long (about 1 h). This type of immunosensor also exhibited a poor selectivity towards other β-lactam antibiotics but a good selectivity towards antibiotics which do not belong to this class: it has therefore been used for the determination of the "pool" of antibiotics of the β-lactam class in common real matrices such as river waste water which can be more or less polluted by these types of antibiotics.

In the present research, we examined the possibility of developing an immunosensor for the direct determination of a β-lactam antibiotic, specifically ampicillin, by using the flow SPR technique, especially in order to shorten the analysis time. The SPR immunosensors are analytical devices capable of detecting, in a selective manner, chemical or biological species, which do not require sample pretreatments and the use of competitive methods.

However, the first results showed that it was not possible to realize an SPR immunosensor using the simplest and most common direct method, as the SPR signal obtained when, for instance, the penicillin G molecule that formed the immunocomplex with the antibody immobilized onto the SPR optical surface, was too low, probably because of the insufficiently high molecular weight of this antibiotic. In addition, the attempt to use a competitive method by immobilizing the antigen (instead of the antibody) and making it compete with the antigen to be determined in order to bind he free antibody in solution, was not successful, as described in this work. Moreover, this competitive method would not show any potential advantage compared to the traditional competitive method with amperometric detection in terms of measurement times, which would have been about the same for both methods. In fact, once the antibody complex is formed, its hydrolytic cleavage, in order to regenerate the optical surface of the SPR (that is the gold plate functionalized with the immobilized and not complexed antigen) to make a subsequent SPR measurement, resulted in being extremely difficult, as described in the "Results" section of the present paper. The research has therefore moved in the direction of the development of an immunosensor for ampicillin detection that is able to operate with a sandwich geometry (1st immobilized antigen molecule—antibody—2nd antigen molecule) that allowed for decreasing the analysis time and simplifying the measurement method.

2. Materials and Methods

2.1. Materials

Sodium dihydrogen phosphate NaH_2PO_4 (⩾99.0%), sodium dibasic phosphate Na_2HPO_4 (⩾99.0%), EtOH (96%), 11-mercaptoundecanoic acid (MUA) (95%), 1-ethyl-3-(3-dimethyl aminopropyl) carbodiimide (EDC), N-hydroxysuccinimide (NHS) (98%), glycine, ethanolamine (⩾99%), ceftriaxone and erythromycin were supplied by Sigma-Aldrich (St. Louis, MO, USA). The SPR plates, composed of a layer of Au of a thickness of 50 nm on a glassy support, were supplied by XanTec bioanalytics GmbH (Dusseldorf, Germany). The oil with a refractive index of 1.6100 ± 0.0002 was supplied by Cargille Laboratories (Cedar Grove, NJ, USA). Sodium Ampicillin was provided by Farmitalia—Carlo Erba (Milan, Italy); anti-Ampicillin was provided by Sigma (St. Louis, MO, USA); penicillin G was produced by Fluka Analyticals (St. Louis, MO, USA); fosfomycin was produced by Crinos S.P.A. (Villa Guardia, Como, Italy).

All solutions were prepared with deionized water ($R = 18.2$ mΩ × cm at 25 °C; TOC (Total Organic Carbon) < 10 g· mL^{-1}) obtained by a Millipore Milli-Q system (Millipore, Molsheim, France).

2.2. Apparatus

SPR flow measurements were realized by using BioSuplar 400T apparatus (Analytical μ-Systems—Department Of Mivitec GmbH, Sinzing, Germany), with a laser diode with low power (630–670 nm) as the light source. This instrument allows for the qualitative analysis of molecules on the basis of the mass of the sandwich antibody formed on the plate, which produces a variation in the resonance angle. This signal is then amplified and transduced. The output signal is successively processed as a function of time in the form of a sensorgram.

3. Results

In this section, we described all the steps carried out during the experimental work in order to develop a sandwich immunosensor for ampicillin detection and to construct the relative calibration curve.

3.1. SPR Immunosensor and Flow Measurements

An SPR immunosensor is an analytical device capable of selectively detecting chemical or biological species without the need of sample pretreatment. It is composed of three main elements: a bioreceptor (or biological component), a transducer, and finally a system for signal processing. The bioreceptor is immobilized on the surface of the optical sensor and is responsible for the variation of the resonance angle, the characteristic parameter of this technique, related to the species to be determined. In fact, we basically measure the variation of the resonance angle, due to the interaction between the analyte and the bioreceptor, in our case the antibody complex, immobilized on a suitably functionalized gold metal film. The "optical" signal generated is transduced into an electric signal, then amplified and processed in the form of a sensorgram (resonance angle *vs.* time).

The SPR flow device (Figure 1) has a prism as the main element, installed on a rotating plate, automatically controlled by a computer. The different samples are introduced into a proper cell by means of a peristaltic pump. The sensor consists of a gold sheet, 50 nm thick, placed on a glassy support. Once functionalized by forming a so-called SAM (Self-Assembled Monolayers), the plate is placed on the prism surface using an oil with a refractive index equal to that of the prism and the support itself, in order to ensure optical continuity. Finally, the plate is fixed with a system for mechanical anchorage. After positioning the SAM on the prism, the assembly of the SPR flow device is completed with a cell suitable for flow analysis. When the software for data processing is ready, it is possible to start the analysis. To observe the SPR phenomenon, the polarized light, emitted by a diode laser at low power, is reflected from the wafer on a detector and monitored as a function of the resonance angle, thanks to the prism rotation [22,23]. Successively, the SPR angle change caused by the formation of the sandwich was recorded, in the form of a sensorgram, as a function of time. The registered variation of resonance angle is proportional to the amount of complexed analyte. The results showed on the sensorgram have several phases (Figure 2) corresponding to the presence of different solutions in the flow cell. The SPR used unit is the Unit of Resonance (r.u.), which corresponds to a change of 0.0001° of the resonance angle.

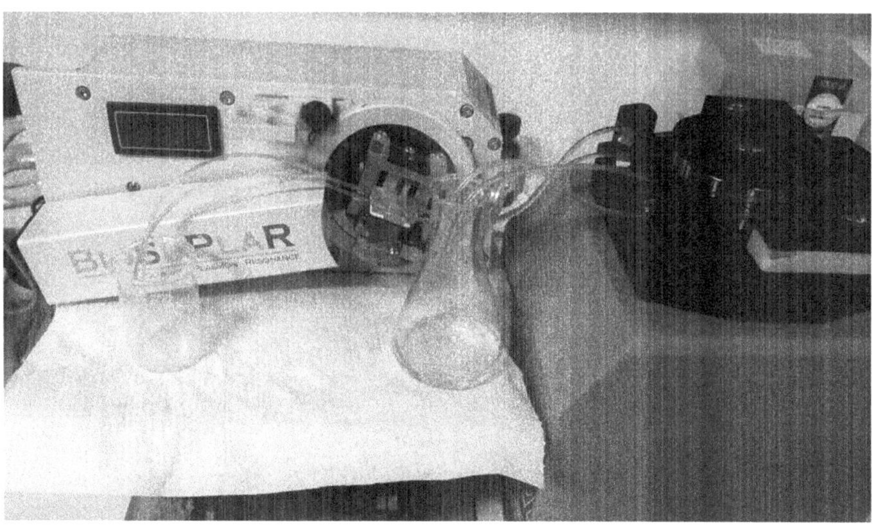

Figure 1. Measurement instrument used for Surface Plasmon Resonance (SPR) operating in flow mode.

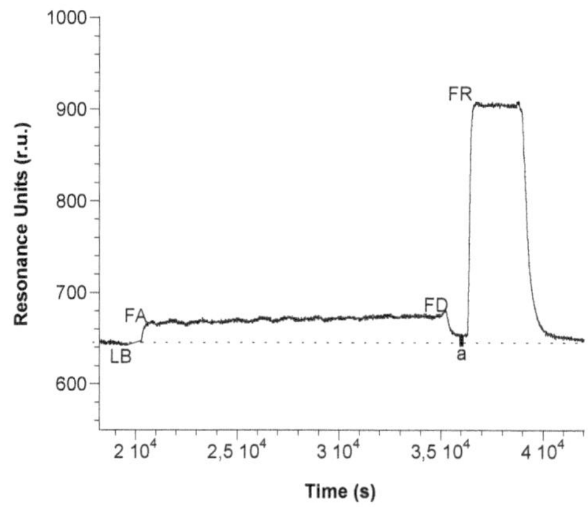

Figure 2. Example of sensorgram obtained with a sandwich format. For each measurement, after checking the original baseline (**LB**) by flowing phosphate buffer 50 mM, pH 7.2, the analyte that flowed into the system upon the steady state has been reached (**FA**); then, the dissociation step (**FD**) started by flowing again phosphate buffer (the small bold line (**a**) indicates the Δ r.u, relative to the formation of the immunocomplex between analyte and bioreceptor); the regeneration step (**FR**) was performed by glycine-HCl solution pH 2.4 inally the phosphate buffer to obtain the baseline.

3.2. Self Assembled Monolayer (SAM)

SAMs are highly ordered structures [24] that form spontaneously. A typical SAM is generally constituted by organosulfur compounds such as the 11-mercaptoundecanoic acid (MUA), which covalently binds to the gold surface of the plate. The preparation is carried out by dipping the plate in a solution of MUA 2 mM in ethanol for about 18 h. A SAM structure is therefore obtained, with the mercapto groups of the MUA able to form Au-S covalent bonds, while the carboxylic groups, which remain free, as shown in Figure 3, are available for subsequent binding with the antibody or the antigen. After 18 h, the plate with SAM is taken away from the solution, washed with ethanol and let to dry. The prism is rinsed with ethanol, then a drop of the oil is placed onto the prism surface and the prepared SAM-modified gold plate.

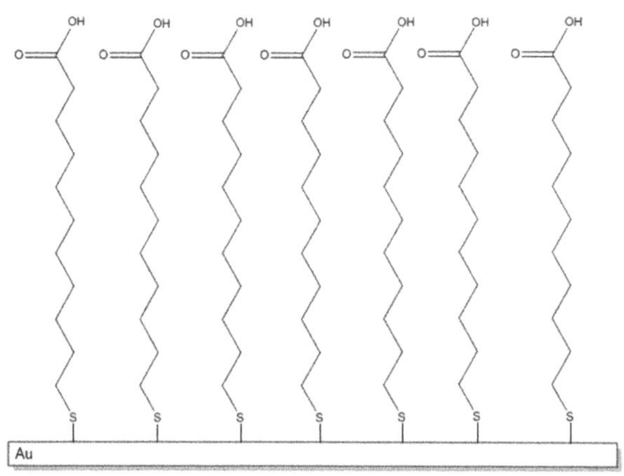

Figure 3. Schematic representation of SAM (Self Assembled Monolayer) with free –COOH and covalent bonds Au-S.

The stabilization of the SPR signal is then carried out by flowing 50 mM phosphate buffer into the cell at pH = 7.2 for about 1 h. This process is crucial as it rehydrates the MUA surface and creates a stable baseline on the sensorgram.

3.3. Choice of the Measurement Format

As mentioned in the Introduction and successively described in the Results and Discussion section, it was found that, after the immobilization of the antigen (ampicillin) on SAM and the association of its antibody (anti-ampicillin), a strong bond is formed, not easy to break through the hydrolysis with the classic eluent solutions normally used for this purpose [21–23]. This suggested the development of a sandwich geometry for the measurement instead of a competitive format type. After the injection of Gly-HCl at pH 2.4, the antibody complex, immobilized on the plate surface, and consisting of the first immobilized antigen—antibody—second antigen is in fact "regenerated" by breaking the bond with the second antigen. This suggests that the bond between the second antigen molecule and the antibody is certainly much weaker than that between the antibody and the first antigen molecule immobilized on the plate, which however is not easily broken by the treatment with the same solvent (Gly-HCl at pH 2.4).

3.4. Immobilization of Ampicillin

The immobilization procedure was studied by monitoring the sensorgram reported in Figure 4. The first operation was the SAM stabilization, which occurred in the cell by the phosphate buffer flowing 50 mM at pH = 7.2 for about 1 h. This allowed for recording a first base line (LB line, Figure 4). Successively, a 1:1 mixture of 0.5 M EDC and 0.1 M NHS is allowed to flow in the cell for about 15 min in order to activate the carboxyl groups of the SAM, with a consequent raising of the signal (A line, Figure 4). The plate is then washed with 50 mM phosphate buffer, pH = 7.2, with a resulting lowering of the signal due to separation from the surface of the excess of reagents (B line, Figure 4). At this point, a solution of ampicillin 10^{-2} M is allowed to flow in the cell for about 40 min (FI line, Figure 4) in order to form the covalent bonds (amidic bonds) between the carboxy groups of the SAM and the antigen (Figure 5). Finally, the cell was washed with phosphate buffer (C line, Figure 4). In order to avoid non-specific interactions with the activated –COOH groups, the latter are blocked by ethanolamine flowing 1 mM (Figure 5) for about 15 min (D line, Figure 4. The cell was then washed with phosphate buffer (E line, Figure 4).

As shown in Figure 4, ampicillin was effectively immobilized on the functionalized surface. In fact, the base line (C), after the step of ampicillin immobilization (FI), is located at r.u. values greater than the base line (B) before the ampicillin immobilization.

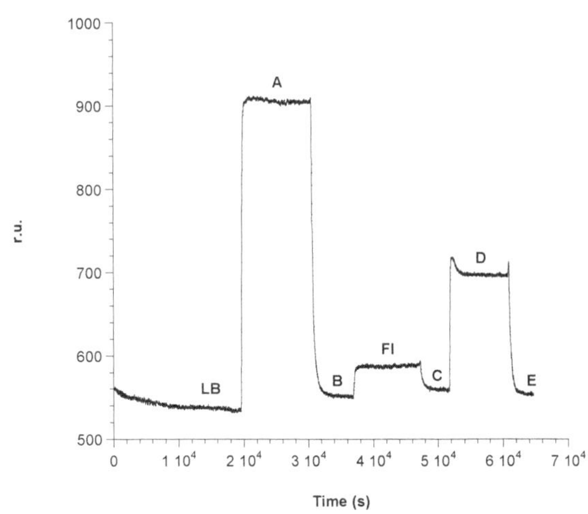

Figure 4. Immobilization of ampicillin: (**LB**) original baseline generated by flowing phosphate buffer; (**A**) activation with **EDC/NHS**; (**B**) washing with phosphate buffer; (**FI**) immobilization of ampicillin 10^{-2} M; (**C**) washing with phosphate buffer; (**D**) inactivation of –COOH groups which may have not reacted with ethanolamine; (**E**) washing with phosphate buffer.

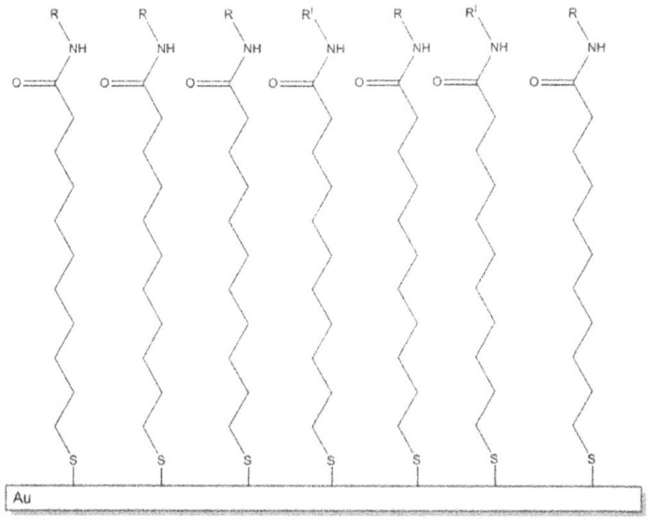

Figure 5. Schematic representation of SAM association with ampicillin 10^{-2} M (**R**) and inactivation of –COOH groups which may have not reacted by ethanolamine (**R'**).

3.5. Association of Anti-Ampicillin

The surface is now ready for the formation of the antibody complex. Subsequent injections of different solutions of antibody at increasing concentrations have been performed. These have been produced from a stock solution with a concentration of 1×10^{-3} M. The first step was to flow 50 mM of phosphate buffer at pH = 7.2 to obtain the base line (LB line, Figure 6). The first antibody solution, at a concentration of 6×10^{-10} M, was introduced into the cell observing the increase of the relative signal until a plateau is reached (A, Figure 6) due to the formation of the antibody complex. At this point, a washing procedure with phosphate buffer was carried out. Then, a solution of Gly-HCl, pH = 2.4 was introduced into the cell, which should, in theory, dissociate the complex between nti-ampicillin and ampicillin (FR line, Figure 6) through a hydrolysis reaction with the consequent regeneration of the activated surface, where only the immobilized antigen is present. The signal was expected to return to the initial reference level, before carrying out a second addition of the antibody. On the contrary, it is easy to see on the sensorgram that the complex between anti-ampicillin and ampicillin immobilized on the gold surface is practically not dissociated after the treatment with Gly-HCl, pH = 2.4. The surface not being regenerated, hence it is impossible to carry out a second measurement with the same plate, so that it would also be impossible to build, for example, a calibration curve using a "competitive" method with the same plate. The experiment was therefore continued with successive additions of further solutions of antibody at increasing concentrations, 8×10^{-10} M (B line, Figure 6) and 1×10^{-9} M (C line, Figure 6), until, for concentration above at least 10^{-3} M, almost all the immobilized antigen molecules had practically reacted with the antibody, by forming the antibody immobilized complex. The Δ r.u. values obtained were plotted against the concentration of anti-ampicillin, obtaining an antibody saturation curve, as shown in Figure 7. The obtained "saturation curve" allowed for evaluating the concentration of antibody solution capable of virtually saturating with the antibody the plate already activated with the antigen, by formation of the antibody complex, immobilized on the plate itself. This concentration is at least higher than 1×10^{-3} M, under the operating suitable conditions. It should be noted that the instrument was able to detect the antibody complex when the increase of its concentration was several orders of magnitude lower, since anti-ampicillin is a molecule with quite a high molecular weight (150 kDa).

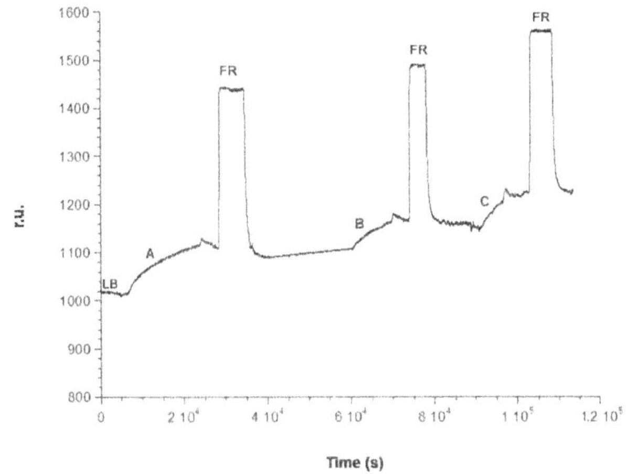

Figure 6. Antibody complexation on the SAM coated with the antygen: (**A**) 6×10^{-10} M; (**B**) 8×10^{-10} M; (**C**) 1×10^{-9} M, anti-ampicillin flowing successive solutions; (**FR**) regeneration step by flowing Gly-HCl at pH 2.4.

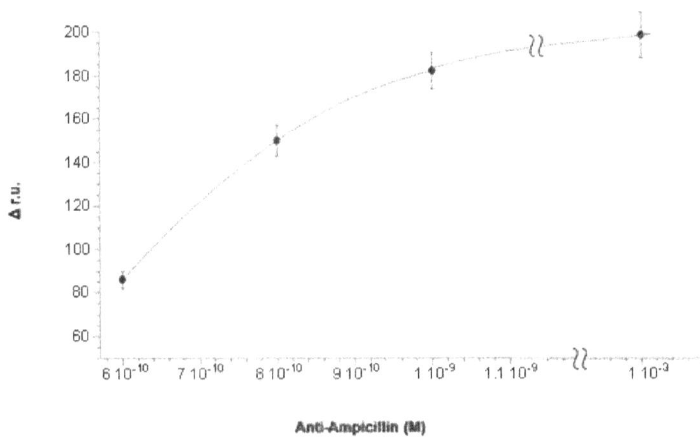

Figure 7. "Saturation curve" with anti-ampicillin, obtained by flowing antibody solutions: 6×10^{-10} M, 8×10^{-10} M, 1×10^{-9} M, 1×10^{-3} M).

3.6. Formation of the Sandwich and Construction of a Calibration Curve for Ampicillin

The experiments described in the previous paragraph confirmed the difficulty with applying a competitive method and therefore suggested the choice to use the sandwich geometry to obtain a calibration curve for ampicillin. Therefore, after completely saturating the plate with a 0.1 M antibody solution and washing it with buffer, as described in the previous paragraph, the experience started by recording the initial baseline when 50 mM phosphate buffer at pH = 7.2 was introduced in the flow cell containing the plate activated with the antibody complex immobilized on its surface. Successively, several injections of solutions at increasing ampicillin concentration, obtained by diluting the same stock solution (1×10^{-1} M), have been carried out. The following parts of the curve were obtained: the flow of the first ampicillin solution at a concentration of 1×10^{-3} M on the antibody immobilized complex caused a small increase of the signal; once a stable signal is reached, phosphate buffer was again injected. A small decrease of the signal was observed, but at the end of the decrease, a positive difference signal (r.u.) compared to the original base line was registered, which proved the sandwich formation. The subsequent injection of a solution of Gly-HCl at pH 2.4 caused a characteristic increase of the signal. Lastly, by flowing again phosphate buffer 50 mM at pH = 7.2, the signal returned to a value of r.u. equal to that of the initial original base line (Figure 2). This showed that the sandwich had broken, but the antibody complex remained fixed on the plate. The same steps were repeated at increasing ampicillin concentrations from 5×10^{-3} M to 1×10^{-1} M. An increasing value for the difference between the signal observed after the washing with phosphate buffer and the initial original base line (example of Figure 8) has been recorded, which demonstrated how the interaction between the 2nd antigen molecule and the antibody was established each time giving rise to the sandwich geometry. A typical example of a recorded measurement for 1×10^{-1} M ampicillin concentration is reported in Figure 8. It was clear, however, that this observation was to be supported by a "blank" test, which is described in the following paragraph. In conclusion, in the described experience, the Δ in r.u. values related to each antigen addition have been determined and the difference, in terms of resonance units, between the final r.u. values (after washing with phosphate buffer), obtained with the association of the second antigen with the antibody and the r.u. values relative to the initial original baseline, was always positive and growing. The so obtained Δ in r.u. values were finally plotted as a function of the relative ampicillin concentration (see calibration line, Figure 9). For ampicillin concentrations lower than 10^{-3} M, it is likely that the sandwich is formed, but the sensitivity of the method does not seem enough to highlight it.

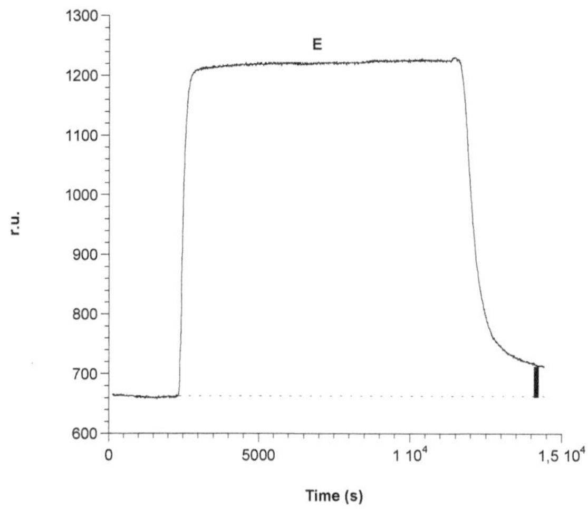

Figure 8. Example of ampicillin detection 1×10^{-1} M with sandwich format. Δ r.u (bold line) is related to the concentration (**E**) 1×10^{-1} M, before and after the association of ampicillin.

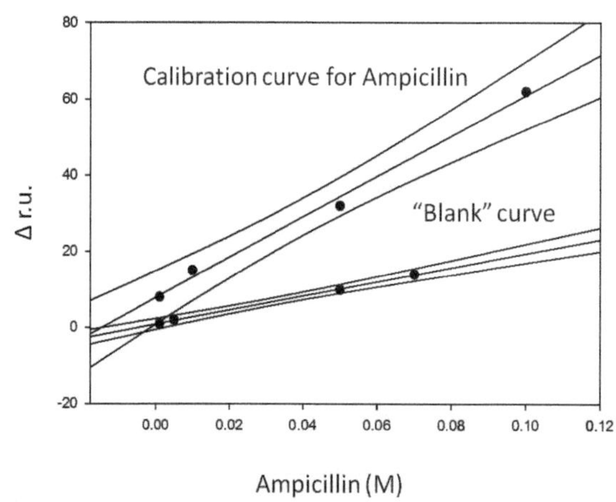

Figure 9. Comparison between blank curve and calibration curve of ampicillin.

3.7. "Blank" Curve for Ampicillin

In order to make a "blank" curve, the usual SAM was prepared by dipping the gold plate for about 18 h in a solution of 2 mM 11-mercaptoundecanoic acid and ethanol. After the fixed time, the SAM was washed with ethanol to remove the excess reagent. Then, the plate was left to dry. The assembly was completed by placing on the prism a drop of oil and then the prepared plate with the SAM. Once obtained, the base line through the flow of phosphate buffer (50 mM at pH = 7.2) for about 1 h, the –COOH groups have been activated with a solution of EDC 0.5 M and NHS 0.1 M at a 1:1 ratio (freshly prepared) for about 15 min, then, the plate was washed with phosphate buffer and finally a solution of ampicillin 10^{-1} M was injected and allowed to flow for about 40 min. The plate was then washed again with 50 mM phosphate buffer at pH = 7.2. In order to be sure that all the sites on the gold plate had been saturated, a solution of 1 mM ethanolamine was injected to block any carboxyl groups that had not reacted. At this point, after removing the excess ethanolamine by washing with phosphate buffer, the following ampicillin solutions at increasing concentrations have been injected: (a) 10^{-3} M; (b) 5×10^{-3} M; (c) 5×10^{-2} M; (d) 7×10^{-2} M. The Δ in r.u. values, determined after each addition, were plotted as a function of increasing concentrations of ampicillin. The "blank" curve thus obtained and the calibration curve described in the previous section were both reported in a single graph (Figure 9) in which each point represents the average of three separate determinations.

The equations of the straight lines obtained and the main analytical data are summarized in Table 1. The fact that the two lines show very different slopes (the slope of the "blank" curve is very low) indicates that the sandwich geometry was actually formed and allowed the construction of the calibration curve, while the immobilization of the antigen alone on the SAM, as in the case of the "blank" curve, gave a signal which is almost zero and barely visible only at the highest antigen concentrations.

Table 1. Analytical data using an SPR device of both calibration and blank curves.

	Equation of the Regression Straight Line	Linearity Range (M)	R^2	Pooled SD (%)	LOD (M)
Calibration straight line (Y = Δ r.u., X = M)	y = 7.89 (± 1.63) + 530.8 (± 29.1)x	1×10^{-3}–1×10^{-1}	0.9940	5.1	10^{-3}
"Blank" curve (Y = Δ r.u., X = M)	y = 0.91 (± 0.15) + 185.3 (± 3.4)x	1×10^{-3}–7×10^{-2}	0.9993	4.4	10^{-3}

3.8. Selectivity Tests

In theory, the response of each immunosensor should be very selective because of the specificity of the antigen-antibody reaction. However, this selectivity should be experimentally verified due to the cross-reactivity, a situation in which it is possible that side reactions occur at the immunosensor due to a chemical compound very similar to the antigen. Consequently, the selectivity was assessed considering both compounds with a structure similar to ampicillin, such as other β-lactam antibiotics (penicillin G and ceftriaxone) and other antibiotics with very different structures (fosfomycin and erythromycin), as possible interferents.

The first selectivity test involved penicillin G (Figure 10), an antibiotic with the same β-lactam ring of ampicillin. Different concentrations of penicillin G have been tested, similar to those used to construct the calibration curve of ampicillin, and injected in succession in the cell as reported in Section 3.6, obtaining the sensorgram shown in Figure 10. It is possible to note that the instrument seems at first to detect the presence of Penicillin G in the cell but also that, after washing with 50 mM phosphate buffer at pH = 7.2, the signal returned to the original base line. This can be ascribed to the fact that the sandwich in the case of penicillin G may not form, or at least it is not detected by the SPR transducer, probably because of the low molecular weight of penicillin G. In other selectivity tests (Figure 11), possible interferences of both β-lactam, such as ceftriaxone, or cephalothin, and non β-lactam antibiotics, such as fosfomycin, or erythromicin, were evaluated by using the same procedure employed for penicillin G.

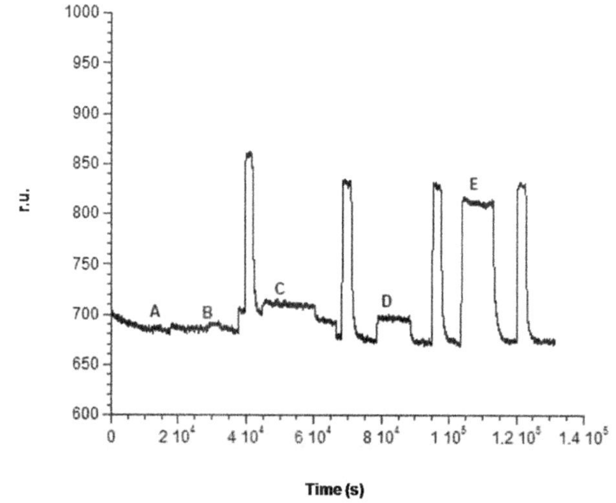

Figure 10. Selectivity: complexation of penicillin G by using sandwich immunosensor format. Penicillin G solutions: (**A**) 5×10^{-4} M; (**B**) 1×10^{-3} M; (**C**) 5×10^{-3} M; (**D**) 1×10^{-2} M; (**E**) 5×10^{-2} M.

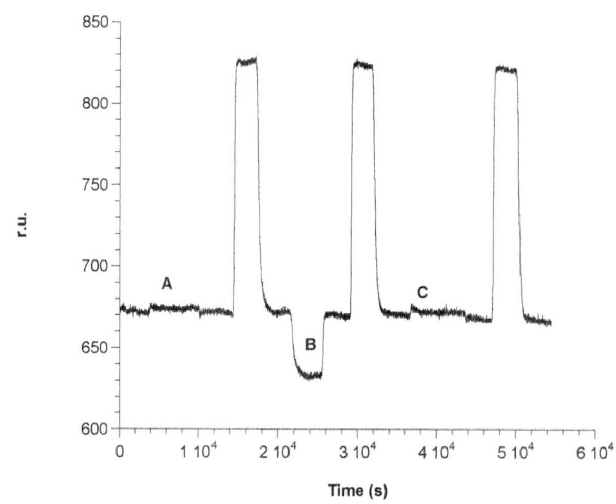

Figure 11. Selectivity test: (**A**) Fosfomycin 1×10^{-3} M; (**B**) Erythromicin 5×10^{-3} M; (**C**) Ceftriaxone 4×10^{-3} M.

Also in the case of ceftriaxone, a cephalosporin, which is a β-lactam antibiotic but does not belong to the same class of ampicillin, the formation of the sandwich was not detected (line C of Figure 11). In the case of fosfomycin, the Δ in r.u. before and after the injection of this antibiotic, resulted in being almost zero (line A of Figure 11). Similar experiments have been carried out with erythromycin, another non β-lactam antibiotic. Its injection resulted in a decreasing signal (line B of Figure 11), as if this addition would cause a partial separation of the antibody complex. However, this assumption does not seem fully explanatory, as both fosfomycin and erythromycin showed Δ in r.u. values equal to zero after the subsequent injection of 50 mM phosphate buffer at pH = 7.2 with a return of the signal to the original baseline on the sensorgram. These results showing that the latter two antibiotics do not create any interference could perhaps be predictable, as they are non β-lactam antibiotics. Based on this evidence, it is possible to conclude that the immunosensor developed for ampicillin detection results in being very selective towards this antibiotic.

4. Conclusions

The purpose of this experimental research was the construction of an immunosensor for the direct determination of ampicillin, using the SPR technique operating in flow conditions. In order to reach the aim of the work, the results obtained suggested the development of a sandwich geometry (first molecule of immobilized antigen—antibody—second antigen molecule) as the best format. The formation of the sandwich was confirmed by comparing the slope value of the calibration curve of ampicillin with the slope of the "blank" curve, which resulted being very low. Furthermore, from the data resulting from the selectivity tests, it was found that none of the other tested antibiotics, both those belonging to very different classes of antibiotics and those structurally similar to the class of β-lactam, resulted in being potential interferents. This is a remarkable result, as it highlights the great selectivity of the SPR immunosensor for ampicillin in the concentration range from 10^{-3} M to 10^{-1} M. A disadvantage of the developed SPR immunosensor, compared to traditional "competitive" immunosensors (non-SPR), is that traditional immunosensors are generally more sensitive devices [21] compared to the SPR immunsensor described in this research, even if they have often proven to be much less selective compared to the SPR immunosensor. However, for certain applications such as the control of commercial pharmaceutical specialties, a high sensitivity is not mandatory. Moreover, good selectivity means that the method could be used in the case of specialties containing different active molecules in association.

Another important positive aspect to be emphasized is the analysis time. In fact, a direct determination of ampicillin in a much shorter time (maximum 20 min) compared to the time required by the traditional competitive methods (which generally require more than 1 h [21] to complete the measure) is possible, thanks to the formation of the sandwich.

Acknowledgments: This work was funded by the Sapienza University of Rome, "Protezione dell'Ambiente e dei Beni Culturali (CIABC)" center and by "Istituto per lo studio dei Materiali Nanostrutturati (ISMN)" of CNR (Consiglio Nazionale delle Ricerche).

Author Contributions: M.T. conceived and designed the experiments; G.C. performed the experiments and prepared the figures; G.S. analyzed the data; L.C. and F.M. contributed reagents/materials/analysis tools; M.T. and R.A. wrote the paper; G.F. gave suggestions on the structure of the manuscript.

Conflicts of Interest: The authors declare no conflict of interest.

Abbreviations

The following abbreviations are used in this manuscript:

SPR	Surface Plasmon Resonance
LOD	Low detection limit
SAM	Self Assembled Monolayer
r.u.	Unit of Resonance
MUA	11-mercaptoundecanoic Acid
Gly	Glycine
EDC	1-ethyl-3-(3-dimethyl aminopropyl) Carbodiimide
NHS	N-hydroxysuccinimide

References

1. Murray, P.R.; Rosenthal, K.S.; Pfaller, M.A. *Microbiologia Medica*, 6th ed.; Edra Masson: Milan, Italy, 2015; pp. 167–169 and 187–190.

2. Benito-Peña, E.; Partal-Rodera, A.I.; Léon-González, M.E.; Moreno-Bondi, M.C. Evaluation of mixed mode solid phase extraction cartridges for the preconcentration of beta-lactam antibiotics in wastewater using liquid chromatography with UV-DAD detection. *Anal. Chim. Acta* **2006**, *556*, 415–422. [CrossRef]
3. Marazuela, M.D.; Bogialli, S. A review of novel strategies of sample preparation for the determination of antibacterial residues in foodstuffs using liquid chromatography-based analytical methods. *Anal. Chim. Acta* **2009**, *645*, 5–17. [CrossRef] [PubMed]
4. Briscoe, S.E.; McWhinney, B.C.; Lipman, J.; Roberts, J.A.; Ungerer, J.P.J. A method for determining the free (unbound) concentration of ten beta-lactam antibiotics in human plasma using high performance liquid chromatography with ultraviolet detection. *J. Chromatogr. B* **2012**, *907*, 178–184. [CrossRef] [PubMed]
5. Samanidou, V.F.; Evaggelopoulou, E.N.; Papadoyannis, I.N. Development of a validated HPLC method for the determination of four penicillin antibiotics in pharmaceuticals and human biological fluids. *J. Sep. Sci.* **2006**, *2*, 1550–1560. [CrossRef]
6. Jin, H.; Kumar, A.P.; Paik, D.H.; Ha, K.C.; Yoo, K.C.; Lee, Y.I. Trace analysis of tetracycline antibiotics in human urine using UPLC–QToF mass spectrometry. *Microchem. J.* **2010**, *94*, 139–147. [CrossRef]
7. Heller, D.N.; Smith, M.L.; Chiesa, O.A. LC/MS/MS measurement of penicillin G in bovine plasma, urine, and biopsy samples taken from kidneys of standing animals. *J. Chromatogr. B* **2006**, *830*, 91–99. [CrossRef] [PubMed]
8. Becker, M.; Zittlau, E.; Petz, M. Residue analysis of 15 penicillins and cephalosporins in bovine muscle, kidney and milk by liquid chromatography–tandem mass spectrometry. *Anal. Chim. Acta* **2004**, *520*, 19–32. [CrossRef]
9. Ohmori, T.; Suzuki, A.; Niwa, T.; Ushikoshi, H.; Shirai, K.; Yoshida, S.; Ogura, S.; Itoh, Y. Simultaneous determination of eight β-lactam antibiotics in human serum by liquid chromatography–tandem mass spectrometry. *J. Chromatogr. B* **2011**, *879*, 1038–1042. [CrossRef] [PubMed]
10. Pikkemaat, M.G.; Rapallini, M.L.; Dijk, S.O.; Elferink, J.W. Comparison of three microbial screening methods for antibiotics using routine monitoring samples. *Anal. Chim. Acta* **2009**, *637*, 298–304. [CrossRef] [PubMed]
11. Musser, M.B.; Anderson, K.L.; Rushing, J.E.; Moats, W.A. Potential for milk containing penicillin G or amoxicillin to cause residues in calves. *J. Dairy Sci.* **2001**, *84*, 126–133. [CrossRef]
12. Brand, U.; Reinhardt, B.; Rüther, F.; Scheper, T.; Schügerl, K. Bio-field-effect transistors as detectors in flow-injection analysis. *Anal. Chim. Acta* **1990**, *238*, 201–210. [CrossRef]
13. Goldfinch, M.J.; Lowe, C.R. Solid-phase optoelectronic sensors for biochemical analysis. *Anal. Biochem.* **1984**, *138*, 430–436. [CrossRef]
14. Adrian, J.; Pasche, S.; Voirin, G.; Adrian, J.; Pinacho, D.G.; Font, H.; Sánchez-Baeza, F.; Marco, J.M.P.; Diserens, J.M.; Granier, B. Wavelength-interrogated optical biosensor for multi-analyte screening of sulfonamide, fluoroquinolone, β-lactam and tetracycline antibiotics in milk. *Trends Anal. Chem.* **2009**, *28*, 769–777. [CrossRef]
15. Thavarungkul, P.; Dawan, S.; Kanatharana, P.; Asawatreratanakul, P. Detecting penicillin G in milk with impedimetric label-free immunosensor. *Biosens. Bioelectron.* **2007**, *23*, 688–694. [CrossRef] [PubMed]
16. Benito-Peña, E.; Moreno-Bondi, M.C.; Orellana, G.; Maquieira, A.; Van Amerongen, A. Development of a novel and automated fluorescent immunoassay for the analysis of β-lactam antibiotics. *J. Agric. Food Chem.* **2005**, *53*, 6635–6642. [CrossRef] [PubMed]
17. Park, E.K.; Jung, W.C.; Lee, H.J. Application of a solid-phase fluorescence immunoassay to determine amoxicillin residues in fish tissue. *Acta Vet. Hung.* **2010**, *58*, 83–89. [CrossRef] [PubMed]
18. Gamella, M.; Campuzano, S.; Conzuelo, F.; Esteban-Torres, M.; De Las Rivas, A.B.; Reviejo, A.J.; Muñoz, R.; Pingarrón, J.M. An amperometric affinity penicillin-binding protein magnetosensor for the detection of β-lactam antibiotics in milk. *Analyst* **2013**, *138*, 2013–2022. [CrossRef] [PubMed]
19. Huth, S.P.; Warholic, P.S.; Devou, J.M.; Chaney, L.K.; Clark, G.H. Parallux™ beta-lactam: A capillary-based fluorescent immunoassay for the determination of penicillin-G, ampicillin, amoxicillin, cloxacillin, cephapirin, and ceftiofur in bovine milk. *J. AOAC Int.* **2002**, *85*, 355–364. [PubMed]
20. Campanella, L.; Tomassetti, M.; Sbrilli, R. Benzylpenicillinate liquid membrane ion-selective electrode: Preparation and application to a real matrix (Drug). *Ann. Chim.* **1986**, *26*, 483–497.
21. Merola, G.; Martini, E.; Tomassetti, M.; Campanella, L. New immunosensor for β-lactam antibiotics determination in river waste waters. *Sens. Actuators B Chem.* **2014**, *199*, 301–313. [CrossRef]

22. Tomassetti, M.; Martini, E.; Campanella, L.; Favero, G.; Sanzò, G.; Mazzei, F. Lactoferrin determination using flow or batch immunosensor surface plasmon resonance: Comparison with amperometric and screen-printed immunosensor methods. *Sens. Actuators B Chem.* **2013**, *179*, 215–225. [CrossRef]
23. Tomassetti, M.; Martini, E.; Campanella, L.; Favero, G.; Sanzó, G.; Mazzei, F. A new surface plasmon resonance immunosensor for Triazine pesticide determination in bovine milk: A comparison with conventional amperometric and screen-printed immunodevices. *Sensors* **2015**, *15*, 10255–10270. [CrossRef] [PubMed]
24. Love, J.C.; Estroff, L.A.; Kriebel, J.K.; Nuzzo, R.G.; Whitesides, G.M. Self-Assembled Monolayers of thiolates on metals as a form of nanotechnology. *Chem. Rev.* **2005**, *105*, 1103–1169. [CrossRef] [PubMed]

9

Single Molecule Bioelectronics and Their Application to Amplification-Free Measurement of DNA Lengths

O. Tolga Gül [1,2,†], Kaitlin M. Pugliese [3,†], Yongki Choi [1,4,†], Patrick C. Sims [1], Deng Pan [1], Arith J. Rajapakse [1], Gregory A. Weiss [3,5,*] and Philip G. Collins [1,*]

1 Department of Physics and Astronomy, University of California at Irvine, Irvine, CA 92697, USA
2 Department of Physics, Polatlı Faculty of Science and Arts, Gazi University, Polatlı 06900, Turkey
3 Department of Chemistry, University of California at Irvine, Irvine, CA 92697, USA
4 Department of Physics, North Dakota State University, Fargo, ND 58108, USA
5 Department of Molecular Biology and Biochemistry, University of California at Irvine, Irvine, CA 92697, USA
* Correspondence: gweiss@uci.edu (G.A.W.); collinsp@uci.edu (P.G.C.)

† These authors contributed equally to this work.

Academic Editor: Prabir Patra

Abstract: As biosensing devices shrink smaller and smaller, they approach a scale in which single molecule electronic sensing becomes possible. Here, we review the operation of single-enzyme transistors made using single-walled carbon nanotubes. These novel hybrid devices transduce the motions and catalytic activity of a single protein into an electronic signal for real-time monitoring of the protein's activity. Analysis of these electronic signals reveals new insights into enzyme function and proves the electronic technique to be complementary to other single-molecule methods based on fluorescence. As one example of the nanocircuit technique, we have studied the Klenow Fragment (KF) of DNA polymerase I as it catalytically processes single-stranded DNA templates. The fidelity of DNA polymerases makes them a key component in many DNA sequencing techniques, and here we demonstrate that KF nanocircuits readily resolve DNA polymerization with single-base sensitivity. Consequently, template lengths can be directly counted from electronic recordings of KF's base-by-base activity. After measuring as few as 20 copies, the template length can be determined with <1 base pair resolution, and different template lengths can be identified and enumerated in solutions containing template mixtures.

Keywords: DNA polymerase; carbon nanotube sensors; single molecule enzymology; DNA sequencing

1. Introduction

In populations of organisms, cells, or molecules, atypical individuals can exert disproportionate roles. In the least consequential cases, these individuals merely nudge the average activity or phenotype of a population; but in more severe cases, they turn on entirely new responses or enable pathways with pathological consequences [1]. For example, a single cancerous cell can initiate a tumor formation or provoke an immune response [2–4]. At an even finer scale, a single errant or mutant biomolecule can disrupt a cell signaling pathway or inappropriately activate transcription [5,6]. Understanding cause and effect in a population is very difficult when single individuals can change the behavior of the overall system, and addressing this challenge requires a detailed study of protein function at the individual level.

Over the past two decades, tremendous progress has been made developing techniques that can address the challenge of characterizing the activity of single molecules. Resolving individual molecules and tracking their dynamic activities has grown into a major subfield at the forefront of biophysical research, leading to a better understanding of the functions of molecular motors, signaling proteins, and pharmaceutical inhibitors [7–11]. Analysis of many individual molecules also provides opportunities to understand heterogeneity within a population and the transition from normal function into malfunction. For example, observation of enzyme catalysis at the single-molecule level has observed that otherwise-identical molecules can have very different turnover rates. By resolving individual chemical events and comparing the reaction trajectories of enzymes, single-molecule techniques reveal the variable dynamics of efficiency, processivity, and kinetics that are all hidden in ensemble averages. Furthermore, details about intramolecular distances and forces [12–14], molecular orientation [15,16], substrate binding and release mechanisms [17–19], and substrate preferences [20–22] can each be revealed.

These underlying motivations have driven the development of a variety of single-molecule experimental techniques. Single-molecule fluorescence has led the way as a versatile method for tracking energy transfer and the relative motions of submolecular domains [23,24], and single-molecule fluorescence is the basis for at least one commercial DNA sequencing technique [25]. In addition, force-based techniques have used magnetic tweezers, optical tweezers, or scanning probes to perturb molecules and measure mechanical responses [26,27]. Although optical and mechanical techniques have been well represented, electronic transduction has generally been missing from the single-molecule toolbox, with the notable exception of patch-clamp techniques for monitoring individual ion channels [28]. However, the recent development of electronic devices with length scales smaller than 10 nm promises to bring electronic measurement modes to this field. Future researchers may be able to choose among optical, mechanical, and electronic transduction methods and select techniques or combinations of complementary techniques, which are best suited to a particular research question.

Achieving this vision of a versatile single-molecule toolkit requires that single-molecule electronic devices become well-controlled and accessible. To be practical for biomolecule research, these devices must operate near room temperature in physiologically relevant, conductive fluids, and have nanometer-scale conduction channels that are well-matched to the size of individual molecules. Nature's elegant solution to these requirements involves transmembrane proteins that fold to define interior, nm-scale pores through which ionic currents can flow [29]. The general idea of ionic currents in nanopores has been successfully extended to synthetic, inorganic barriers like SiN or polymer films [30,31]; a DNA sequencing technology based on arrays of nanopores has been commercialized by Oxford Nanopore Technologies [32,33]. Aside from ionic currents, the scanning tunneling microscope provides one example of a conduction channel for electrons that has single-molecule sensitivity. Although arrays of tunneling microscopes have proven impractical, precision deposition of thin insulating films has helped extend the principle of tunneling to arrays of stable, solid state devices that can compete with nanopores for sensitivity [34,35]. Another competing new technology is based on nanoscale transistors made from Si nanowires [36–40] or carbon nanotubes [41–46], conducting wires that are sensitive enough to transduce the motions of single molecules and their dynamics.

For this special issue on carbon nanotube sensing, we review the fabrication and operation of single-molecule carbon nanotube-based biosensing devices. Abundant research over the past decade has demonstrated the biosensing capabilities of carbon nanotubes, and recently this sensitivity has been extended to single-molecule electronics. Specifically, experiments have attached single enzymes to single-walled carbon nanotube field-effect transistors (SWNT-FETs, Figure 1a) and demonstrated the versatile ability of tracking an enzyme's conformational states and revealing distributive and processed enzyme movements. The electronic nature of the FET technique has immediate benefits such as microsecond time resolution and long-duration capabilities, which are both advantages over fluorescence for studying the conformational dynamics and processivity of a single molecule. SWNT-FETs functionalized with T4 lysozyme [21,46,47], cAMP-dependent protein kinase A [48], and the Klenow Fragment of DNA Polymerase I (KF) [49,50] have all been successfully used to study each enzyme's dynamic variability and demonstrate the capabilities of the SWNT-FET approach.

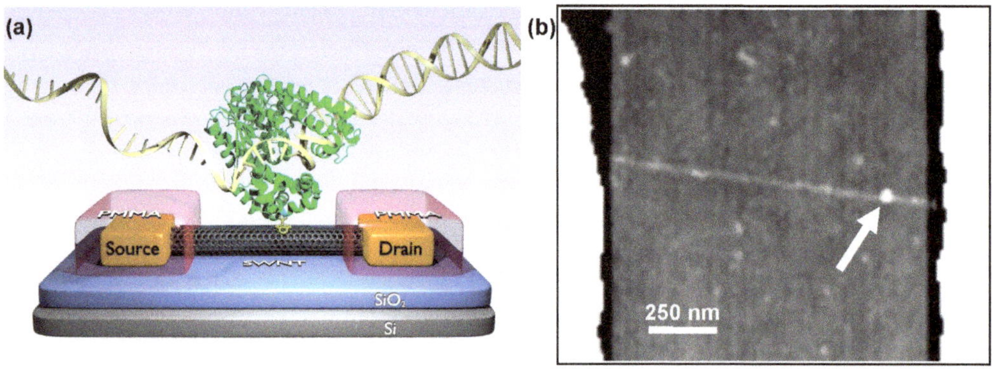

Figure 1. (**a**) Schematic of a single-walled carbon nanotube field effect transistor (SWNT-FET) functionalized with a single copy of a protein. This device depicts the Klenow Fragment of DNA polymerase I converting a single-stranded DNA template into a double-stranded helix. A pyrene-maleimide (**yellow**) is shown linking the protein to the SWNT. (**b**) Atomic force microscopy image of a typical SWNT-FET device after functionalization confirms attachment of a single protein (**arrow**).

The remainder of the paper is organized into three sections. Section 2 describes methods of fabricating SWNT-FETs and labeling them with single active molecules like enzymes. Section 3.1 summarizes example results from SWNT-FETs sensing the activity of DNA polymerases processing single-stranded DNA templates. As an illustrative example of the general SWNT-FET technique, the DNA polymerase devices are particularly useful for two reasons. First, the range of possible DNA templates and both native and chemically modified starting materials for DNA polymerization make this a rich and complex experimental system. Second, accurate sensing of DNA polymerase activity has practical applications in DNA sequencing; nearly all single-molecule techniques have been applied to this challenge, and published data is thus available for direct comparison with the SWNT-FET results. Section 3.2 describes new analysis of the accuracy of the SWNT-FET technique and the challenges that must be overcome for these devices to be successfully deployed in DNA sequencing.

2. Materials and Methods

2.1. Fabrication and Functionalization of SWNT-FETs

The initial demonstration of field-effect transistors based on SWNTs [51,52] and silicon nanowires [36] laid the foundation for the later development of hybrid devices incorporating biomolecules. Early research revealed the general sensitivity of these one-dimensional (1-D) FETs [41,42], which could then be coated with sensitizing agents to produce a variety of chemoresistive responses for biosensing [36,53]. However, continuous coatings fail to take advantage of the unique properties that make 1-D FETs unmatched by other types of chemical sensors. Namely, 1-D channels allow scattering at a single location to be communicated to distant electrodes. The intrinsic amplification of a scattering site in an otherwise pristine, 1-D channel allows single molecular events to produce output signals that can be monitored by relatively simple control electronics.

Taking advantage of this unique sensitivity requires a strategic functionalization approach. To avoid ensemble averaging of the signals from multiple independent molecules, sensitization should be limited to one active site. The success of this strategy was first demonstrated by introducing single point defects into SWNT-FETs, which imbued each device with a chemical degree of freedom while also localizing sensitivity to the modified position [54]. Researchers have monitored the kinetics of individual molecular reactions [44] and DNA binding events [45,55] using defect sites; however, these defects enhance sensitivity without substantial benefits in signal-to-noise and at the cost of damaging the carbon lattice. Consequently, non-covalent surface functionalization remains preferable if it can be controlled with single-site precision. As described below, non-covalent schemes have been successfully diluted to the point that SWNT-FETs have either zero or one sensitizing molecule, according to Poisson statistics [21,46]. These techniques are the focus of this review.

Aside from functionalization, the fabrication of single-molecule devices follows protocols for SWNT-FETs that have become standard in the field. SWNTs can be deposited onto surfaces by spin coating or spraying from solutions, by dry transfer from other substrates, or by direct synthesis in place. The latter technique exposes SWNTs to the least chemical processing, manipulation, and damage; so it is advantageous for achieving precise control of single active sites. We spin coat a water-soluble solution of $Fe_{30}Mo_{84}$ catalyst nanoparticles [56] onto 4″ silicon wafers, diluted to achieve the desired SWNT density. The wafers are then processed in a chemical vapor deposition (CVD) furnace [57]. The particles are oxidized to remove their stabilizing ligands (air, 5 min at 700 °C), reduced to a catalytically active form (10% H_2 in Ar, 5 min at 940 °C), and then exposed to a carbon source that initiates SWNT growth (15% CH_4 and 10% H_2 in Ar, 5 min at 940 °C). The catalyst density is set to achieve a uniform density of ~0.01 SWNTs/μm^2, so that arrays of electrodes patterned on the wafer by photolithography will contact, on average, only one SWNT.

In our process, three-terminal FETs are achieved by using degenerately doped (p++) silicon wafers with a 250 nm thermal oxide. The SiO_2 is a good promoter of catalyst activity and SWNT growth, and it serves as a gate dielectric between the SWNTs and the underlying wafer. Source and drain contacts are defined on top of the SWNTs using a bilayer undercut resist (S-1808 on LOR-1A, Microchem), followed by electron beam evaporation of a thin sticking layer (0.7 nm Ti) and electrode metal (30 nm Pt). After liftoff, the exposed FETs are coated with passivating layers of Al_2O_3 and/or polymer resist (poly(methyl methacrylate), PMMA in Figure 1a) to protect the SWNTs and SWNT-metal interfaces from the environment. After fabrication, the entire wafer is mapped to determine the resistance, transconductance, and type of each electrical connection. For the purposes of successful prototyping, extra care is taken to investigate devices individually. Stable, noise-free devices with resistances <5 MΩ are selected for investigation by scanning electron microscopy and atomic force microscopy (AFM) to ensure that each is comprised of an individual SWNT free from particles or other obvious contaminants.

Biofunctionalization of the SWNT-FETs is a three-step process. First, a small window is opened in the protective passivation layer over the SWNT-FET channel. Using either optical or electron-beam lithography, a small portion (~1 μm) midway between the source and drain electrodes is removed to expose the SWNT sidewall to the environment while keeping the rest of the device protected. Next, the devices are soaked in a solution of a non-covalent linker molecule like *N*-(1-pyrenyl)maleimide (saturated solution in EtOH, Sigma-Aldrich, St. Louis, MO, USA). The linker is chosen to have a pyrene or other aromatic polycyclic functional group to adhere to the SWNT sidewall via π-π stacking. After rinsing (phosphate-buffered saline, 0.1% Tween-20, Acros Organics, Geel, Belgium) to remove excess linkers, the device is soaked in a buffered aqueous solution containing the biomolecule to be attached to the SWNT. Numerous bioconjugation chemistries are possible, including attachments through unnatural amino acids [58], HaloTags [59], or even the terminal His tags used for protein purification [60]. We have selected a linker containing a maleimide group to take advantage of stable thioether bond formed with the thiol of a surface-exposed cysteine [61,62]. With the help of mutagenesis, proteins with a single exposed cysteine can be designed, expressed, and purified for attachment to the SWNT using pyrene-maleimides; often several single cysteine variants must be prepared to identify an appropriate site for bioconjugation to the SWNT.

The successful creation of single-molecule devices occurs by preparing multiple SWNT devices in parallel and tailoring the final bioconjugation step to yield only 0.2 to 0.3 molecules per device. Protein incubation is performed for 15 to 60 min using protein concentrations of 50 to 500 nM, where the optimum conditions for a particular protein are determined empirically using AFM to directly image the conjugation yield. An example image of one protein attachment is shown in Figure 1b. The optimum incubation parameters are specific to each protein due to the accessibility of the cysteine attachment site, the protein's tendency to aggregate, and the concentration dependence of undesirable nonspecific adsorption. Alternate conjugation chemistries would involve additional considerations. After a final rinse to remove unbound protein, the devices are ready for measurement or storage. After successful measurements, devices are always imaged by AFM to verify the presence of one active protein.

The fabrication of SWNT-FETs is an active field that continues to be refined. In addition to the methods described here, investigators are successfully parallelizing large arrays of SWNT-FETs for digital electronics applications [63,64] and solving the interfacial materials problems that cause excess noise and resistance [65,66]. The non-covalent biofunctionalization scheme described here is easily modified to other linkage schemes and readily adapted to surfaces containing many devices; with automated microfluidic dispensers it can be expanded to arrays of devices having different proteins or protein variants. Thus, many opportunities exist for combining best practices and expanding proof-of-principle single-molecule devices into functional arrays for different commercial uses.

2.2. *Operation of Single-Molecule SWNT-FETs*

After fabrication, chemical activity of the attached protein is transduced into fluctuations in the source-drain current $I(t)$ flowing in the SWNT channel (Figure 2). $I(t)$ measurements are usually performed with the active portion of the device submerged in a buffered aqueous solution containing the protein's binding partners and other reaction co-factors. Typical $I(t)$ values of 10 to 100 nA require a current preamplifier with an appropriate bandwidth. For example, a Keithley 428 amplifier has a 15 μs rise time at 10^7 V/A gain, which is a suitable choice for resolving dynamics down to 100 μs.

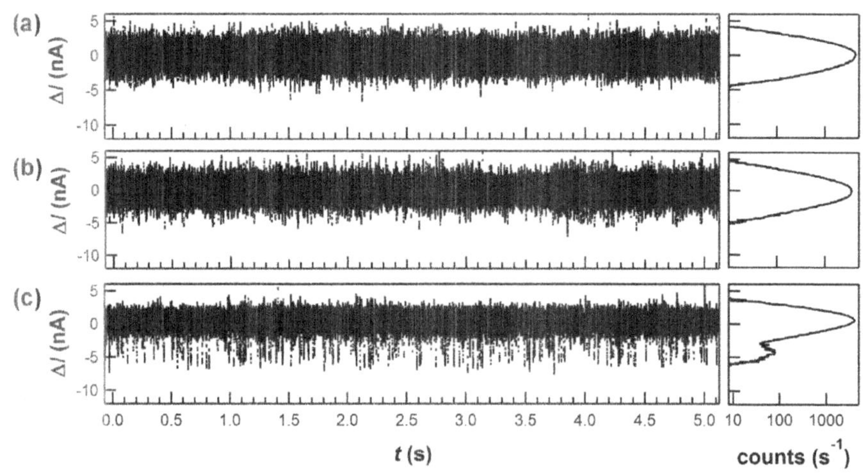

Figure 2. Example $\Delta I(t)$ signals and signal histograms generated by KF in a solution containing: (**a**) 1 nM poly(dA)$_{42}$ homopolymer template; (**b**) template with 10 μM non-complementary dGTP; and (**c**) template with 10 μM complementary dTTP. Both (**a**) and (**b**) are indistinguishable from the baseline noise fluctuations observed from a SWNT, either with or without KF attachments. Only combinations of a successful KF attachment and a solution containing template and complementary dNTPs produced the type of additional excursions shown here.

Successful measurements also require stable control of the electrode and electrolyte potentials. An electrochemical bipotentiostat can provide complete control of the three-terminal FET and its electrolyte gate, but simpler methods are sufficient. We typically use DC sources to apply up to 100 mV to the drain electrode, 0 V to the Si wafer back gate, and a modest biasing voltage (−0.3 to +0.3 V) to the electrolyte using a Pt wire as a counter electrode. Except for the Pt wire, the electrical connections are wirebonds or probing needles located outside the electrolyte.

$I(t)$ signals from the current amplifier are digitized and saved for real-time or offline analysis. Typical data sets of 10 min are usually sufficient to determine the average kinetics of a single molecule, though data may be collected for much longer durations. To test a molecule with different analyte concentrations or combinations as shown in Figure 2, it is important to rinse a device with buffer until molecular activity appears to cease. Depending on the degree of nonspecific surface adsorption, a device may need to sit in buffer for up to 10 min before rinsing returns the device to its baseline current $I(t)$. Testing a molecule with many analytes, and performing proper control measurements for each case, usually involves dozens of rinses that benefit from integrating the data acquisition with an automated fluid delivery system (e.g., SmartSquirt, Automate Scientific). Presumably, nonspecific adsorption could be further reduced by surface blocking techniques used in other biosensing or surface analytical techniques, but these methods and their effects on single-molecule sensitivity have not yet been explored with SWNT-FET devices.

Finally, data analysis is an important part of the proper operation of these devices. One advantage of the SWNT-FET technique is its ability to continuously monitor the full reaction trajectory of a molecule over minutes, hours, or days. However, SWNT-FETs generate noise with a 1/f spectrum [67,68], meaning that long-duration measurements also exhibit large-magnitude baseline fluctuations. AC coupling or other highpass filtering successfully eliminates the lowest-frequency wanderings and emphasizes just the deviations $\Delta I(t)$ from the DC average. Figure 3a illustrates the typical noise levels after filtering, and it depicts the threshold level used to distinguish fluctuations that are attributable to KF with certainty. The filter cutoff must be chosen carefully to avoid biasing the analysis of protein activity. For example, substantial 1/f noise in the 0.1 to 10 Hz frequency band directly overlaps with the enzymatic activity of DNA polymerase, which has average turnover rates of 20 to 40 s^{-1} amid stochastic pauses lasting 1 s or more. The overlap of the desired signal with SWNT noise requires more sophisticated filtering techniques such as the open source analysis solutions vbFRET [69] and NoRSE [70] or, for the most challenging analyses, other nonlinear, machine learning techniques [71,72]. At present, reliable enumeration of enzyme information from long data records remains a challenging task that has only been partly automated.

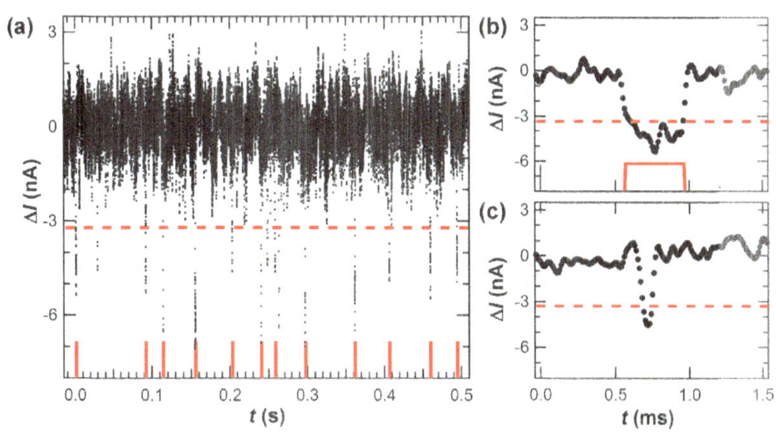

Figure 3. (**a**) $\Delta I(t)$ excursions and event enumeration (**red**) at higher magnification. Individual excursions were counted as dNTP incorporations if they exceeded a threshold determined by the baseline 1/f noise (dashed lines) and if their duration exceeded 100 μs (*i.e.*, 10 data points). (**b**,**c**) Magnified plots of the first two $\Delta I(t)$ excursions in (**a**) demonstrate examples of: (**b**) a base incorporation event; and (**c**) an excursion rejected for having a short, unresolved duration. A 40 μs amplifier rise time limited analysis to the longer events, but better time resolution might reliably identify brief $\Delta I(t)$ excursions caused by noncatalytic KF motions.

To provide a specific example, Section 3 is focused on single-molecule measurements of the Klenow Fragment (KF) of DNA polymerase I, a moderately processive and well-characterized polymerase from *E. coli.* For these experiments, a single-cysteine variant of exonuclease-defective KF (D355A/E357A/L790C/C907S) [73] was engineered using site-directed mutagenesis followed by overexpression and purification from *Escherichia coli* (*E. coli*) [49,50]. KF was attached to SWNT-FETs as described above using 500 nM protein in a standard DNA polymerase I activity buffer (20 mM Tris, 50 mM NaCl, 10 mM $MgCl_2$, 100 μM TCEP, pH 8.0). Separately, a fluorescence-based ensemble assay confirmed activity of this variant.

To measure KF activity, devices were submerged in an activity buffer containing 10 μM of dNTPs (Fisher Scientific) and 0.5 to 100 nM of DNA templates. The templates were synthesized by fusing an M13 priming site to different sequences of overhanging bases. The M13 priming site of each template was hybridized to an M13 forward primer in a 1:1 stoichiometric ratio by heating to 95 °C for 5 to 10 min followed by slow-cooling to room temperature. Following hybridization, overhanging bases for each template were composed of homopolymeric sequences as short as 10 bases and more varied sequences as long as 104 bases. Most of the measurements reported here are focused on the repeating patterns $(CTTT)_9$, $(CTTT)_{10}$, and $(CTTT)_{11}$.

3. Results

3.1. Single-Molecule Activity of DNA Polymerase (KF)

The primary function of DNA polymerases like KF is the replication or repair of DNA. Under the direction of a single-stranded DNA template, the polymerase incorporates dNTPs into a complementary template strand. The nascent strand lengthens base-by-base as the polymerase accepts an incoming dNTP and catalyzes its addition to the new strand's 3′-hydroxyl terminus [74]. A minimum scheme [75] for each cycle of this process requires multiple kinetic steps and checkpoints. In the first step, the enzyme's so-called "thumb" domain binds a primer-template DNA to form a binary open complex $E \cdot DNA_n$. Successful recognition and binding of a complementary dNTP allows the enzyme's "fingers" subdomain to snap closed on the activated ternary complex $E^* \cdot DNA_n \cdot dNTP$. This conformational transition has been directly observed by numerous smFRET-based experiments [76–83] and inferred from co-crystal X-ray structures [84,85]. As it completes incorporation of the new base, the polymerase translocates one position along the template to begin a new cycle or else dissociates from the template [86,87].

This complex cycle makes monitoring KF activity an excellent test of the SWNT-FET single-molecule technique. Many of KF's critical steps have remained hidden, including dNTP recognition, error checking, and translocation, though the enzyme has been investigated using a range of techniques [88]. The precise timing of KF's reopening, the variability of KF's kinetic rates, and its dissociation probabilities each remains unknown or contested [89–91]. Part of this problem arises from the fact that the most common single-molecule method, Förster resonance energy transfer (smFRET), has limited time resolution for very fast events [92] and no capacity for long-duration monitoring of a single, FRET-labeled molecule [93]. The SWNT-FET technique, on the other hand, has been demonstrated with 2 μs resolution [72]; the approach can also be used to observe long, time-varying reaction trajectories [21,48] because the enzyme of interest is essentially permanently attached to the device. In a typical 10-min measurement, a single KF will incorporate thousands of dNTPs into many template molecules, whereas no smFRET measurement has measured more than three successive replications by the same KF molecule [77].

To be especially sensitive to dNTP incorporation events, KF was engineered to attach to SWNT-FETs on the back side of the active fingers subdomain (Figure 1a), using the single-cysteine bioconjugation protocol described above [85]. After attachment, KF activity was monitored electronically by placing the device in different solutions of DNA template and dNTPs. Figure 2 shows example $I(t)$ records acquired under various experimental conditions. Stochastic excursions

$\Delta I(t)$ occurred at 10 to 40 s^{-1} when template and complementary dNTPs were both present in the measurement solution, consistent with smFRET measurements of KF replication [78]. $\Delta I(t)$ excursions of this type disappeared when the complementary dNTPs were absent or replaced by non-complementary dNTPs [49], or when template was removed from the solution. These types of control experiments helped to confirm that $\Delta I(t)$ excursions like these were unique fluctuations associated with the incorporation of new bases and not simply the random motions of KF in solution.

In addition, detailed measurements in low template concentrations proved a one-to-one correspondence between each $\Delta I(t)$ excursion and one dNTP incorporation. The dissociation constant K_D for the KF-template complex is 5 nM [94,95], and template concentrations below 1 nM increase the likelihood for KF to be unbound. Under these conditions, $\Delta I(t)$ showed quiet periods in which KF waited for template association interrupted by a cluster of continuous $\Delta I(t)$ excursions (Figure 4a). Still lower concentrations like 0.1 nM reduced KF's average rate one hundred fold; in this limit, diffusional waiting times grew to many seconds but the instantaneous processing rate within a cluster of events remained 20 s^{-1}. Thus, $\Delta I(t)$ was determined to accurately identify the arrival, processing, and dissociation of individual template strands.

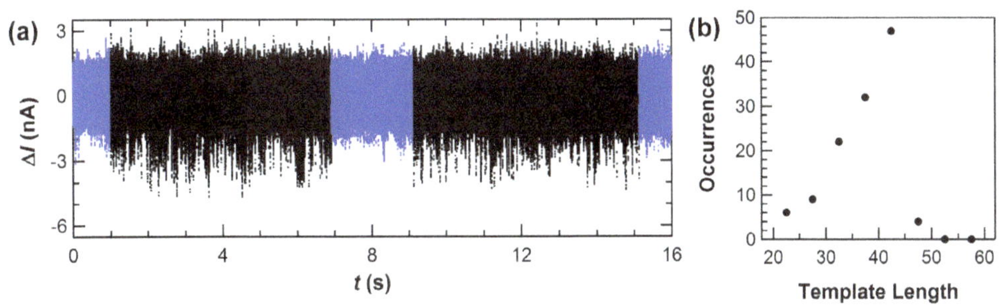

Figure 4. (**a**) Template concentrations below 5 nM introduced additional pauses (**blue**) in the records of KF activity. The pauses represent diffusional waiting times for template arrival and association. Each uninterrupted sequence of $\Delta I(t)$ excursions (**black**) represents the processing of one template strand. (**b**) Distribution of apparent lengths observed using a low concentration of the homopolymer $(dC)_{42}$ template, as determined by counting the individual $\Delta I(t)$ excursions in a 10-min data set containing 135 uninterrupted sequences.

In this low-concentration limit, the number of $\Delta I(t)$ excursions observed for each template molecule could be enumerated and compared to the template's overhang length. Figure 4b illustrates a low-resolution histogram of such counts peaked around 42 $\Delta I(t)$ excursions for a homopolymer template $(dC)_{42}$ [49]. Some template molecules dissociate before KF reaches the end of the strand, giving clusters with fewer than 42 counts; but very few clusters registered more than 42 counts, indicating that the event filtering in Figure 3 correctly identifies the base incorporation events. $\Delta I(t)$ can therefore be interpreted as a direct record of KF as it waits for template to arrive, processes the template base-by-base at its normal rate, and then dissociates from the template.

Having determined that individual $\Delta I(t)$ excursions correspond to single nucleotide incorporations, the individual low- and high-current levels in $I(t)$ can be assigned to two portions of KF's catalytic cycle. Since nucleotide incorporation occurs during a brief closing of the fingers subdomain [80], the $\Delta I(t)$ excursion is assigned to some portion of the fingers-closed conformation. The baseline $I(t)$ level, on the other hand, is associated with KF's rate-limiting open conformation. According to X-ray crystallography, the fully-closed conformation can only be accessed when template and complementary nucleotide are both bound to KF [85]; this selectivity helps explain why $\Delta I(t)$ excursions correctly enumerate template lengths without erroneous extra counts from random fluttering motions or the rejections of non-complementary nucleotides.

The X-ray crystal structures also reveal the precise motions of charged amino acid residues surrounding the 790C attachment site. The allosteric motions of these charges, which are essentially adjacent to the SWNT-FET, are primarily responsible for electrostatically gating the sensitized region of the SWNT and inducing the observed $\Delta I(t)$ signal. The motions of KF's more distant charges and charged domains are screened by the surrounding buffer, which has a Debye screening length of 1 nm [96]. In similar single-molecule SWNT-FET measurements using T4 lysozyme instead of KF, charged residues near the attachment site were varied by mutagenesis to prove their role in signal transduction [47]. Therefore, the SWNT-FET is not merely a precise transducer of enzyme motion; the system can be designed to probe selected subdomain motions with appropriate design of the attachment site and nearby charged residues.

Identifying the levels in $I(t)$ as open and closed conformations enabled a statistical analysis of KF's single-nucleotide incorporation kinetics. Each dNTP incorporation was represented by one ΔI excursion, which had a duration τ_{closed} and a waiting time τ_{open} during which KF was in its open conformation. Figure 5 shows τ_{closed} and τ_{open} probability distributions from thousands of incorporation events for each of the four homopolymeric DNA templates measured with a significant excess (10 μM) of complementary dNTPs. The combination of eight τ distributions gives a sense of the information density of the SWNT-FET technique and the opportunities for revealing new information about molecular processes and molecule-to-molecule variation. The distributions are summarized in Table 1 for one typical KF molecule.

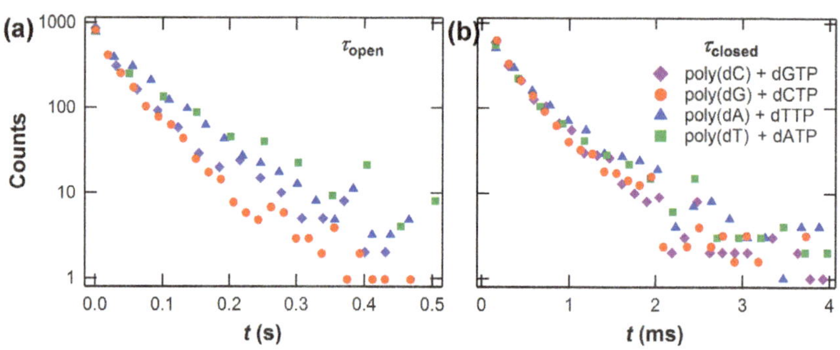

Figure 5. Example distributions of (**a**) τ_{open} and (**b**) τ_{closed} acquired for all four native nucleotides using a single KF molecule. The different slopes for τ_{open} represent different average processing rates for the four nucleotides. The portion of the cycle represented by τ_{closed}, in which catalytic incorporation of the nucleotide occurs, is insensitive to the nucleotide species. The exact value of $<\tau_{open}>$ varies from one molecule to another and can be 50% to 300% of the values shown here. However, each different copy of KF follows the trends shown here.

Table 1. Single-nucleotide processing rates with homopolymeric templates [1].

Template	Nucleotide	τ_{closed} (ms)	τ_{open} (ms)	k (1/s)
poly(dT)$_{42}$	dATP	0.33 ± 0.08	71.4 ± 1.4	14.4 ± 2.9
poly(dA)$_{42}$	dTTP	0.42 ± 0.09	63.7 ± 1.1	16.0 ± 2.9
poly(dG)$_{42}$	dCTP	0.32 ± 0.07	39.0 ± 5.6	26.2 ± 4.4
poly(dC)$_{42}$	dGTP	0.33 ± 0.05	38.0 ± 5.8	28.5 ± 3.5

[1] Average values ± one standard deviation.

The kinetic results showed that the rate-limiting duration $<\tau_{open}>$ was much longer than $<\tau_{closed}>$, averaging 50 ms. In addition, $<\tau_{open}>$ was sensitive to the specific nucleotide, being nearly twice as long for dTTP and dATP incorporations than for dCTP and dGTP incorporations. The longer duration for A·T base pairs compared to C·G base pairs, regardless of which nucleotide is being incorporated into the single-stranded template, suggests that the formation of A·T pairs may involve a mechanism that is distinct from the formation of C·G pairs. Two different conformations, for example, could be relevant for dNTP recognition and processive fidelity. Unlike $<\tau_{open}>$, the mean duration $<\tau_{closed}>$ was insensitive to dNTP identity with values of 0.3 to 0.4 ms. Thus, the events sensed by the SWNT-FET represent a brief, efficient part of the enzyme's closure or closed configuration [87], occurring with a timing that is independent of the specific nucleotide. When averaged together to produce an effective replication rate $k = (<\tau_{closed}> + <\tau_{open}>)^{-1}$, the SWNT-FET measurements are consistent with other published values for KF's activity [77,78,91].

In addition to durations and kinetics, one more independent aspect of the $\Delta I(t)$ excursions is the signal amplitude. Since $\Delta I(t)$ is transduced by motions of the protein's charge residues, differences in $\Delta I(t)$ are an indirect means of probing the conformational differences associated with the formation of different base pairs. On average, A·T base pairs produced larger $\Delta I(t)$ excursions than C·G base pairs. As with the timing, however, differences did not distinguish dATP incorporations from dTTP incorporations.

Even larger conformational effects were observed when a native dNTP was replaced with a synthetic, unnatural dNTP analog. Long-duration measurements of the same KF molecule allowed direct comparisons of dCTP incorporation against dCTP analogs such as α-thio-dCTP or 2-thio-dCTP, molecules for which slight alterations slowed down or sped up KF's average kinetics, respectively (Figure 6) [50]. The $\Delta I(t)$ amplitude for 2-thio-dCTP also revealed a bistability in which KF adopts one of two different conformations during fidelity checking of the nucleotide incorporation. This effect was even more pronounced with 6-chloro-2-aminopurine-drTP (6-Cl-2-APTP), a pseudo-analog of dGTP that replaces the 6-amino group with chlorine to dramatically decrease the hydrogen bonding of the new base pair. During 6-Cl-2-APTP incorporations into homopolymeric poly(dC) templates, $\Delta I(t)$ excursions had τ_{closed} durations similar to the native dGTP but with reversed magnitudes, as shown in Figure 6c [50]. The reversal of $\Delta I(t)$ indicated different motions of charged residues as KF accommodated the unnatural analog. We have proposed that the active site O-helix may twist in two different directions for dGTP and 6-Cl-2-APTP. Rotations of Y766 and F762 in the active site, depicted in Figure 6d, can allosterically propagate to charged residues adjacent to the SWNT-FET and cause the observed signals. In fact, a brief conformational change has been observed by smFRET when KF moves the nascent base pair to a post-insertion site [77], and this motion may be the conformation sensed during τ_{closed}. A twisting O-helix mechanism would also account for the larger $\Delta I(t)$ excursions for A·T base pairs, which bury deeper in KF's active site [97] and allow greater motions of the O-helix.

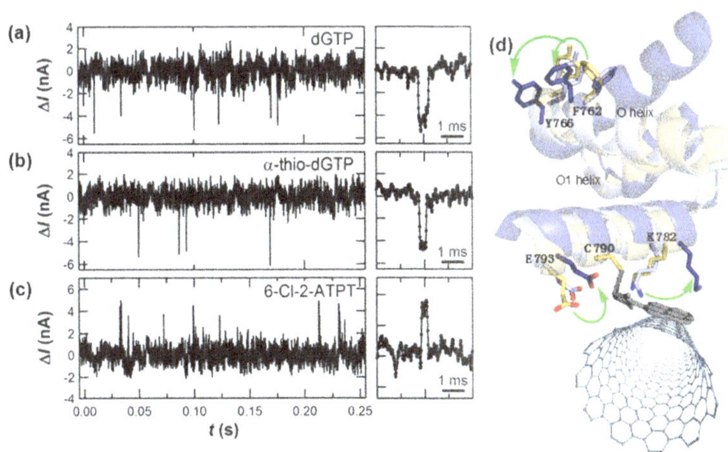

Figure 6. Direct comparison of nucleotide incorporation events into poly(dC)$_{42}$ templates using: (**a**) native dGTPs; (**b**) α-thio-dGTP; and (**c**) 6-Cl-2-APTP. (**d**) Reversal of the excursion direction suggests that conformational accommodation of the latter analog is allosterically transmitted to the SWNT, perhaps through motions of the O-helix depicted here.

3.2. *Accuracy of Amplification-Free Measurements of DNA Template Lengths*

The previous section described how SWNT-FET devices have provided detailed recordings of DNA polymerase activity. Despite being densely informative, the $\Delta I(t)$ signals are currently insufficient for DNA sequencing applications because they do not fully differentiate between the four base pairs. Successful differentiation will require additional work tailoring the transduction to be more sensitive to small differences between the bases. Nucleotide analogs already show the promise of this strategy in Figure 6, and targeted point mutations may further enhance the SWNT-FET's sensitivity to specific nucleotide-recognition mechanisms of KF.

To justify further work in those directions, experiments revisited the conclusion that $\Delta I(t)$ successfully records every base incorporation. Accurate base enumeration, after all, is a critical precondition to successful sequencing, and the first counting experiments using $(dC)_{42}$ were not designed to determine the method's accuracy. To investigate base enumeration in greater detail, we repeated the diffusion-limited length counting experiments described for Figure 4 using DNA templates designed to assess the challenges of a $(CTTT)_n$ repeating motif. $(CTTT)_n$ occurs with 80 different alleles on chromosome 4 of the human alpha fibrinogen gene, and this variety is potentially useful for human identification from DNA [98]. In fact, traditional DNA sequencing-by-synthesis technologies have difficulty determining the correct length of this and other repeated motifs in the human genome, and accurate base-by-base readout with SWNT-FETs represents a new opportunity to correctly enumerate these segments. In addition, in vivo errors by polymerase as it replicates repeating motifs lead to disease and cellular malfunction; so, accurate base-by-base readout might reveal the causes of such errors.

Improved counting experiments used four templates designed with 9, 10, 11, and 26 repeats of the sequence CTTT. For comparison, experiments also used random sequences with the same length like $(B_{10}A)_4$, in which B_{10} represents a random sequence of G, T, and C. As described above, KF-functionalized SWNT-FETs were measured for 10 min in template solutions diluted to 0.5 nM to produce diffusion-limited waiting times of multiple seconds, on average, between each template strand. At the end of each idle waiting time, template association initiated a cluster of stochastic $\Delta I(t)$ excursions that occurred at an average rate of 20 s^{-1}. The events in each cluster were enumerated and binned into histograms, and the template concentration was kept low enough that no double-length clusters from two, back-to-back template molecules were observed.

To minimize bias in the data processing, a semi-automated routine was used to identify and count $\Delta I(t)$ excursions. After smoothing the raw data to remove baseline fluctuations, the routine determined the standard deviation σ of the $I(t)$ baseline noise and then counted events that met two criteria: magnitudes greater than 3σ and durations longer than 100 μs (10 data points at 100 kHz sampling rates). Figure 3 illustrates an $\Delta I(t)$ record with example events accepted and rejected by these dual criteria. Small-magnitude and short-duration fluctuations that were rejected by the filter may have represented real motions of KF intermediates, but studying such transients accurately and in greater detail will require future measurements with higher bandwidths. This work focused exclusively on events accepted by the filter and, specifically, identifying the long pauses used to define clusters of events. The pause between two adjacent events within a cluster was only 80 ms on average, so idle baseline lasting >0.5 s was deemed an extraordinary duration indicative of template dissociation.

Figure 7 shows new length-enumeration histograms obtained with the SWNT-FET technique. A template like $(CTTT)_{11}$ produced 44 stochastic events over a duration of 2 to 4 s, followed by one or more seconds of idle baseline noise (Figure 7d). Over the course of 10 min acquisition periods, fewer than 40 templates were typically bound, processed, and released by KF. Despite the low number of molecules, the distribution could be fit by a single Gaussian peak. Furthermore, measurements with template mixtures produced enumeration histograms having separately resolved peaks. Results from a 1:1 molar ratio of $(CTTT)_9$ with $(CTTT)_{10}$ are shown in Figure 7b, and the mixture of $(CTTT)_{10}$ with $(CTTT)_{11}$ is shown in Figure 7c. In both pairs, the templates differ by just one repeat unit of four base pairs (bp). The total template concentration was kept constant in each experiment, so the distributions with template mixtures contained fewer than 20 molecules of each template in most data records. The uncertainty in peak position was ≤0.3 bp in each fit, and other fitting results are summarized in Table 2. With template mixtures, the peak position errors were no worse than in the single-template case, indicating that template molecules did not interfere with each other at these concentrations. In Figure 7d, a data record shows a $(CTTT)_{10}$ template and then a $(CTTT)_9$ being processed in succession to illustrate how KF's processing of one molecule in a mixture was independent of the next.

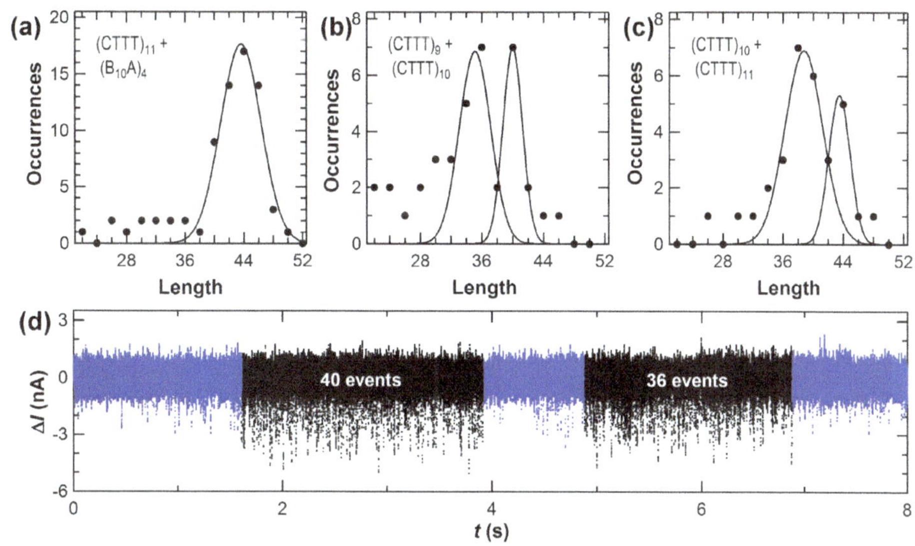

Figure 7. Base-enumeration distributions obtained from 0.5 nM concentrations of the templates: (**a**) $(CTTT)_{11}$ and $(B_{10}A)_4$ measured separately; (**b**) $(CTTT)_9$ mixed with $(CTTT)_{10}$; and (**c**) $(CTTT)_{10}$ mixed with $(CTTT)_{11}$. Solid curves are Gaussian curve fits to each peak and fitting results are summarized in Table 2. Mixing two templates together led to fewer that 25 template molecules being counted in a typical data record, but the accuracy of peak fitting was not substantially reduced. (**d**) Example $\Delta I(t)$ record collected with the $(CTTT)_9$ + $(CTTT)_{10}$ mixture, illustrating a cluster of 40 dNTP incorporations, a 1-s pause, and a cluster of 36 incorporations.

Table 2. Gaussian fitting parameters from length-counting experiments.

Template Sequence	Length(s)	N [2]	Peak Position(s) (bp)	FWHM (bp)
$(CTTT)_{11}$	44	27	42.3 ± 0.3	7.6 ± 0.8
$(B_{10}A)_4$	44	45	44.2 ± 0.1	6.4 ± 0.4
$(CTTT)_{11}$ and $(B_{10}A)_4$	44 and 44	72	43.6 ± 0.2	7.8 ± 0.6
$(CTTT)_9$ and $(CTTT)_{10}$	36 and 40	38	34.5 ± 1.1 40.0 ± 0.2	10.1 ± 3.6 3.6 ± 0.4
$(CTTT)_{10}$ and $(CTTT)_{11}$	40 and 44	31	38.8 ± 0.3 43.5 ± 0.3	7.1 ± 1.0 4.0 ± 1.0

[2] Total number of template molecules observed in the distribution.

Two main sources of error were identified during the analysis of these measurements. First, the peak positions determined by Gaussian fitting were systematically smaller than the actual template length, with an average of −0.6 bp. This error resulted from the 2-bp width of the bins needed for analyzing so few counts. Second, the peaks exhibited a full-width at half maximum (FWHM) of 6 to 8 bp. The FWHM primarily arose from isolated events occurring during the 0.5 s before and after each cluster. These events, which could not be conclusively associated with a template, led to uncertainties as large as ± 2 bp in the enumeration of the worst-case data clusters. In other words, the overall accuracy in peak position reached <1 bp after as few as 20 template reads, but the length of any single template molecule included errors of ± 2 bp.

Accuracy can be improved somewhat with larger data sets. Our experimental protocol flushed or rinsed the devices with buffer every 10 min to avoid excess contamination from non-specific adsorption. However, consecutive data sets from a single device were no better nor worse than nonconsecutive data from different days or data appended from two or more different SWNT-FET devices. Consequently, several data sets could be accumulated to compile larger numbers of template reads for improved analysis of template mixtures. For example, the repeating motif $(CTTT)_{11}$ was read just as accurately as the semi-random sequence $(B_{10}A)_4$, so these two distributions have been combined in Figure 7a. The single peak indicates that the SWNT-FET technique was insensitive to the repeating sequence, though the peak width is slightly larger than peaks shown in Figure 7b,c. In another experiment, a similar distribution was accumulated from 200 min of single-molecule signal containing nearly 1000 template reads. With a bin size reduced to 1 bp, the systematic error in peak position was reduced from -0.6 bp to -0.2 bp and the uncertainty in the Gaussian fit reduced from 0.3 bp to 0.2 bp. Even with these larger data sets, the FWHM only reduced to 4 bp because the errors associated with correct identification of the beginning and end of each template molecule do not average out. Better accuracy in single-molecule enumeration will require better identification of these endpoints, either by lowering the template concentration further or by developing techniques that create other distinguishing features in $I(t)$.

The measurements focused on templates shorter than 50 base pairs, but there was no evidence suggesting that longer templates would fare worse. In fact, the FWHM was not proportional to template length since it primarily arose from the template endpoints. Thus, long templates could be read with the same accuracy as short templates, and improving the analysis methodology might further reduce the FWHM without requiring longer data records. On the other hand, we note a tendency of shorter templates to associate with KF more readily than longer templates. In the 1:1 mixtures depicted in Figure 7b,c, the different areas under each peak suggest that shorter templates were counted nearly twice as often as longer templates. The exact magnitude of this difference also depended on the sequences used. The reduction may reflects different diffusion and KF-association constants for the two template molecules; it also illustrates that this technique can be inaccurate for determining molecular ratios.

In general, the templates described here were chosen to be shorter than KF's maximum processivity. Previous ensemble measurements have estimated this processivity limit to be 50 ± 5 bp [89,90], but the value is very difficult to determine precisely. The SWNT-FET technique provides a new, direct method for measuring processivity. Using the $(CTTT)_{26}$ template with an overhang length of 104 bp, we have observed rare sequences of up to 94 $\Delta I(t)$ excursions but none as long as the template. Instead, the distribution of cluster lengths had no peak and averaged only 70 bases, indicating that KF dissociates from the template before reaching its end. The distributions in Figure 7 provide a good measurement of this dissociation probability because the non-zero background on the left of each histogram peak represents those cases where KF dissociated mid-template before reaching its end. Within the limits of the available statistics, this background was constant from the template length down to ~5 bp (below which it becomes difficult to distinguish short templates from random noise and spurious events), indicating a constant dissociation probability after each base incorporation. Based on the fraction of background events in each bin of the histogram, we calculate this probability to be $1.8\% \pm 0.2\%$. A probability of ~2% agrees with the ensemble processivity of about 50 bp [89,90], while also allowing for the rarer 70 and 80 bp runs observed with $(CTTT)_{26}$. It is also possible that enhanced processivity results from an unintended stabilization of the template-KF complex by the SWNT. In all other respects, the SWNT-FET measurements agree with ensemble measurements of KF activity.

Note that the background counts used for estimating the dissociation rate were not observed to the right of each peak, since the templates had a finite length. In fact, the absence of excess counts illustrates the efficiency of dNTP incorporations with each closure. If more than one closure was needed for KF to successfully position the template strand and incorporate a nucleotide, then the histograms shown in Figure 7 would extend well beyond the template's actual length. Other than the peak's FWHM, extra counts beyond the template length have not been observed. Thus, the inefficient steps of recognizing the correct dNTP and rejecting mismatched ones do not register as events in this SWNT-FET signal, and such mechanisms must be occurring during τ_{open}. The same conclusion has been reached by smFRET studies and it has been used to explain why τ_{open} is the rate-limiting portion of the catalytic cycle [80,83].

4. Conclusions

Single-molecule enzymology provides many new opportunities to understand complex biochemical mechanisms. While single-molecule optics have become a well-established characterization method, single-molecule electronics have only recently been demonstrated. Here, we have summarized one successful method for building and using single-molecule electronic devices. Using KF as a model enzyme with a complex catalytic cycle, we have demonstrated high resolution, long-duration electronic recording that reveal KF's sensitivity to native and analog nucleotides and its processivity limits. Selection of an appropriate attachment site maximized the device's sensitivity to nucleotide incorporations over other protein movements, enabling error-free base-pair enumeration unaffected by nucleotide mismatch rejections. While these particular results with KF have been described in relation to DNA sequencing applications, they represent a much more general method for single-molecule enzymology that is readily extended to other processive enzymes.

In that sense, single-molecule electronics is likely to be complementary to traditional single-molecule fluorescence. The electronic technique was well-suited to the question of processivity, for example, and it was straightforward to continuously monitor one molecule's activity in many different conditions. More general benefits of the solid state platform include new opportunities for parallelization in arrays and high bandwidth detection of brief fluctuations. In addition, new research becomes possible for proteins that do not readily incorporate fluorophores or which are especially sensitive to photo-oxidation. The availability of single-molecule electronics is unlikely to replace other single-molecule techniques, but it does provide a new tool for addressing difficult research questions. In fact, since the electronic readout is independent of optical excitation, future devices may even provide opportunities to combine the electronic and fluorescent channels for dual, simultaneous readout of two subdomains of the same molecule. That type of synergetic combination prompts hope that creative researchers will find many uses for single-molecule electronics as a research platform.

Acknowledgments: This research was supported financially by the NIH NCI (R01 CA133592-01), the NIH NIGMS (1R01GM106957-01) and the NSF (DMR-1104629 and ECCS-1231910).

Author Contributions: †O.T.G., K.M.P. and Y.C. all contributed equally to this work and shared in the design, execution, and analysis of the experiments, data, and conclusions. O.T.G., P.C.S., A.J.R. and P.G.C. developed the techniques for dilute SWNT synthesis; A.J.R., D.P. and P.G.C. designed and fabricated the devices; and K.M.P. and G.A.W. expressed and purified the KF protein. O.T.G., K.M.P. and P.G.C. contributed equally to writing the paper and preparing the figures.

Conflicts of Interest: The authors declare no conflict of interest.

Abbreviations

The following abbreviations are used in this manuscript:

KF	Klenow Fragment of DNA polymerase I
DNA	deoxyribonucleic acid
smFRET	single-molecule Förster resonance energy transfer
SWNT	single-walled carbon nanotube
FET	field effect transistor
dNTP	deoxynucleoside triphosphate

References and Notes

1. Casas-Selves, M.; Degregori, J. How cancer shapes evolution, and how evolution shapes cancer. *Evolution* **2011**, *4*, 624–634. [CrossRef] [PubMed]
2. Hanahan, D.; Weinberg, R.A. Hallmarks of cancer: The next generation. *Cell* **2011**, *144*, 646–674. [CrossRef] [PubMed]
3. Hanahan, D.; Weinberg, R.A. The hallmarks of cancer. *Cell* **2000**, *100*, 57–70. [CrossRef]
4. Weinberg, R.A. *One Renegade Cell: The Quest for the Origins of Cancer*; Basic Books: New York, NY, USA, 1999.
5. Wu, Z.Q.; Brabletz, T.; Fearon, E.; Willis, A.L.; Hu, C.Y.; Li, X.Y.; Weiss, S.J. Canonical wnt suppressor, axin2, promotes colon carcinoma oncogenic activity. *Proc. Natl. Acad. Sci. USA* **2012**, *109*, 11312–11317. [CrossRef] [PubMed]
6. Dravis, C.; Spike, B.T.; Harrell, J.C.; Johns, C.; Trejo, C.L.; Southard-Smith, E.M.; Perou, C.M.; Wahl, G.M. Sox10 regulates stem/progenitor and mesenchymal cell states in mammary epithelial cells. *Cell Rep.* **2015**, *12*, 2035–2048. [CrossRef] [PubMed]
7. Xie, S.N. Single-molecule approach to enzymology. *Single Mol.* **2001**, *2*, 229–236. [CrossRef]
8. Min, W.; English, B.; Luo, G.; Cherayil, B.; Kou, S.; Xie, X. Fluctuating enzymes: Lessons from single-molecule studies. *Acc. Chem. Res.* **2005**, *38*, 923–931. [CrossRef] [PubMed]
9. Hohlbein, J.; Gryte, K.; Heilemann, M.; Kapanidis, A.N. Surfing on a new wave of single-molecule fluorescence methods. *Phys. Biol.* **2010**, *7*, 031001. [CrossRef] [PubMed]
10. Lim, D.K.; Jeon, K.S.; Hwang, J.H.; Kim, H.; Kwon, S.; Suh, Y.D.; Nam, J.M. Highly uniform and reproducible surface-enhanced raman scattering from DNA-tailorable nanoparticles with 1-nm interior gap. *Nat. Nanotechnol.* **2011**, *6*, 452–460. [CrossRef] [PubMed]
11. Song, S.; Qin, Y.; He, Y.; Huang, Q.; Fan, C.; Chen, H.Y. Functional nanoprobes for ultrasensitive detection of biomolecules. *Chem. Soc. Rev.* **2010**, *39*, 4234–4243. [CrossRef] [PubMed]
12. Yang, H.; Luo, G.B.; Karnchanaphanurach, P.; Louie, T.M.; Rech, I.; Cova, S.; Xun, L.Y.; Xie, X.S. Protein conformational dynamics probed by single-molecule electron transfer. *Science* **2003**, *302*, 262–266. [CrossRef] [PubMed]
13. Pudney, C.R.; Lane, R.S.K.; Fielding, A.J.; Magennis, S.W.; Hay, S.; Scrutton, N.S. Enzymatic single-molecule kinetic isotope effects. *J. Am. Chem. Soc.* **2013**, *135*, 3855–3864. [CrossRef] [PubMed]
14. Jagannathan, B.; Marqusee, S. Protein folding and unfolding under force. *Biopolymers* **2013**, *99*, 860–869. [CrossRef] [PubMed]
15. Rosenberg, S.A.; Quinlan, M.E.; Forkey, J.N.; Goldman, Y.E. Rotational motions of macromolecules by single-molecule fluorescence microscopy. *Acc. Chem. Res.* **2005**, *38*, 583–593. [CrossRef] [PubMed]
16. Vrtis, K.B.; Markiewicz, R.P.; Romano, L.J.; Rueda, D. Carcinogenic adducts induce distinct DNA polymerase binding orientations. *Nucleic Acids Res.* **2013**, *41*, 7843–7853. [CrossRef] [PubMed]
17. Lieberman, K.R.; Dahl, J.M.; Mai, A.H.; Cox, A.; Akeson, M.; Wang, H. Kinetic mechanism of translocation and dNTP binding in individual DNA polymerase complexes. *J. Am. Chem. Soc.* **2013**, *135*, 9149–9155. [CrossRef] [PubMed]
18. Zheng, D.S.; Lu, H.P. Single-molecule enzymatic conformational dynamics: Spilling out the product molecules. *J. Phys. Chem. B* **2014**, *118*, 9128–9140. [CrossRef] [PubMed]
19. Rivas-Pardo, J.A.; Alegre-Cebollada, J.; Ramirez-Sarmiento, C.A.; Fernandez, J.M.; Guixe, V. Identifying sequential substrate binding at the single-molecule level by enzyme mechanical stabilization. *ACS Nano* **2015**, *9*, 3996–4005. [CrossRef] [PubMed]

20. Craig, D.B.; Eggertson, M.J.; Chikamatsu, M.; Horwood, C.A. Single molecule assay of *Escherichia coli* beta-galactosidase using two competing substrates simultaneously, ddao-beta-d-galactoside and resorufin-beta-d-galactoside. *Anal. Lett.* **2011**, *44*, 1835–1841. [CrossRef]
21. Choi, Y.; Moody, I.S.; Sims, P.C.; Hunt, S.R.; Corso, B.L.; Seitz, D.E.; Blaszcazk, L.C.; Collins, P.G.; Weiss, G.A. Single molecule dynamics of lysozyme processing distinguishes linear and cross-linked peptidoglycan substrates. *J. Am. Chem. Soc.* **2012**, *134*, 2032–2035. [CrossRef] [PubMed]
22. Betous, R.; Couch, F.B.; Mason, A.C.; Eichman, B.F.; Manosas, M.; Cortez, D. Substrate-selective repair and restart of replication forks by DNA translocases. *Cell Rep.* **2013**, *3*, 1958–1969. [CrossRef] [PubMed]
23. Joo, C.; Balci, H.; Ishitsuka, Y.; Buranachai, C.; Ha, T. Advances in single-molecule fluorescence methods for molecular biology. *Annu. Rev. Biochem.* **2008**, *77*, 51–76. [CrossRef] [PubMed]
24. Blank, K.; De Cremer, G.; Hofkens, J. Fluorescence-based analysis of enzymes at the single-molecule level. *Biotechnol. J.* **2009**, *4*, 465–479. [CrossRef] [PubMed]
25. Eid, J.; Fehr, A.; Gray, J.; Luong, K.; Lyle, J.; Otto, G.; Peluso, P.; Rank, D.; Baybayan, P.; Bettman, B.; et al. Real-time DNA sequencing from single polymerase molecules. *Science* **2009**, *323*, 133–138. [CrossRef] [PubMed]
26. Neuman, K.C.; Nagy, A. Single-molecule force spectroscopy: Optical tweezers, magnetic tweezers and atomic force microscopy. *Nat. Methods* **2008**, *5*, 491–505. [CrossRef] [PubMed]
27. Deniz, A.A.; Mukhopadhyay, S.; Lemke, E.A. Single-molecule biophysics: At the interface of biology, physics and chemistry. *J. R. Soc. Interface* **2008**, *5*, 15–45. [CrossRef] [PubMed]
28. Martina, M.; Taverna, S. *Patch-Clamp Methods and Protocols*, 2nd ed.; Humana Press: New York, NY, USA, 2014; p. 403.
29. Iqbal, S.M.; Bashir, R. *Nanopores*; Springer US: New York, NY, USA, 2011; p. 369.
30. Healy, K.; Schiedt, B.; Morrison, A.P. Solid-state nanopore technologies for nanopore-based DNA analysis. *Nanomedicine* **2007**, *2*, 875–897. [CrossRef] [PubMed]
31. Venkatesan, B.M.; Bashir, R. Nanopore sensors for nucleic acid analysis. *Nat. Nanotechnol.* **2011**, *6*, 615–624. [CrossRef] [PubMed]
32. Branton, D.; Deamer, D.W.; Marziali, A.; Bayley, H.; Benner, S.A.; Butler, T.; Di Ventra, M.; Garaj, S.; Hibbs, A.; Huang, X.H.; et al. The potential and challenges of nanopore sequencing. *Nat. Biotechnol.* **2008**, *26*, 1146–1153. [CrossRef] [PubMed]
33. Feng, Y.; Zhang, Y.; Ying, C.; Wang, D.; Du, C. Nanopore-based fourth-generation DNA sequencing technology. *Genom. Proteom. Bioinform.* **2015**, *13*, 4–16. [CrossRef] [PubMed]
34. Huang, S.; He, J.; Chang, S.; Zhang, P.; Liang, F.; Li, S.; Tuchband, M.; Fuhrmann, A.; Ros, R.; Lindsay, S. Identifying single bases in a DNA oligomer with electron tunnelling. *Nat. Nanotechnol.* **2010**, *5*, 868–873. [CrossRef] [PubMed]
35. Zhao, Y.; Ashcroft, B.; Zhang, P.; Liu, H.; Sen, S.; Song, W.; Im, J.; Gyarfas, B.; Manna, S.; Biswas, S.; et al. Single-molecule spectroscopy of amino acids and peptides by recognition tunnelling. *Nat. Nano* **2014**, *9*, 466–473. [CrossRef] [PubMed]
36. Cui, Y.; Wei, Q.Q.; Park, H.K.; Lieber, C.M. Nanowire nanosensors for highly sensitive and selective detection of biological and chemical species. *Science* **2001**, *293*, 1289–1292. [CrossRef] [PubMed]
37. Patolsky, F.; Zheng, G.; Hayden, O.; Lakadamyali, M.; Zhuang, X.; Lieber, C.M. Electrical detection of single viruses. *Proc. Natl. Acad. Sci. USA* **2004**, *101*, 14017–14022. [CrossRef] [PubMed]
38. Patolsky, F.; Zheng, G.F.; Lieber, C.M. Nanowire-based biosensors. *Anal. Chem.* **2006**, *78*, 4260–4269. [CrossRef] [PubMed]
39. Patolsky, F.; Zheng, G.F.; Lieber, C.M. Fabrication of silicon nanowire devices for ultrasensitive, label-free, real-time detection of biological and chemical species. *Nat. Protoc.* **2006**, *1*, 1711–1724. [CrossRef] [PubMed]
40. Zheng, G.F.; Gao, X.P.A.; Lieber, C.M. Frequency domain detection of biomolecules using silicon nanowire biosensors. *Nano Lett.* **2010**, *10*, 3179–3183. [CrossRef] [PubMed]
41. Kong, J.; Franklin, N.R.; Zhou, C.W.; Chapline, M.G.; Peng, S.; Cho, K.J.; Dai, H.J. Nanotube molecular wires as chemical sensors. *Science* **2000**, *287*, 622–625. [CrossRef] [PubMed]
42. Collins, P.G.; Bradley, K.; Ishigami, M.; Zettl, A. Extreme oxygen sensitivity of electronic properties of carbon nanotubes. *Science* **2000**, *287*, 1801–1804. [CrossRef] [PubMed]

43. Guo, X.; Small, J.P.; Klare, J.E.; Want, Y.; Purewal, M.S.; Tam, I.W.; Hong, B.H.; Caldwell, R.; Huang, L.; O'Brien, S.; et al. Covalently bridging gaps in single-walled carbon nanotubes with conducting molecules. *Science* **2006**, *311*, 356–359. [CrossRef] [PubMed]
44. Goldsmith, B.R.; Coroneus, J.G.; Kane, A.A.; Weiss, G.A.; Collins, P.G. Monitoring single molecule reactivity on a carbon nanotube. *Nano Lett.* **2008**, *8*, 189–194. [CrossRef] [PubMed]
45. Sorgenfrei, S.; Chiu, C.-Y.; Gonzalez, R.L.; Yu, Y.-J.; Kim, P.; Nuckolls, C.; Shepard, K.L. Label-free single-molecule detection of DNA-hybridization kinetics with a carbon nanotube field-effect transistor. *Nat. Nanotechnol.* **2011**, *6*, 126–132. [CrossRef] [PubMed]
46. Choi, Y.; Moody, I.S.; Sims, P.C.; Hunt, S.R.; Corso, B.L.; Weiss, G.A.; Collins, P.G. Single-molecule lysozyme dynamics monitored by an electronic circuit. *Science* **2012**, *335*, 319–324. [CrossRef] [PubMed]
47. Choi, Y.; Olsen, T.J.; Sims, P.C.; Moody, I.S.; Corso, B.L.; Dang, M.N.; Weiss, G.A.; Collins, P.G. Dissecting single-molecule signal transduction in carbon nanotube circuits with protein engineering. *Nano Lett.* **2013**, *13*, 625–631. [CrossRef] [PubMed]
48. Sims, P.C.; Moody, I.S.; Choi, Y.; Dong, C.; Iftikhar, M.; Corso, B.L.; Gul, O.T.; Collins, P.G.; Weiss, G.A. Electronic measurements of single-molecule catalysis by camp-dependent protein kinase A. *J. Am. Chem. Soc.* **2013**, *135*, 7861–7868. [CrossRef] [PubMed]
49. Olsen, T.J.; Choi, Y.; Sims, P.C.; Gul, O.T.; Corso, B.L.; Dong, C.; Brown, W.A.; Collins, P.G.; Weiss, G.A. Electronic measurements of single-molecule processing by DNA polymerase I (klenow fragment). *J. Am. Chem. Soc.* **2013**, *135*, 7855–7860. [CrossRef] [PubMed]
50. Pugliese, K.M.; Gul, O.T.; Olsen, T.J.; Choi, Y.; Collins, P.G.; Weiss, G.A. Incorporation of deoxynucleoside triphosphate analogs by single-molecule DNA polymerase I (klenow fragment) nanocircuits. *J. Am. Chem. Soc.* **2015**, *137*, 9587–9594. [CrossRef] [PubMed]
51. Martel, R.; Schmidt, T.; Shea, H.R.; Hertel, T.; Avouris, P. Single- and multi-wall carbon nanotube field-effect transistors. *Appl. Phys. Lett.* **1998**, *73*, 2447–2449. [CrossRef]
52. Tans, S.J.; Verschueren, A.R.M.; Dekker, C. Room-temperature transistor based on a single carbon nanotube. *Nature* **1998**, *393*, 49–52.
53. Star, A.; Gabriel, J.C.P.; Bradley, K.; Gruner, G. Electronic detection of specific protein binding using nanotube fet devices. *Nano Lett.* **2003**, *3*, 459–463. [CrossRef]
54. Goldsmith, B.R.; Coroneus, J.G.; Khalap, V.R.; Kane, A.A.; Weiss, G.A.; Collins, P.G. Conductance-controlled point functionalization of single-walled carbon nanotubes. *Science* **2007**, *315*, 77–81. [CrossRef] [PubMed]
55. Sorgenfrei, S.; Chiu, C.-Y.; Johnston, M.; Nuckolls, C.; Shepard, K.L. Debye screening in single-molecule carbon nanotube field-effect sensors. *Nano Lett.* **2011**, *11*, 3739–3743. [CrossRef] [PubMed]
56. Müller, A.; Das, S.K.; Kogerler, P.; Bogge, H.; Schmidtmann, M.; Trautwein, A.X.; Schunemann, V.; Krickemeyer, E.; Preetz, W. A new type of supramolecular compound: Molybdenum-oxide-based composites consisting of magnetic nanocapsules with encapsulated keggin-ion electron reservoirs cross-linked to a two-dimensional network. *Angew. Chem. Int. Ed.* **2000**, *39*, 3413–3417. [CrossRef]
57. An, L.; Owens, J.M.; McNeil, L.E.; Liu, J. Synthesis of nearly uniform single-walled carbon nanotubes using identical metal-containing molecular nanoclusters as catalysts. *J. Am. Chem. Soc.* **2002**, *124*, 13688–13689. [CrossRef] [PubMed]
58. Kim, C.H.; Axup, J.Y.; Schultz, P.G. Protein conjugation with genetically encoded unnatural amino acids. *Curr. Opin. Chem. Biol.* **2013**, *17*, 412–419. [CrossRef] [PubMed]
59. England, C.G.; Luo, H.; Cai, W. Halotag technology: A versatile platform for biomedical applications. *Bioconj. Chem.* **2015**, *26*, 975–986. [CrossRef] [PubMed]
60. Hoffmann, A.; Roeder, R.G. Purification of his-tagged proteins in non-denaturing conditions suggests a convenient method for protein interaction studies. *Nucleic Acids Res.* **1991**, *19*, 6337–6338. [CrossRef] [PubMed]
61. Chen, R.J.; Zhan, Y.G.; Wang, D.W.; Dai, H.J. Noncovalent sidewall functionalization of single-walled carbon nanotubes for protein immobilization. *J. Am. Chem. Soc.* **2001**, *123*, 3838–3839. [CrossRef] [PubMed]
62. Hermanson, G.T. *Bioconjugate Techniques*, 2nd ed.; Academic Press, Inc.: Chicago, IL, USA, 2008.
63. Shulaker, M.M.; Hills, G.; Patil, N.; Wei, H.; Chen, H.-Y.; Wong, H.S.P.; Mitra, S. Carbon nanotube computer. *Nature* **2013**, *501*, 526–530. [CrossRef] [PubMed]

64. Franklin, A.D.; Tulevski, G.S.; Han, S.-J.; Shahrjerdi, D.; Cao, Q.; Chen, H.-Y.; Wong, H.S.P.; Haensch, W. Variability in carbon nanotube transistors: Improving device-to-device consistency. *ACS Nano* **2012**, *6*, 1109–1115. [CrossRef] [PubMed]
65. Liu, W.; Hierold, C.; Haluska, M. Electrical contacts to individual swcnts: A review. *Beilstein J. Nanotechnol.* **2014**, *5*, 2202–2215. [CrossRef] [PubMed]
66. Cao, Q.; Han, S.-J.; Tersoff, J.; Franklin, A.D.; Zhu, Y.; Zhang, Z.; Tulevski, G.S.; Tang, J.; Haensch, W. End-bonded contacts for carbon nanotube transistors with low, size-independent resistance. *Science* **2015**, *350*, 68–72. [CrossRef] [PubMed]
67. Collins, P.G.; Fuhrer, M.S.; Zettl, A. 1/f noise in carbon nanotubes. *Appl. Phys. Lett.* 2000, *76*, 894–896. [CrossRef]
68. Lin, Y.-M.; Appenzeller, J.; Zhihong, C.; Avouris, P. Electrical transport and 1/f noise in semiconducting carbon nanotubes. *Phys. E* **2007**, *37*, 72–77. [CrossRef]
69. Bronson, J.E.; Fei, J.; Hofman, J.M.; Gonzalez, R.L., Jr.; Wiggins, C.H. Learning rates and states from biophysical time series: A bayesian approach to model selection and single-molecule fret data. *Biophys. J.* **2009**, *97*, 3196–3205. [CrossRef] [PubMed]
70. Reuel, N.F.; Bojo, P.; Zhang, J.; Boghossian, A.A.; Ahn, J.-H.; Kim, J.-H.; Strano, M.S. Norse: Noise reduction and state evaluator for high-frequency single event traces. *Bioinformatics* **2012**, *28*, 296–297. [CrossRef] [PubMed]
71. Chung, S.H.; Kennedy, R.A. Forward-backward nonlinear filtering technique for extracting small biological signals from noise. *J. Neurosci. Methods* **1991**, *40*, 71–86. [CrossRef]
72. Akhterov, M.V.; Choi, Y.; Olsen, T.J.; Sims, P.C.; Iftikhar, M.; Gul, O.T.; Corso, B.L.; Weiss, G.A.; Collins, P.G. Observing lysozyme closing and opening motions by high-resolution single molecule enzymology. *ACS Chem. Biol.* **2015**, *10*, 1495–1501. [CrossRef] [PubMed]
73. Derbyshire, V.; Freemont, P.; Sanderson, M.; Beese, L.; Friedman, J.; Joyce, C.; Steitz, T. Genetic and crystallographic studies of the 3′,5′-exonucleolytic site of DNA polymerase I. *Science* 1988, *240*, 199–201. [CrossRef] [PubMed]
74. Aposhian, H.V.; Kornberg, A. Enzymatic synthesis of deoxyribonucleic acid 9. The Polymerase formed after T2 bacteriophage infection of *Escherichia coli*—A new enzyme. *J. Biol. Chem.* **1962**, *237*, 519–525. [PubMed]
75. Joyce, C.M. Techniques used to study the DNA polymerase reaction pathway. *Biochim. Biophys. Acta Proteins Proteom.* **2010**, *1804*, 1032–1040. [CrossRef] [PubMed]
76. Allen, D.J.; Benkovic, S.J. Resonance energy-transfer measurements between substrate binding-sites within the large (klenow) fragment of *Escherichia-coli* DNA-polymerase-I. *Biochemistry* 1989, *28*, 9586–9593. [CrossRef] [PubMed]
77. Christian, T.D.; Romano, L.J.; Rueda, D. Single-molecule measurements of synthesis by DNA polymerase with base-pair resolution. *Proc. Natl. Acad. Sci. USA* **2009**, *106*, 21109–21114. [CrossRef] [PubMed]
78. Schwartz, J.J.; Quake, S.R. Single molecule measurement of the "speed limit" of DNA polymerase. *Proc. Natl. Acad. Sci. USA* **2009**, *106*, 20294–20299. [CrossRef] [PubMed]
79. Torella, J.P.; Holden, S.J.; Santoso, Y.; Hohlbein, J.; Kapanidis, A.N. Identifying molecular dynamics in single-molecule fret experiments with burst variance analysis. *Biophys. J.* **2011**, *100*, 1568–1577. [CrossRef] [PubMed]
80. Santoso, Y.; Joyce, C.M.; Potapova, O.; Le Reste, L.; Hohlbein, J.; Torella, J.P.; Grindley, N.D.F.; Kapanidis, A.N. Conformational transitions in DNA polymerase I revealed by single-molecule fret. *Proc. Natl. Acad. Sci. USA* **2010**, *107*, 715–720. [CrossRef] [PubMed]
81. Markiewicz, R.P.; Vrtis, K.B.; Rueda, D.; Romano, L.J. Single-molecule microscopy reveals new insights into nucleotide selection by DNA polymerase I. *Nucleic Acids Res.* **2012**, *40*, 7975–7984. [CrossRef] [PubMed]
82. Gill, J.P.; Wang, J.; Millar, D.P. DNA polymerase activity at the single-molecule level. *Biochem. Soc. Trans.* **2011**, *39*, 595–599. [CrossRef] [PubMed]
83. Berezhna, S.Y.; Gill, J.P.; Lamichhane, R.; Millar, D.P. Single-molecule förster resonance energy transfer reveals an innate fidelity checkpoint in DNA polymerase I. *J. Am. Chem. Soc.* **2012**, *134*, 11261–11268. [CrossRef] [PubMed]
84. Kohlstaedt, L.A.; Wang, J.; Friedman, J.M.; Rice, P.A.; Steitz, T.A. Crystal-structure at 3.5 angstrom resolution of HIV-1 reverse-transcriptase complexed with an inhibitor. *Science* **1992**, *256*, 1783–1790. [CrossRef] [PubMed]

85. Johnson, S.J.; Taylor, J.S.; Beese, L.S. Processive DNA synthesis observed in a polymerase crystal suggests a mechanism for the prevention of frameshift mutations. *Proc. Natl. Acad. Sci. USA* **2003**, *100*, 3895–3900. [CrossRef] [PubMed]
86. Polesky, A.H.; Steitz, T.A.; Grindley, N.D.F.; Joyce, C.M. Identification of residues critical for the polymerase-activity of the klenow fragment of DNA-polymerase-I from *Escherichia-coli*. *J. Biol. Chem.* **1990**, *265*, 14579–14591. [PubMed]
87. Purohit, V.; Grindley, N.D.F.; Joyce, C.M. Use of 2-aminopurine fluorescence to examine conformational changes during nucleotide incorporation by DNA polymerase I (klenow fragment). *Biochemistry* **2003**, *42*, 10200–10211. [CrossRef] [PubMed]
88. Delagoutte, E. DNA polymerases: Mechanistic insight from biochemical and biophysical studies. *Front. Biosci. Landmark* **2012**, *17*, 509–544. [CrossRef]
89. Bryant, F.R.; Johnson, K.A.; Benkovic, S.J. Elementary steps in the DNA-polymerase-I reaction pathway. *Biochemistry* **1983**, *22*, 3537–3546. [CrossRef] [PubMed]
90. Kaushik, N.; Pandey, V.N.; Modak, M.J. Significance of the O-helix residues of *Escherichia coli* DNA polymerase I in DNA synthesis: Dynamics of the dNTP binding pocket. *Biochemistry* **1996**, *35*, 7256–7266. [CrossRef] [PubMed]
91. Joyce, C.M.; Potapova, O.; DeLucia, A.M.; Huang, X.; Basu, V.P.; Grindley, N.D.F. Fingers-closing and other rapid conformational changes in DNA polymerase I (klenow fragment) and their role in nucleotide selectivity. *Biochemistry* **2008**, *47*, 6103–6116. [CrossRef] [PubMed]
92. Johnson, S.; Cain, S. Bound on range precision for shot-noise limited ladar systems. *Appl. Opt.* **2008**, *47*, 5147–5154. [CrossRef] [PubMed]
93. Kong, X.; Nir, E.; Hamadani, K.; Weiss, S. Photobleaching pathways in single-molecule fret experiments. *J. Am. Chem. Soc.* **2007**, *129*, 4643–4654. [CrossRef] [PubMed]
94. Kuchta, R.D.; Mizrahi, V.; Benkovic, P.A.; Johnson, K.A.; Benkovic, S.J. Kinetic mechanism of DNA-polymerase-I (klenow). *Biochemistry* **1987**, *26*, 8410–8417. [CrossRef] [PubMed]
95. Dahlberg, M.E.; Benkovic, S.J. Kinetic mechanism of DNA-polymerase-I (klenow fragment)—Identification of a 2nd conformational change and evaluation of the internal equilibrium-constant. *Biochemistry* **1991**, *30*, 4835–4843. [CrossRef] [PubMed]
96. The fast motion of ions in the surrounding electrolyte contribute to the overall noise measured in dNTP-free buffer, but they do not produce $\Delta I(t)$ excursions in defect-free SWNTs.
97. Bermek, O.; Grindley, N.D.F.; Joyce, C.M. Prechemistry nucleotide selection checkpoints in the reaction pathway of DNA polymerase I and roles of glu710 and tyr766. *Biochemistry* **2013**, *52*, 6258–6274. [CrossRef] [PubMed]
98. Butler, J.M. *Forensic DNA Typing: Biology, Technology, and Genetics of Str Markers*, 2nd ed.; Academic Press: San Diego, CA, USA, 2010; p. 688.

10

Integrating Nanostructured Artificial Receptors with Whispering Gallery Mode Optical Microresonators via Inorganic Molecular Imprinting Techniques

G. Denise Hammond, Adam L. Vojta, Sheila A. Grant and Heather K. Hunt *

Department of Bioengineering, University of Missouri, Columbia, MO 65211, USA;
gdh52b@mail.missouri.edu (G.D.H.); alv5y2@mail.missouri.edu (A.L.V.); grantsa@missouri.edu (S.A.G.)
* Correspondence: hunthk@missouri.edu

Academic Editor: Ibrahim Abdulhalim

Abstract: The creation of label-free biosensors capable of accurately detecting trace contaminants, particularly small organic molecules, is of significant interest for applications in environmental monitoring. This is achieved by pairing a high-sensitivity signal transducer with a biorecognition element that imparts selectivity towards the compound of interest. However, many environmental pollutants do not have corresponding biorecognition elements. Fortunately, biomimetic chemistries, such as molecular imprinting, allow for the design of artificial receptors with very high selectivity for the target. Here, we perform a proof-of-concept study to show how artificial receptors may be created from inorganic silanes using the molecular imprinting technique and paired with high-sensitivity transducers without loss of device performance. Silica microsphere Whispering Gallery Mode optical microresonators are coated with a silica thin film templated by a small fluorescent dye, fluorescein isothiocyanate, which serves as our model target. Oxygen plasma degradation and solvent extraction of the template are compared. Extracted optical devices are interacted with the template molecule to confirm successful sorption of the template. Surface characterization is accomplished via fluorescence and optical microscopy, ellipsometry, optical profilometry, and contact angle measurements. The quality factors of the devices are measured to evaluate the impact of the coating on device sensitivity. The resulting devices show uniform surface coating with no microstructural damage with Q factors above 10^6. This is the first report demonstrating the integration of these devices with molecular imprinting techniques, and could lead to new routes to biosensor creation for environmental monitoring.

Keywords: molecularly imprinted polymers; Whispering Gallery Mode optical microresonators; optical biosensors; nanostructured thin films

---

1. Introduction

Environmental pollutants, and, in particular, emerging environmental pollutants, such as agricultural contaminants (pesticides, herbicides, *etc.*) and veterinary pharmaceutical by-products, represent one of the largest and most challenging classes of pollutant chemicals that can have a significant, detrimental impact on human health and the environment. For example, pesticides and herbicides are classified by Environmental Protection Agency as two of the most toxic classes of environmental pollutants [1–3]. One of the most dangerous effects of these pollutants is that they are capable of causing serious health problems, such as bone marrow disease, increased infertility, and increased instances of immunological and respiratory diseases, at relatively low prevalence [2–5]. Hence, it is essential to have an accurate method that is capable of trace detection of these pollutants in food and water systems. Currently, the primary method for detecting and identifying these pollutants is chromatography, including GC-MS and HPLC, which can accurately detect and identify these compounds from water samples extracted from the environment [6]. However, there are significant disadvantages to these methods that can interfere with adequate monitoring: for instance, the requirement for a library of data from high purity standards of all possible pollutants, the extensive sample preparation time needed, and the high equipment costs, in addition to the general lack of portability of these methods. Therefore, significant improvement is needed to address the ever-increasing complexity and pervasiveness of environmental pollutants in food and water systems.

Recently, biosensors, and in particular, optical biosensors, have been suggested as a possible alternative to chromatography-based techniques [7–9]. Optical biosensors have shown tremendous promise for numerous applications in medical diagnostics, and more recently, national security, and environmental monitoring applications [10–12]. In general, their utility arises from their non-destructive sample interrogation methods, their ability to perform extremely sensitive detection in liquid environments, and their high signal-to-noise ratios compared to other signal transduction methods, due to their relative immunity to the environment or system noise from electrical and mechanical sources [13]. Traditional optical sensors are typically labeled devices, which detect a label on the target of interest (such as fluorophores, enzymes, nanoparticles, *etc.*), rather than the target itself [14]. Label-free optical sensors can offer better device stability, quicker response, and potentially enhanced performance, particularly when tracking molecules whose behavior may change due to the presence of the label. Labels are typically used to increase the signal-to-noise ratio; label-free sensors have an inherently high signal-to-noise ratio, negating the need for a label. Many label-free optical sensors are refractometric sensors; that is, they function by detecting small changes in the effective refractive index of their optical field, which allows them to perform fast detection of minute changes in the refractive index of the optical field at the sensor surface/sample interface. These sensors, which include optical fiber sensors, Surface Plasmon Resonance (SPR) devices, and Whispering Gallery Mode (WGM) devices, have become increasingly popular due their speed, sensitivity, and label-free sensing properties [15,16]. Recently, a biosensing platform using an ultrahigh-Q microcavity has been reported for the detection of the Influenza A virus and polystyrene nanobeads. Although this method used a microtoroid platform, it can be applied to other type of WGM devices, such as silica microdisks and microspheres [17]. In this study, we focus specifically on silica microsphere WGM optical microresonators as the device of interest.

WGM optical microresonators are a type of circular resonant cavity device that confines light around their periphery via total internal reflection. WGM optical microresonators can be fabricated in a number of geometries, such as spheres, toroids, disks, and rings, both on-chip and free-standing [18]. In this study, we use silica microspheres of approximately 100 μm in diameter as the optical microresonator. Because of the low sorption of light by silica and their atomically smooth surface, these devices typically have very low loss, so that when light is coupled into these devices, it can circulate around these microspheres over 100,000 times [19,20]. While the light is reflected around the periphery of the device, it is not totally confined, but instead extends into the surrounding environment through the process of evanescence, allowing the field to interact with both the device surface and the surrounding environment [20]. Each time the optical field circulates around the device, it has an opportunity to interact with the environment, resulting in the amplification of the single-pass sensitivity that would be present if the device was linear. The photon lifetime in the resonator is measured by the Quality (Q) Factor of the device. A longer photon lifetime results in higher Q Factors. In sensing, the adsorption of an analyte onto the device's surface causes the circulating optical field to undergo a change in its effective refractive index, thus inducing a rapid and measurable shift in the resonant frequency of the circulating field. This is the fundamental basis for the sensing capabilities of WGM optical microresonators, as well as their inherently high sensitivity [21].

When these devices are paired with an appropriate recognition element, they are also capable of high *selectivity* detection and target identification [21–24]. Typically, these recognition elements will target a compound of interest through biological molecular recognition processes, such as antibody-antigen binding, hormone-receptor binding, *etc.* Previously, a number of routes to adding selectivity to label-free optical biosensors, such as WGM optical microresonators, has been explored. These routes include physical adsorption, the generation of self-assembled monolayers, the use of covalent binding (or other grafting-type approaches, including the use of inorganic-organic coupling agents, such as silane molecules, polymer brushes, *etc.*), and the generation of sandwich-type attachment using the streptavidin- biotin complex [21,24]. These have resulted in surfaces modified to present a number of different receptors, including nanoparticles [25–28], polymers [19], and a host of biological substances, including proteins, antibodies, oligonucleotides, *etc.* [21,29–32]. These devices, when integrated with the appropriate recognition element, have performed ultra-low detection of trypsin, thrombin, DNA, and streptavidin, among many others [24,33]. Recently, another method that includes a WGM-nanoshell hybrid resonator has been used to detect MS2, which is the smallest RNA virus. Further, the detection of the thyroid cancer marker, Thyroglobulin, and bovine serum albumin has been demonstrated with WGM-h microcavities that were created by adding a single gold nanoshell to the equator of the WGM resonator [34].

However, many biologically relevant compounds, including many emerging environmental pollutants, do not have correspondingly specific biorecognition elements. Fortunately, biomimetic chemistries, such as molecular imprinting, allow for the design of nanostructured, artificial receptors, based on shape, size, and functional group selectivity, that have greater stability than most biological recognition elements and the potential for very high selectivity [35,36]. The molecular imprinting technique offers a promising alternative to the use of traditional biorecognition elements, and has been used extensively for the development of high selectivity optical biosensors [23,35,37]. In general, artificial receptors created via the molecular imprinting of a target molecule are stable at a wide range of temperatures and pH, are typically less costly to create than natural biorecognition elements and easier to process, can be produced for almost any compound, and are significantly more compatible with the typical inorganic surfaces that comprise most label-free optical sensor surfaces than traditional biorecognition elements [36].

The first attempt of using Molecularly Imprinted Polymers (MIPs) as a recognition element for biosensors was made in 1992 [36]. Since that time, MIPs have become an important class of synthetic, nanostructured material whose ability to selectively adsorb and otherwise interact with a variety of compounds has seen use not only in sensing applications but also in chemical and biological separations [38,39]. The term molecular imprinting refers to Fischer's 'lock and key concept' [40], which explains the specific action of an enzyme with a single substrate, where the lock is the enzyme and key is the substrate. This theory helps to illustrate the specificity of enzymes towards a certain substrate. In addition, Pauling's 'production of antibodies *in vitro*' [41] and Dickey's 'specific adsorbents' [28] influenced the initial design of MIPs structures. However, "modern molecular imprinting was clearly established by Wulff and Mosbach, and their pioneering work has led to the current flourishing of molecular imprinting" [42]. Since then, the molecular imprinting technique has proven to be an effective technique for the creation of specific recognition sites in polymeric matrices.

The molecular imprinting technique is accomplished by polymerizing (typically organic) monomers in the presence of the target compound, which acts as a template around which the polymer network forms, and with which the network interacts. After polymerization, the template is removed from the polymer host network, resulting in a three-dimensional, nanostructured, porous polymeric network that theoretically is capable of reabsorbing the template molecule—and only the template molecule, due to the strong interactions between the template and host matrix. This process creates artificial recognition sites that have a high affinity for the template molecule [43].

MIPs created in this fashion can then be prepared in a variety of physical forms [44]. The traditional approach is to synthesize MIPs in bulk, then grind the resulting polymer and successively sieve the particles into the desired size ranges according to the specific application. Although this method is simple, the overall process is time-consuming and often produces non-uniform particles in terms or size or shape. Moreover, the grinding process might result in the destruction of some interaction sites, which reduces the material's loading capacity [45]. Generally, macro, micro, and nano-sized interaction sites are formed from the monomers simultaneously as a result of this process. Therefore, it is hard to optimize the binding properties of bulk MIPs [46]. An alternative approach is the creation of MIPs in thin layers (such as conformal coatings or thin films). Although both methods provide an imprinting effect, and result in reasonable specificity, and selectivity, thin layer MIPs result in significantly better outcomes in all areas [47]. Recently, the literature has reported the creation of membranes, *in situ* prepared monoliths, surface imprinting, and monolayers through a thin layer approach [48]. Additionally, bulk MIPs are challenging to appropriately integrate with a high-sensitivity optical signal transducer, which is usually quite sensitive to the impact of surface treatments on its overall performance. Therefore, if MIPs are to be integrated with a high sensitivity, label-free optical signal transducer, such as a Whispering Gallery Mode optical microresonator, a thin layer MIPs procedure will be required to obtain a well-adhered, conformal coating that does not negatively impact the underlying device performance. Previously, there have been studies demonstrating the coating of single layer of molecular gain media on WGM optical resonators [49,50]. However, this study represents a coating that is nanostructured and theoretically able to act as an artificial receptor and therefore able to respond selectively to various target molecules.

However, there are some challenges that exist in terms of integrating surface coatings with micro/nanoscale, often fragile, optical devices. Surface coatings applied to WGM optical microresonators may decrease the sensitivity due to damage the coating process may cause to their glass structure. In general, these devices do not respond well to traditional wet chemistry techniques, which significantly limits the approaches that may be taken to create a conformal coating of a nanostructured, polymeric network that can act as a source of artificial receptors. Furthermore, they often require inorganic-organic linkers in order to be bound to the surface to ensure good adhesion between the surface and the recognition element or the coating. Hence, in this study, the possibility of creating of an artificial receptor via the molecular imprinting technique using *inorganic silane* polymer precursors, which can covalently bond to the underlying silica device surface, is examined. The expected (and achieved) result is the creation of nanostructured, inorganic polymer that is compatible with and capable of good adhesion to the underlying device.

The choice of a target molecule (and, therefore, MIPs templating agent) was based upon the need to easily confirm its presence or absence using well-accepted techniques, such as microscopy and spectroscopy, and upon the requirement that it be reasonably sized, such that it can act as a model target for common environmental pollutants. Therefore, fluorescein isothiocyanate (FITC) was chosen as the target molecule, as it satisfies the aforementioned conditions. In order to promote adhesion and conformal coating to form an inorganic polymer network around the template, silane precursors were used. To ensure high quality coatings, different types of coating methods were examined, including dip coating by hand and via automation. In addition, different types of extraction methods were studied to determine an appropriately effective route to template removal. Optical performance of the devices was measured in term of Q factors, both before and after coating and template removal, which allowed the quantification of the impact of the coatings on the devices. This study represents the first example of pairing silica microsphere WGM optical resonators with molecularly imprinted polymers, and, in particular, an inorganic polymeric network. Therefore, it should serve as an initial guide for designing appropriate solutions for the detection of emerging environmental pollutants using artificial receptors.

2. Materials and Methods

2.1. Preparation of Whispering Gallery Mode Optical Microresonators and Control Surfaces

Microspheres were created by gravimetrically melting the tip of a stripped, single-mode optical fiber with a 25 W CO_2 laser (Synrad, 48-2) operating at 7%–10% power. Microspheres should be above 40 μm in diameter to minimize diffraction losses; typically, they are between 100 and 200 μm in diameter. The primary advantage of using the CO_2 laser for the fabrication of microspheres is that the resulting microsphere has an atomically smooth surface that is free of defects [51]. To achieve this, a small section of optical fiber (F-SC, Newport, CA, USA) is sliced to obtain a 4–7 cm length of fiber. On one end of the fiber, 1 cm of the protective coating is stripped off using a fiber stripper (No-Nik). The stripped portion is then cut down to approximately 2 mm with using a bare fiber cleaver. The prepared section of optical fiber is then cleaned with methanol using a Kimwipe to remove any loose protective coating. The optical fiber sample is then placed vertically into the path of the CO_2 laser by attaching the fiber to a 3-axis stage. The fiber is then located in the cameras used to image the microsphere screen by moving the stage via the Z-axis motor controller (ThorLabs, Newton, NJ, USA). When the stripped end of the fiber appears in the center of the screen, the laser is fired. Approximately 3 s into the lasing process, the tip of the fiber starts forming a liquid droplet. When the ideal shape is obtained, and no air bubbles are present inside the droplet, lasing is stopped, and the droplet solidifies into a microsphere (Figure 1).

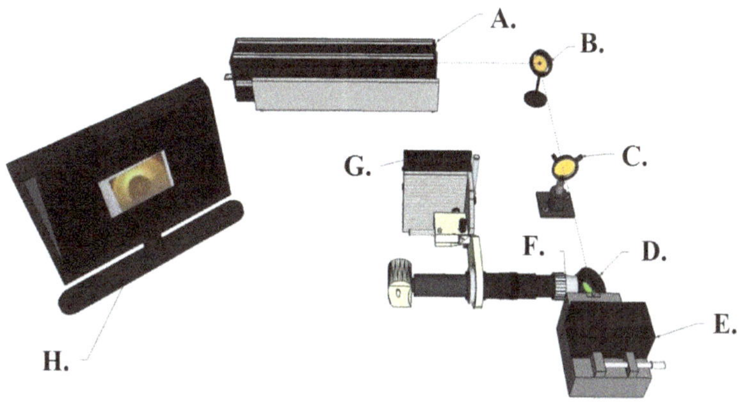

Figure 1. Schematic of the CO_2 laser setup used to produce silica microspheres of approximately 100 μm diameters. **A**—CO_2 Laser; **B**—Mirror; **C**—Focusing Lens; **D**—Beam Splitter; **E**—Sample Stage; **F**—Microscope; **G**—Microscope Alignment Block (2-axis Stage); **H**—Computer.

The fabricated microspheres are placed into Petri dishes that contain a glass slide prepared for microsphere storing. Double-sided scotch foam tape is cut and placed horizontally on one end of the normal-sized microscopic glass slide. The stems of the microspheres are then carefully placed onto the tape. Since the tape has a thickness about 1.5 mm, the stripped end/microsphere end of the optical fiber is lifted above the glass surface, preventing the microsphere from touching the container. This reduces the contamination or surface damage that might occur. The Petri dishes are then covered and placed in a humidity- and dust-controlled cabinet until further use [52].

Silica-on-silicon wafers served as controls to determine the quality of the resulting thin layer for techniques that do not work well with silica microspheres, such as ellipsometry. Prior to treatment, the silica surface was cleaned by submersion in a beaker containing C_3H_6O that was placed for 20 min in an ultrasonic bath (Elma, LC20H); this method of cleaning proved more effective than wiping the wafers with KimWipes using DDI H_2O (Fisher Scientific, Pittsburgh, PA, USA) and acetone (Fisher Scientific, 99.5%). After this initial cleaning, the silica surface of both the wafers and the as-fabricated silica microspheres was terminated with hydroxyl groups to improve adhesion and binding to the MIPs thin layer using literature procedures using either an O_2 plasma treatment (Plasma Etch, PE-50, 202 mTorr, 15 and 30 min) or a 70:30 H_2SO_4 (fuming, Sigma-Aldrich, St. Louis, MO, USA): H_2O_2 (30 wt %, Sigma-Aldrich) piranha etch for 45 min [53–55]. Immediately after the hydroxylation step, the samples were cleaned with DDI H_2O (Fisher Scientific, f.w. 18.02) and air-dried at room temperature for 1–24 h to remove water from the sample surface. Following drying, each silica wafer or microsphere was coated according to Section 2.3.

2.2. Characterization of the Optical Devices

Evaluation of the effect of the added artificial receptor coating on the device's Q factor is essential to determining the utility of coating and the coated device. In order to achieve this, the Q factors of the devices are measured before coating, after coating, and after template removal. To do this, light is coupled into the devices from a narrow linewidth, CW tunable laser centered at 980 nm (New Focus) via a tapered optical fiber waveguide. During testing, the device is monitored simultaneously with side and top view cameras ((Moticam 1000, 1.3 M pixel) to enable for precise coupling between the microresonator and the optical fiber waveguide. The device itself is held within a microsphere holder attached to a 3-axis nanopositioning stage (Optosigma, Santa Ana, CA, USA) used to control the position of the microsphere relative to the tapered optical fiber waveguide (Figure 2). Resonance linewidth data that are obtained from this test are recorded using a digitizer/oscilloscope card that is integrated with the computer; this data are then input into a custom LabVIEW program, which simultaneously controls the laser system and the oscilloscope. The quality factor of the WGM microresonator under study is calculated from the recorded data by performing a Lorentzian fit to the resonance peak and abstracting the center wavelength and full-width at half-maximum from the peak. The Q factor is then calculated via the formula $Q = \lambda/\Delta\lambda$. The Q-factor data are obtained three times for each device: prior to coating, after coating, and post extraction.

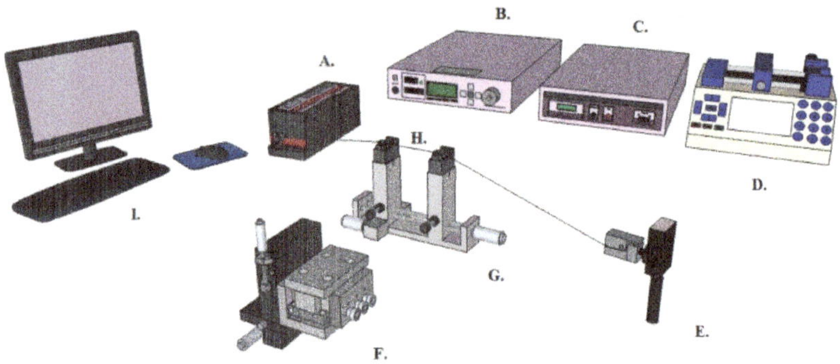

Figure 2. A model for the experimental setup used to determine the Q factors of the microspheres. **A**—Laser; **B**—Laser Controller; **C**—Stage Controller; **D**—Syringe Pump; **E**—Photo Detector; **F**—Nano-Positioning Stage; **G**—Taper Holder; **H**—Taper; **I**—Computer. Used with permission from Ref. [56].

2.3. Synthesis of MIPs

The molecular imprinting technique results in the production of a nanostructured, polymeric network that is formed around the template molecule. This process is composed of three main steps. The first step includes choosing the monomer based on its potential interactions with a template molecule. Afterward, these monomers are polymerized in the presence of template molecules as the second step. The final step involves removal of the template molecule from this complex leaving the molecularly imprinted polymer with a pocket or binding site of the relative shape and size of that template molecule (Figure 3). Intermolecular interactions like hydrogen bonding, dipole–dipole bonding, and ionic interactions between the template molecule and functional groups present in the final polymer matrix drive the molecular recognition phenomena [45]. Thus, the resultant polymeric network "recognizes" and binds selectively to the template molecules. Most of the time, acrylate and methacrylic monomers are used for the preparation of molecularly imprinted polymers [36].

In this study, FITC is used to identify the key points of making the desired artificial receptor that is compatible with the material, geometry, and transduction mechanism of the proposed sensing system. The procedure for synthesizing a molecularly imprinted silica network is generally as follows: silica sol-gels are created by mixing 5 mL ethanol (95%), 440 μL methyltriemethoxysilane (Sigma-Aldrich,

St. Louis, MO, USA, 99%), 14 μL aminopropyltriethoxysilane (Sigma-Aldrich, 98%), and 25 μL hydrochloric acid (HCL, 1 M, Sigma-Aldrich, 37%) in a glass beaker; the solution is stirred for 30 min at room temperature. 1.5 μL of a solution containing the template molecule is prepared by dissolving 1 mg FITC (Thermo Scientific) in 1 mL Dimethyl Sulfoxide (DMSO, Fisher Scientific, 99.9%), is then added to the solution, which is stirred for additional 1–2 min. The resulting sol is then coated onto either silica-on-silicon wafers or onto silica microspheres, via manual dip coating or automated dip coating (Thor Labs). The coating is followed by aging at room temperature, under darkened conditions (so as to reduce photobleaching) for a certain amount of days, ranging from 1 to 10, to yield a thin layer of polymer adhered to the surface of either the control wafers or the silica microspheres.

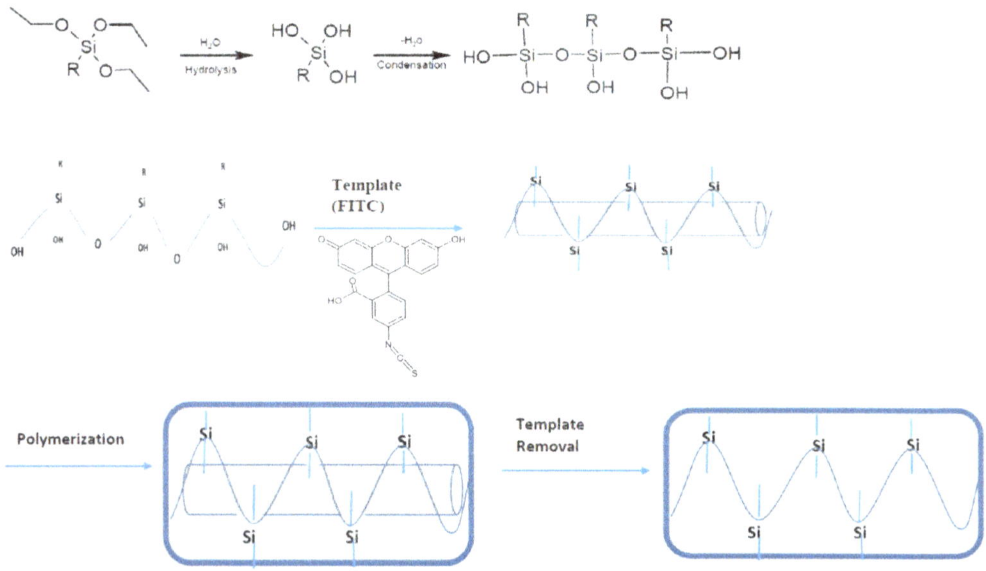

Figure 3. Molecularly Imprinting Technique using inorganic silanes as polymer precursors, and FITC as the template molecule. The silane precursors polymerize through hydrolysis and condensation reactions to form a three-dimensional, interconnected polymer network around the template.

2.4. Optimization of Microspheres

During this study, the sol-gel formation parameters were varied to obtain high quality thin films on the surface, while minimizing the structural damage to the WGM resonators. The two main parameters were the coating techniques and the aging times, as shown in Table 1. Two different coating methods were tested: automated dip coating and manual dip coating. The coating time, 45–50 s, was kept the same for both coating methods. One dip was used for each method, as multiple dips resulted in coating thicknesses beyond 100 nm, which has the potential to exceed the thickness of the coating that enables the entire coating to be within the evanescent tail region of the circulating optical field of the device.

Table 1. Summary of optimization parameters tested in order to maximize the performance of the WGM optical resonators.

Optimization Parameters	Tested Methods	
Coating	Automated dip coating	Manual dip coating
Aging Times	1–3 days aging	1–10 days aging
Extraction	Chemical extraction	Oxygen Plasma extraction

Another important parameter tested was the aging times of the silica sol-gels after they were coated onto the surface of interest. Fabricated optical devices were placed in Petri dishes as a group of 5. In the interest of observing the effect of aging time on the quality of the resulting coating on the devices, a range of aging times, from 1 day to 10 days, was tested. A total of 10 sets of silica microspheres was fabricated and then coated with molecularly imprinted silica sol-gels. Starting from day 1, each group was examined daily using Fluorescence Microscopy. Fluorescent images and measurements were obtained for each set of microspheres to determine the best aging time within the given range. Normalized Intensity values were obtained by the division of the average intensity value of the sphere to its area.

2.5. Extraction Procedure

As mentioned previously, the most important property of molecularly imprinted polymers is having specific binding sites for the target molecule. Typically, chemical extraction is the template removal method used with MIPs. Several chemical extraction parameters were tested and fluorescence intensity measurements were used to confirm extraction. Extraction Solution 1 was synthesized by combining the following chemicals: 4 mL Ethanol (95%), 1 mL Chloroform (Sigma-Aldrich, 99.5%), and 0.5 mL Acetic Acid (Sigma-Aldrich, 99.7%). An alternative solution (Solution 2) was prepared with 8 mL Ethanol (95%), 2 mL Acetonitrile (Sigma-Aldrich, 99.8%), and 1 mL Acetic Acid (Sigma-Aldrich, 99.7%). As shown in Table 2, two different extraction solutions, Solution 1 and Solution 2, as well as different stage conditions (stationary *versus* run on a tilt-tray) were analyzed.

Table 2. Summary of the type of extraction solutions used and the parameters tested for each solution.

Extraction Solution	Chemicals Used	Extraction Stage	Extraction Time
Solution 1	4 mL Ehanol, 1 mL Chloroform, 0.5 mL Acetic Acid	Tilt-tray, Stationary	24 h
Solution 2	8 mL Ethanol, 2 mL Acetonitrile, 1 mL Acetic Acid	Tilt-tray, Stationary	24 h

A total of 4 Petri dishes were used (20 microspheres) in the extraction analysis. For each Petri dish, a different extraction solution and a stage condition was tested, resulting in a total of four extraction methods that were examined. Table 3 summarizes this information.

Table 3. Summary of extraction procedure. Dish 10, Dish 21, Dish 18 and Dish 19 were used for this procedure. Extraction time, 24 h, and extraction temperature, room temperature was kept constant for all conditions.

Petri Dish ID	Sphere	Stage Condition	Extraction Solution
Dish 10	1–5	Tilt-Tray	1
Dish 18	1–5	Stationary	2
Dish 19	1–5	Stationary	2
Dish 21	1–5	Tilt-Tray	1

It was essential for the tips of the microspheres to be submersed in the extraction solution without touching the bottom of the container (to avoid microstructural damage). Thus, microsphere holders were used for stabilizing the positions of microspheres. A microsphere holder was made by inserting 8 very thin metal tubes (1–2 cm length) into a rubber stopper (Figure 4). After inserting microspheres through this tube, the rubber stopper was placed on top of the Erlenmeyer flask containing the extraction solution of interest; the flask was covered with aluminum foil.

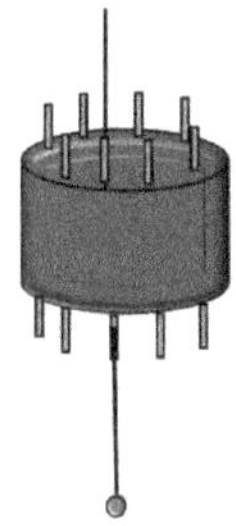

Figure 4. Schematic of a microsphere holder holding a single microsphere. This rubber stopper may then be placed inside a glass jar, suspending the microspheres in the solution without touching the side of the jars. This minimizes the possibility of damaging the microspheres due to handling. Up to eight microspheres may be suspended at once, although only one is shown here.

2.6. Characterization of the Surface Coatings

Surface characterization of the coated wafers and silica microspheres was carried out using an Olympus IX70 inverted fluorescence microscope with an ORCA digital camera (Hamahatsu), before coating, after coating, post-template removal, and post-re-uptake of the template. Surface roughness of the thin layers on the wafers was evaluated using a Vecco NT 9109 optical profilometer using a PSI scan at 40× magnification and 0.5× field of view. To confirm the thickness of the coating on the wafers, ellipsometry was performed using a J. A. Woollam ellipsometer. A scan from 500 to 600 nm in intervals of 2 nm at angles of 65 and 75 degrees was performed; modeling via the Cauchy equations yielded an average thickness of the layer. Lastly, contact angle measurements were gathered from the wafers using a Ramé-Hart Model 200 Standard Contact Angle Goniometer for each the cleaned, hydroxylated, and coated wafers.

Further analysis of the microsphere coatings, and in particular, the loading capacity for FITC, was made with Ultraviolet-Visible Spectroscopy (Shimadzu, Columbia, MD, USA UV-2401). To be able to understand the coating chemistry, the initial sol-gel solution containing the template molecule FITC was analyzed before and after coating the microspheres to determine the concentration of FITC on the microspheres using the Beer-Lambert relation.

A set of 5 microspheres were fabricated and the silica sol-gel solution containing the template molecule was also synthesized. The calculated concentration for the MIPs solution containing the template was 15.2 M. In the first step, 1–1.5 mL of ethanol (Fisher Scientific, 95%) was added to the reference cuvette and the sample cuvette. This step was needed to create the baseline for the background, and ethanol was chosen as the baseline due to having a relatively high concentration in the solution mixture. After the initial spectra of the background solution was obtained, the second cuvette was emptied, cleaned, and refilled with 1–1.5 mL of the aforementioned MIPs solution. This step provided the spectroscopic data for the solution prior to coating. Next, the microspheres were coated using the MIPs solution, and after the coating was complete, MIPs solution that remained after the coating was analyzed in the second cuvette as before.

3. Results

In this study, we have used a series of microspheres to test different coating parameters and conditions. Table 4 below, shows a summary of samples utilized and the coating parameters to which they were subjected.

Table 4. Summary of spheres used in this study and their identifications along with tested parameters. All the spheres in a Petri dish were treated exactly the same way as the other spheres in the particular Petri dish.

Microsphere ID		Coating Conditions		Extraction Conditions			
Petri Dish	Spheres	Coating Method	Aging Time	Extraction Method	Extraction Solution	Extraction Stage	Extraction Time
Dish 1	1–5	Manual	3 days	NA	NA	NA	NA
Dish 3	1–5	Manual	8 days	NA	NA	NA	NA
Dish 4	1–5	Manual	9 days	NA	NA	NA	NA
Dish 5	1–5	Manual	10 days	NA	NA	NA	NA
Dish 9	1–3	Uncoated	NA	NA	NA	NA	NA
Dish 10	1–5	Automated	3 days	Chemical	Solution 1	Tilt-Tray	24 h
Dish 12	1–3	Manual	10 days	O_2 Plasma	NA	NA	2 h
Dish 13	1–5	Automated	1 days	NA	NA	NA	NA
Dish 14	1–5	Automated	1 days	NA	NA	NA	NA
Dish 17	1–5	Manual	5 days	NA	NA	NA	NA
Dish 18	1–5	Manual	6 days	Chemical	Solution 2	Stationary	24 h
Dish 19	1–5	Manual	7 days	Chemical	Solution 2	Stationary	24 h
Dish 20	1–5	Manual	3 days	NA	NA	NA	NA
Dish 21	1–5	Manual	3 days	Chemical	Solution 1	Tilt-tray	24 h
Dish 22	1–5	Manual	3 days	O_2 Plasma	NA	NA	15 min
Dish 23	1–5	Manunal	3 days	O_2 Plasma	NA	NA	30 min

Please note: NA: not applicable.

3.1. *Characterization of the Uncoated Optical Devices*

The microspheres in Dish 9 were tested to obtain typical Q-factor values of the bare spheres used in the project; these spheres were considered controls. All three microspheres had a Q factor value of 10^7 magnitude, as expected, with an average Q factor of 1.241×10^7. An example Q factor result for Dish 9, Sphere 1 is shown in Figure 5. It is important for optical devices to have high Q factor values before applying the MIPs coating so that, even if the coating decreases the Q factor, a good Q factor (typically defined as $>10^6$, the lower limit for performing single molecule detection [57]) can still be obtained. Note that, with precise control of intrinsic device losses, such as material absorption (which is set when the wavelength and material are chosen), scattering (based on the quality of the surface and the presence of scattering sites), radiation (due to the curvature of the devices), *etc.*, intrinsic Q factors above 10^7 can be attained [18]. In this study, the extrinsic Q factors devices were in the 10^7 range, likely due to extrinsic losses from coupling.

3.2. *Optimization of Microsphere Coating*

Devices fabricated in this study were initially designed to target the FITC molecule. In order to create artificial receptors for this fluorescent dye, which exhibits a polyaromatic ring structure, we adapted the well-understood methods that are used to create MIPs for nitroaromatic explosives, which are of similar size and polyaromaticity. These methods were analyzed and transformed to allow for the production of inorganic silica sol-gel nanostructured coatings [58,59].

Here, we used two different silane monomers, and we evaluated the impacts of aging time and coating methods on the resulting quality of the coatings, as determined by Fluorescence Microscopy. Once the coating method was optimized, the aging time was analyzed. The aging window was expanded from 1 to 3 days to 1 to 10 days. The best aging time within this range was found according to the best normalized fluorescence intensity results (normalized as intensity per area under analysis, to allow for more accurate comparison between spheres and methods), which is discussed in Section 3.2.2. The template removal procedure was then investigated. Two different removal methods were tested: chemical extraction and oxygen plasma degradation. While chemical extraction is the typical template removal process for MIPs devices, it is a wet procedure, which can damage the microspheres. Template removal via oxygen plasma degradation, on the other hand, has been shown to work well with these devices, and does not require wet chemistry techniques [60]. Moreover, since oxygen plasma typically only degrades the organic molecule for the short time periods we evaluated, it is able to leave the silica coating intact, although it is likely that it will increase the formation of silanol groups on the surface. For the chemical extraction procedure, two different stage conditions and two different solutions were analyzed. Once the parameters were optimized, the best procedures for coating, aging, and extraction were applied to the control group of microspheres, which were tested at each coating step for their Q factor, as discussed previously.

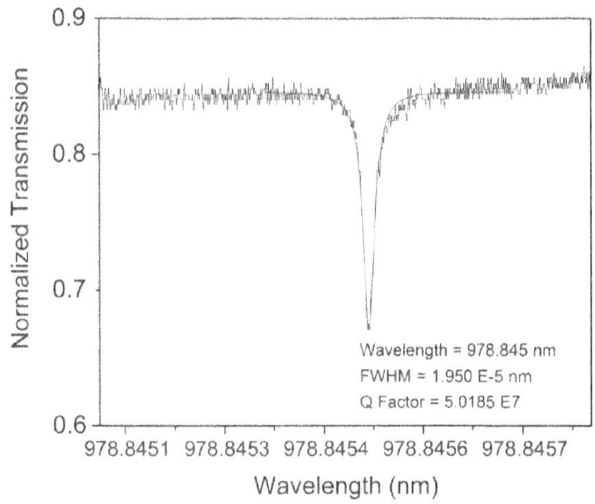

Figure 5. Q factor results of Dish 9 Sphere 1 (uncoated). Q Factors for the Dish 9 Spheres yielding consistent and high results above 10^6 Q-factor measurements. The figure depicts a peak with the Lorentzian fit (**red** line) used to determine the center wavelength and full-width at half-maximum of the peak.

3.2.1. Coating Methods

We first evaluated the coating method (automated *versus* manual dip coating) to determine which resulted in higher-quality conformal coatings. Interestingly (and unexpectedly), switching from automated dip coating to manual dip coating led to a significant improvement in the coating results, as quantified by the optical and fluorescence microscopy images obtained. We surmise this was due to the rough/jerky start and stop of the coating equipment used, compared to the ability to finesse the coating by hand. Using manual dip coating, we were able to thoroughly control and consistently apply a conformal coating to the surfaces of the microspheres.

The results of this method are shown in Figure 6, which displays the uneven coating around the optical device (Figure 6a). On the other hand, manual dip coating results in a much better finish and even coating (Figure 6b). Images are taken with Olympus Widefield Fluorescence Microscopy. Therefore, the manual dip coating provides significantly better coating around the device than automated dip coating.

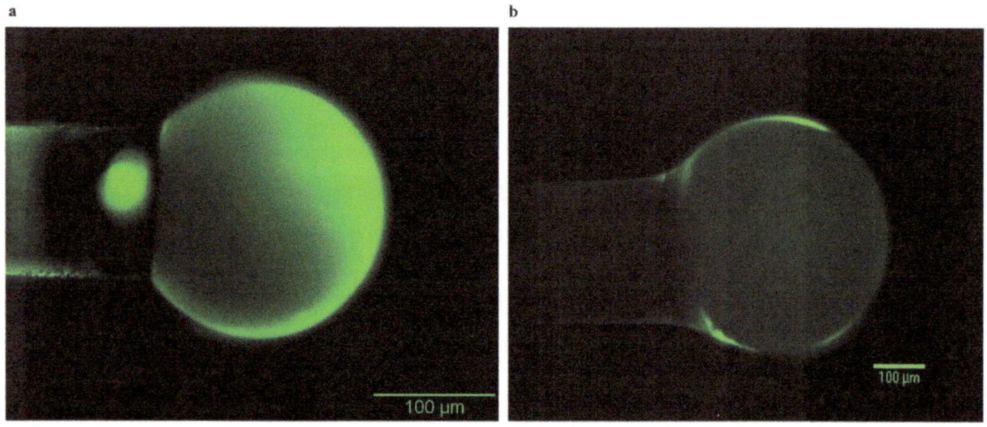

Figure 6. Dip coating methods applied to coat molecularly imprinted solution on the optical devices. (**a**) The result of the automated dip coating method, showing uneven saturation, and some microstructural damage (image from Dish 14 Sphere 30); (**b**) The result of the manual dip coating method shows uniform coating around the device (image taken from Dish 20 Sphere 4).

3.2.2. Aging Times

The result of this study showed that the optimum aging times for the microspheres was either 3 or 10 days (Figure 7). The fluorescence intensity measurements were the most important factors to determine the aging time. It was also observed that the fluorescence intensity generally decreased over the time until day 7 and then increased thereafter. Three days of aging was selected as the best parameter, due to its consistency and its shorter time-frame.

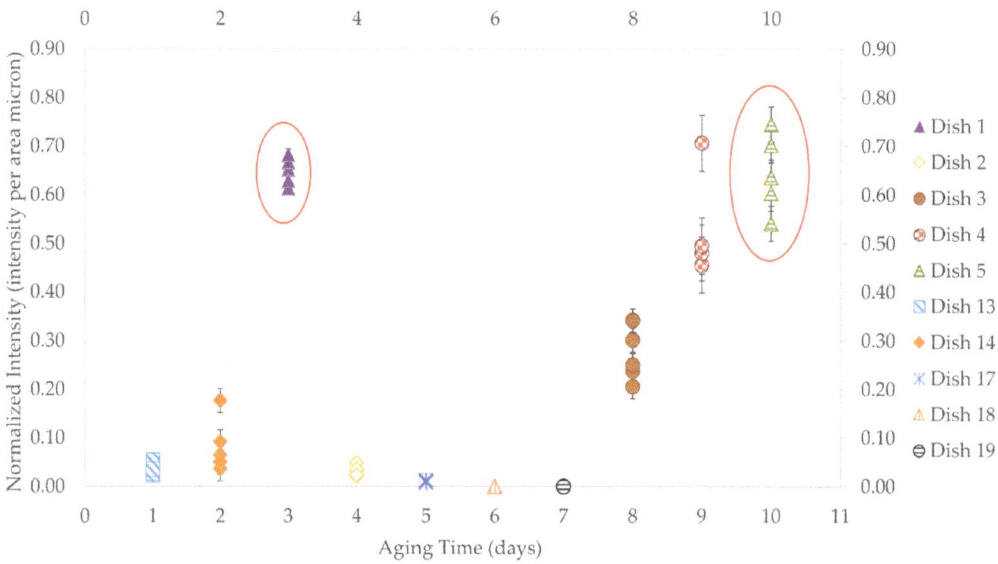

Figure 7. Normalized intensity *vs.* aging time. Each analyzed day includes a Petri dish that contains five coated microspheres. Day 3 and Day 10 shows the optimum results for MIPs coating procedure. Day 3 was chosen as it resulted in a more consistent normalized intensity and a shorter time-frame.

3.2.3. Template Removal Procedure

It is expected that after the template removal, the fluorescence intensity exhibited by the coated microspheres will decrease. Early tests using Solutions 1 and 2 showed poor extraction results.

Therefore, different parameters were tested to determine if the results could be improved. Two different extraction solutions, as well as two different stage conditions, were analyzed. Dish 10 was extracted with using Solution 1 and was placed on the tilt-tray (VWR incubating rocker), whereas, Dish 18, which was placed in the same extraction solution, was kept stationary. Moreover, Dish 21 was extracted using Solution 2 and was kept on the tilt tray during the extraction time. On the other hand, Dish 19 was kept stationary while being extracted with Solution 2 as well. Extraction time, 24 h, and reaction temperature, room temperature, were held constant for all conditions. The results, shown in Figure 8, suggest that there is an increase in the fluorescence intensity after the extraction procedure, which indicates that the extraction was not successful. This might have resulted from contamination that could have occurred during wet chemistry techniques (for instance, the molecules could have been extracted, and then re-absorbed onto the surface). Any extra residue that cannot be extracted via extraction solutions can cause increase in the fluorescent intensity. No significant difference was observed between Solution 1 and Solution 2 extractions.

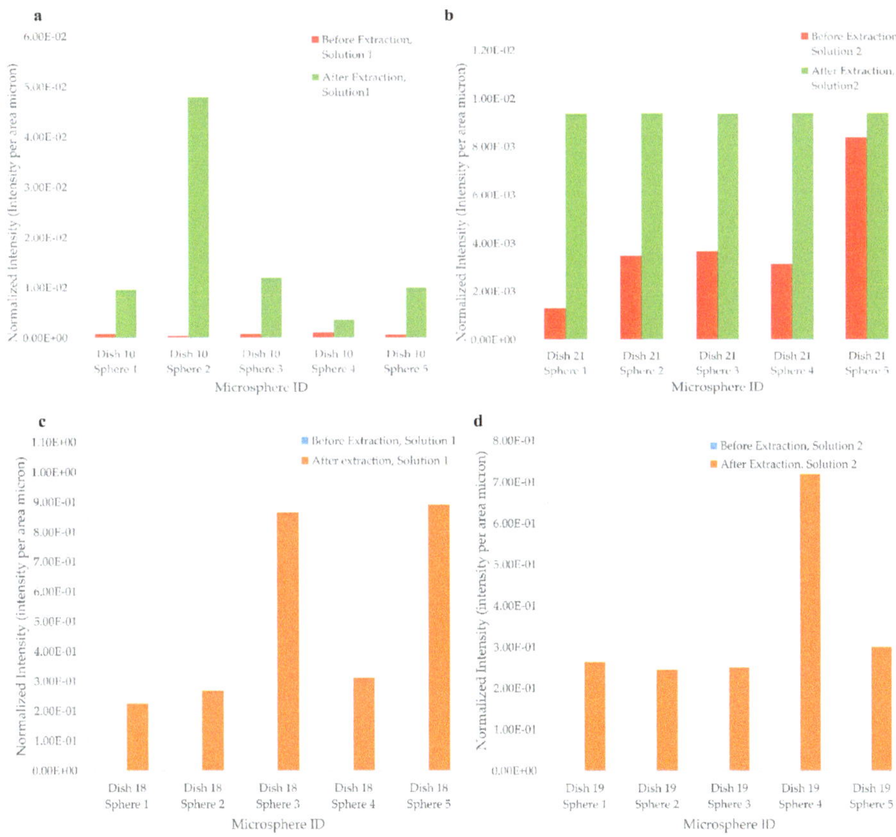

Figure 8. Results of the template removal via chemical extraction. Two different parameters, stage condition, and different solutions were tested. (**a**) and (**b**) shows the results for the tilt tray condition applied to Dish 10 and Dish 21; (**c**) and (**d**) shows the results for the stationary condition applied to Dish 18 and Dish 19. Chemical extraction results were not as expected; in fact, an increase in the fluorescence intensity measurements was observed. Therefore, several extraction parameters and different extraction methods were analyzed. Please note that, in figures (**c**) and (**d**), the pre-extraction data were so low in comparison, they do not show on the graphs.

The next step was to perform a template removal procedure using O_2 plasma treatment. During this treatment, oxygen gas is introduced into the chamber. Like other forms of plasma, oxygen cleans organics and is capable of surface modification. Fortunately, the template molecule will be able to leave the MIPs complex intact, since it does not interact with inorganic surfaces as it does with organic materials.

Oxygen plasma treatment, on the other hand, yielded better results, with significantly less risk of microstructural damage. Treatment parameters were varied until the best removal extent was measured; these parameters are presented in the Materials and Methods section. Figures 9 and 10 show the results of this study. Although some FITC is still present in the template-removed coating, that is expected, as it is likely that the FITC closest to the sphere in the coating may be difficult to access via the oxygen plasma treatment, since the network of "pockets" for the template is not necessarily interconnected. Regardless, removal of the surface FITC will allow open pockets for template/target reabsorption.

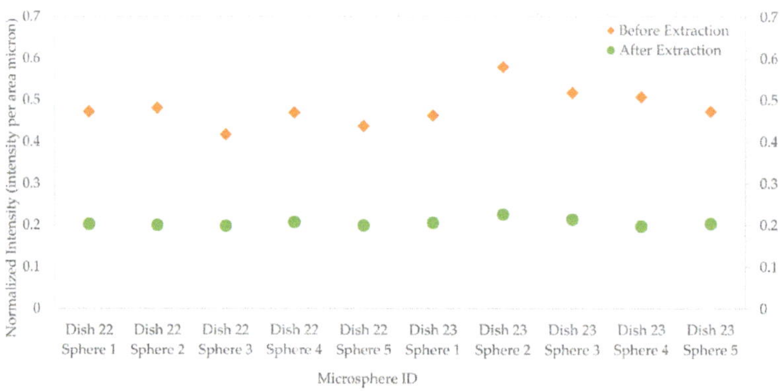

Figure 9. The result of normalized intensity values before and after the Oxygen plasma treatment taken from two Petri dishes, 22 and 23. Each Petri dish contains 5 spheres that are labeled with numbers for identification. A decrease in the normalized intensity is observed after the treatment suggesting that the template has been removed.

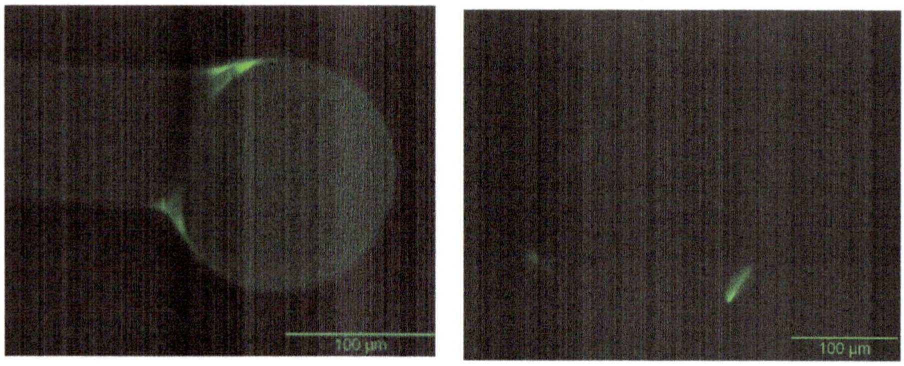

(a) (b)

Figure 10. Images were taken from Dish 23 Sphere 3. Visible difference in the fluorescence intensity between two phases. (**a**) Pre-extraction; (**b**) Post-extraction. This particular image showed 59% loss in the intensity value after the extraction. The average intensity loss for this data set was calculated as 58%.

3.2.4. Q Factor Measurements

Quality factors of the devices also represent significant evidence about the potential device performance. Previously, Q-factor values of uncoated spheres are presented which were recorded to be on average on the order of 10^7. Figure 11 represents a sample Q-factor taken from coated microspheres both before and after template removal. Both graphs had a Q-factor that was higher than 10^6 magnitude. These results show promising data in terms of using these devices in the further analysis. Figure 12 shows the results over all the spheres tested with the selected "best" parameters, and the impact of the coating on the Q factors.

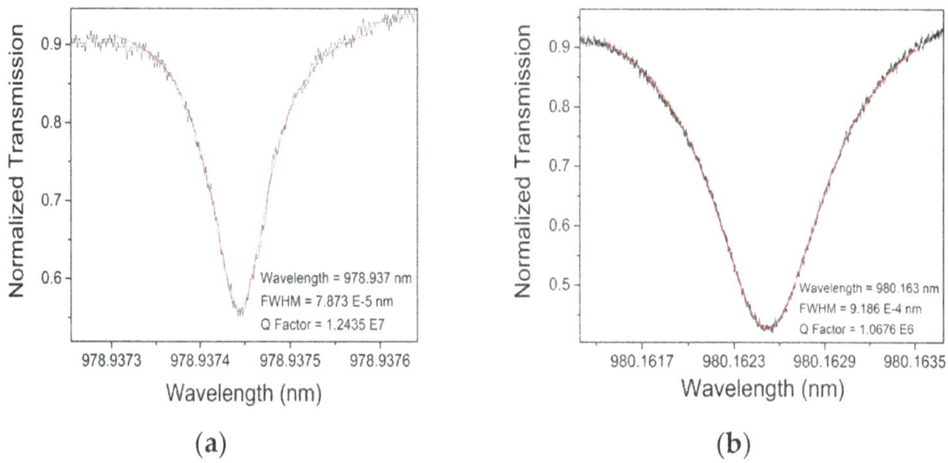

Figure 11. Q Factor graphs taken from a coated sphere before and after the extraction process. (**a**) depicts the fundamental peak of a coated sphere with a Lorentzian fit curve; the Q factor obtained was 1.243×10^6; (**b**) depicts a similar peak on the same sphere following extraction via O_2 plasma; its Q factor was 1.006×10^6. Please note that the values given on the graph represent the direct output of the fitting and do not take into account the precision of the equipment. Transmission data (mW) were normalized based on the initial transmission of the laser.

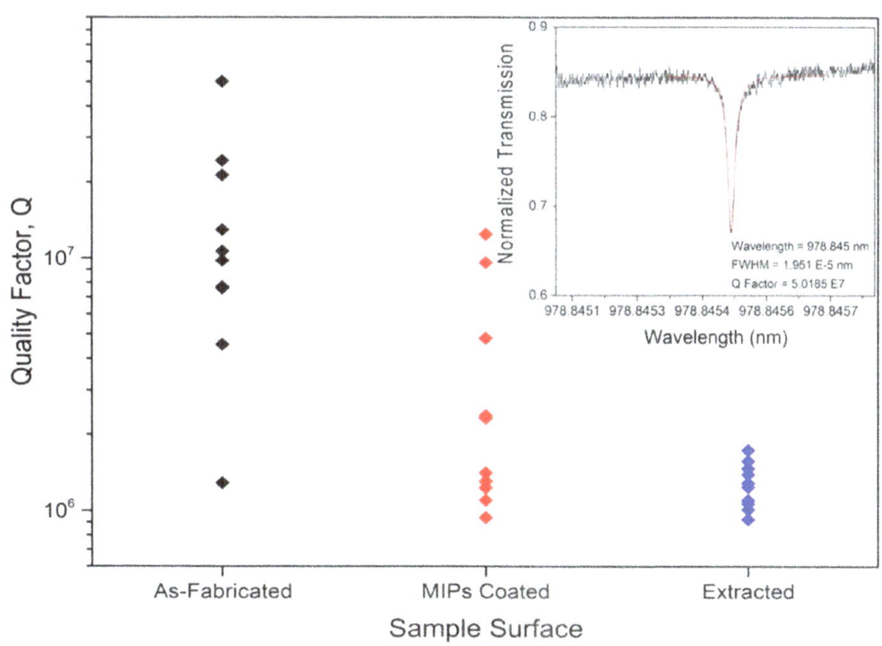

Figure 12. Q factors of all 10 spheres from Dish 22 and 23 taken as-fabricated, MIPs coated, and after the extraction process. The inset depicts the fundamental peak of an as-fabricated sphere with a Lorentzian fit curve; the Q factor was 5.0185×10^7. As you can see the Q factor decreases at with each step in the procedure; and interestingly with a decrease in Q factor but less deviation after extraction.

3.3. UV-VIS Analysis

Through calculations of the absorption spectra, it was calculated that there was a 0.0008244-mole difference between pre and post-coating. This coating procedure involved 10 spheres in total, thus, the number of molecules ending up in the polymer network coating each sphere was approximately 4.965×10^{19} molecules of FITC, which represents the total FITC loading in the coating. On average, 58% template removal was obtained. One particular set, Dish 12, showed 73% template loss, resulting in uptake capacity of 3.62×10^{19} molecules of FITC per device. It is important to note that some of the MIPs coating also binds to a small portion of the microsphere stem, and thus the number of molecules coating each sphere itself would be some factor smaller. From fluorescence imaging, the normalized intensity could be found for all the parameters including the background intensity of the MIPs coating without the FITC template, the 3 and 10-day aging sets, post extraction, and finally reuptake of the template. Each set of measurements were averaged and their differences used to draw conclusions about the behavior and effect of the coating, extraction, and reuptake process (Table 5). This particular set, Dish 12 was extracted for 2 h using Oxygen plasma treatment.

Table 5. Summary of different fluorescence parameters tested and their results.

Fluorescence Parameters	Normalized Intensity
Autofluorescence	0.193
3 Day Aging	0.648
10 Day Aging	0.645
Post Extraction	0.031
Reuptake	0.332

These results show the normalized intensity for each step. Of note is the autofluorescence intensity from the MIPs solution without the FITC template and then the near total loss of fluorescence after O_2 plasma extraction. The reuptake average is much lower than the initial coating measurements; however the loss of the autofluorescence intensity could be a large factor in this decrease.

3.4. Control Groups—Surface Quality of the Conformal Coatings

Surface roughness was calculated using a Vecco NT 9109 optical profilometer. Tests yielded consistent results across all parameters with an average surface roughness of 44 nm (Figure 13). Ellipsometry was performed to confirm the thickness of the coating on the wafers and an average of 70 nm was observed. Note that any increase in roughness of the microresonator's surface will result in a direct decrease in the intrinsic quality factor that can be obtained from that microresonator. According to the work of Rahachou and Zozoulenko, quality factor reductions from theoretical values may arise due to geometrical imperfection, inhomogeneity in the microresonator in terms of material properties, *etc.* They focus specifically on the impact of surface roughness as an aspect of geometrical imperfection, showing that in the roughness range we report, high Q resonances will typically decrease by half an order of magnitude, which is similar to what is seen in this work [61]. Moreover, contact angle measurements were used and consistent measurements were obtained across all aging and hydroxylation parameters with an average contact angle of $73.16° \pm 6.06°$.

Piranha treatment has the possibility of being too harsh in terms of temperature and acid strength with respect to the structural and surface integrity of the devices. As an alternative, O_2 plasma, which is typically used for cleaning residue from surfaces, is simple, minimizes device handling, and does not require post-treatment to remove excess water from the surface. On the other hand, O_2 plasma treatment might not yield as high of a surface hydroxyl density as piranha etching, causing a lower adhesion of the coating to the surface. Therefore, it was important to identify which route is most compatible. In the end, O_2 plasma treatment was chosen for such ease as no significant difference in measurements occurred between it and piranha etching.

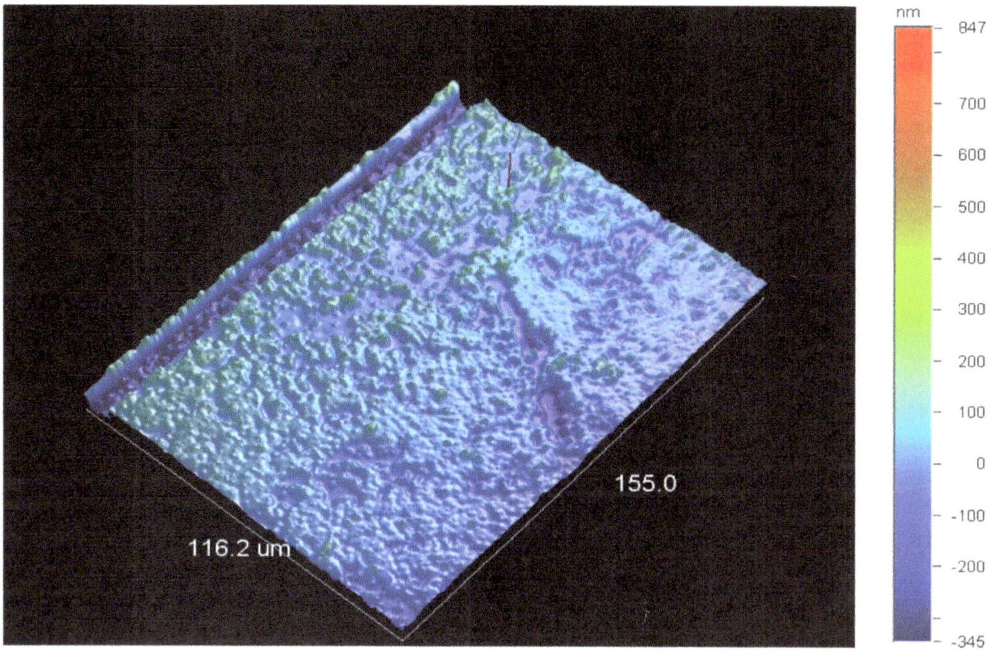

Figure 13. 3D Image is taken using optical profilometry with 40.89 magnification and PSI measurement mode. Surface statistics for the sample shown: Ra = 50.14 nm, Rq = 75.29 nm, 1192.44 nm.

4. Discussion and Conclusions

Whispering Gallery Mode optical devices fabricated in this study were initially designed to target the FITC molecule. In order to create artificial receptors for this fluorescent dye, a molecular imprinting technique was used. Integration of the artificial receptors with WGM resonators was the primary challenge; therefore, the primary goal of this study was to demonstrate the creation of a thin, uniform coating on the surface of the microresonators that was templated by and for FITC, while keeping underlying transducer undamaged. To achieve this goal, a thin film (<100 nm) is necessary to ensure that the coating, and any sorption interactions that could occur, remain within the evanescent tail of the device. The active region of the evanescent tail for devices that have a diameter of 50–100 μm is around 100 nm [62,63].

One of the challenges in this study was the selection of appropriate solvents in order to create the inorganic polymer network. However, by using prior literature results for both the creation of silica sol-gels and for the creation of organic MIPs for explosives detection, we were able to identify both good pre-cursors as well as solvents that interacted well and allowed the FITC molecule to still fluoresce. Once the solvents were selected as silica precursors, molecularly imprinted polymer synthesis studies were established. Artificial receptors with on-chip silica microsphere WGM resonators are created by gravimetrically melting the tip of an optical fiber with CO_2 laser. Two of the most important key points during the microspheres production were having no air bubbles inside the device and obtaining a high Q factor. Several parameters were observed and tested during MIPs procedure in order to acquire the best quality coatings. The results showed that manually dip coating was the best selection in order to obtain a uniform coating around the sphere. The optimum aging time was determined as 3 days and 10 days; 3 days was selected due to its shorter time-frame. The template extraction method that gave the desired results was the oxygen plasma treatment, varying from 15 min to 2 h. Oxygen plasma treatment successfully removed a significant portion of the template molecule, which is confirmed by the difference between pre-extraction and post-extraction fluorescence intensity values. Furthermore, early extraction results suggested that the non-templated MIPs solution tends to auto-fluoresce. Therefore, it is important to take intensity readings without giving much time for the polymerization complex to auto-fluoresce. Otherwise, the extraction result is not verifiable since post-extraction intensity values might be higher than the pre-extraction values, which indicate that extraction might have been unsuccessful. Uptake of the template molecule after the extraction was confirmed via fluorescence intensity measurements. Finally, silica wafers were used as control groups to support the findings of the optimization studies. The results of the same procedures applied on silica wafers also proved that selected factors were the most appropriate.

The fundamental goal of this work is the creation of novel, highly sensitive and highly selective label-free optical sensor platforms that can be used to detect harmful environmental chemicals in trace quantities. The long-term goal of this work is to develop a generic, robust biosensor platform that can be arrayed to address multiple environmental pollutants, such as herbicides and pesticides, through minor adjustments to the artificial receptors.

Acknowledgments: The authors would like to acknowledge Alexander Jurkevich for his assistance with the Olympus Widefield Microscopy and Cherian Mathai for his assistance with ellipsometry, optical profilometry, and contact angle measurements. All the fluorescence images, as well as the intensity measurements, were taken at Molecular Cytology Core at Bond Life Sciences Center, University of Missouri-Columbia.

Author Contributions: H.K.H. and S.A.G. conceived and designed the experiments; G.D.H. and A.L.V. performed the experiments; H.K.H. and G.D.H. analyzed the data; G.D.H., H.K.H., and S.A.G. wrote the paper.

Conflicts of Interest: The authors declare no conflict of interest.

Abbreviations

The following abbreviations are used in this manuscript:

MIP	Molecularly Imprinted Polymer
WGM	Whispering Gallery Mode
FITC	Fluorescein isothiocyanate
HCL	Hydrochloric Acid
DMSO	Dimethyl Sulfoxide

References

1. Barceló, D. Environmental protection agency and other methods for the determination of priority pesticides and their transformation products in water. *J. Chromatogr. A* **1993**, *643*, 117–143. [CrossRef]
2. Simcox, N.J.; Fenske, R.A.; Wolz, S.A.; Lee, I.C.; Kalman, D.A. Pesticides in household dust and soil: Exposure pathways for children of agricultural families. *Environ. Health Perspect.* **1995**, *103*, 1126–1134. [CrossRef] [PubMed]
3. Kolpin, D.W.; Furlong, E.T.; Meyer, M.T.; Thurman, E.M.; Zaugg, S.D.; Barber, L.B.; Buxton, H.T. Pharmaceuticals, hormones, and other organic wastewater contaminants in U.S. Streams, 1999–2000: A national reconnaissance. *Environ. Sci. Technol.* **2002**, *36*, 1202–1211. [CrossRef] [PubMed]
4. Dich, J.; Zahm, S.H.; Hanberg, A.; Adami, H.-O. Pesticied and cancer. *Cancer Causes Control* **1997**, *8*, 420–443. [CrossRef] [PubMed]
5. Stackelberg, P.E.; Furlong, E.T.; Meyer, M.T.; Zaugg, S.D.; Henderson, A.K.; Reissman, D.B. Persistence of pharmaceutical compounds and other organic wastewater contaminants in a conventional drinking-water-treatment plant. *Sci. Total Environ.* **2004**, *329*, 99–113. [CrossRef] [PubMed]
6. Yang, G.; White, I.M.; Fan, X. An opto-fluidic ring resonator biosensor for the detection of organophosphorus pesticides. *Sens. Actuators B Chem.* **2008**, *133*, 105–112. [CrossRef]
7. Frense, D.; Müller, A.; Beckmann, D. Detection of environmental pollutants using optical biosensor with immobilized algae cells. *Sens. Actuators B Chem.* **1998**, *51*, 256–260. [CrossRef]
8. Mulchandani, A.; Chen, W.; Mulchandani, P.; Wang, J.; Rogers, K.R. Biosensors for direct determination of organophosphate pesticides. *Biosens. Bioelectron.* **2001**, *16*, 225–230. [CrossRef]
9. Viveros, L.; Paliwal, S.; McCrae, D.; Wild, J.; Simonian, A. A fluorescence-based biosensor for the detection of organophosphate pesticides and chemical warfare agents. *Sens. Actuators B Chem.* **2006**, *115*, 150–157. [CrossRef]
10. Fang, Y. Label-free cell-based assays with optical biosensors in drug discovery. *Assay Drug Dev. Technol.* **2006**, *4*, 583–595. [CrossRef] [PubMed]

11. Bhatta, D.; Stadden, E.; Hashem, E.; Sparrow, I.J.G.; Emmerson, G.D. Multi-purpose optical biosensors for real-time detection of bacteria, viruses and toxins. *Sens. Actuators B Chem.* **2010**, *149*, 233–238. [CrossRef]
12. Long, F.; Zhu, A.; Shi, H. Recent advances in optical biosensors for environmental monitoring and early warning. *Sensors* **2013**, *13*, 13928–13948. [CrossRef] [PubMed]
13. Luppa, P.B.; Sokoll, L.J.; Chan, D.W. Immunosensors—Principles and applications to clinical chemistry. *Clin. Chim. Act Int. J. Clin. Chem.* **2001**, *314*, 1–26. [CrossRef]
14. Sassolas, A.; Blum, L.J.; Leca-Bouvier, B.D. Optical detection systems using immobilized aptamers. *Biosens. Bioelectron.* **2011**, *26*, 3725–3736. [CrossRef] [PubMed]
15. Abbas, A.; Linman, M.J.; Cheng, Q. New trends in instrumental design for surface plasmon resonance-based biosensors. *Biosens. Bioelectron.* **2011**, *26*, 1815–1824. [CrossRef] [PubMed]
16. Dudak, F.C.; Boyacı, İ.H. Rapid and label-free bacteria detection by surface plasmon resonance (SPR) biosensors. *Biotechnol. J.* **2009**, *4*, 1003–1011. [CrossRef] [PubMed]
17. Lu, T.; Lee, H.; Chen, T.; Herchak, S.; Kim, J.-H.; Fraser, S.E.; Flagan, R.C.; Vahala, K. High sensitivity nanoparticle detection using optical microcavities. *PNAS* **2011**, *108*, 5976–5979. [CrossRef] [PubMed]
18. Vahala, K.J. Optical microcavities. *Nature* **2003**, *424*, 839–846. [CrossRef] [PubMed]
19. Nguyen, D.T.; Norwood, R.A. Label-free, single-object sensing with a microring resonator: FDTD simulation. *Opt. Express* **2013**, *21*, 49–59. [CrossRef] [PubMed]
20. Vollmer, F.; Arnold, S. Whispering-gallery-mode biosensing: Label-free detection down to single molecules. *Nat. Methods* **2008**, *5*, 591–596. [CrossRef] [PubMed]
21. Hunt, H.K.; Armani, A.M. Label-free biological and chemical sensors. *Nanoscale* **2010**, *2*, 1544–1559. [CrossRef] [PubMed]
22. McDonagh, C.; Burke, C.S.; MacCraith, B.D. Optical chemical sensors. *Chem. Rev.* **2008**, *108*, 400–422. [CrossRef] [PubMed]
23. Li, H.; Fan, X. Characterization of sensing capability of optofluidic ring resonator biosensors. *Appl. Phys. Lett.* **2010**, *97*, 011105. [CrossRef]
24. Fan, X.; White, I.M.; Shopova, S.I.; Zhu, H.; Suter, J.D.; Sun, Y. Sensitive optical biosensors for unlabeled targets: A review. *Anal. Chim. Acta* **2008**, *620*, 8–26. [CrossRef] [PubMed]
25. Charlebois, M.; Paquet, A.; Verret, L.S.; Boissinot, K.; Boissinot, M.; Bergeron, M.G.; Allen, C.N. Toward automatic label-free whispering gallery modes biodetection with a quantum dot-coated microsphere population. *Nanoscale Res. Lett.* **2010**, *5*, 524–532. [CrossRef] [PubMed]
26. Himmelhaus, M.; Krishnamoorthy, S.; Francois, A. Optical sensors based on whispering gallery modes in fluorescent microbeads: Response to specific interactions. *Sensors* **2010**, *10*, 6257–6274. [CrossRef] [PubMed]
27. Li, H.; Guo, Y.; Sun, Y.; Reddy, K.; Fan, X. Analysis of single nanoparticle detection by using 3-dimensionally confined optofluidic ring resonators. *Opt. Express* **2010**, *18*, 25081–25088. [CrossRef] [PubMed]
28. Swaim, J.D.; Knittel, J.; Bowen, W.P. Detection of nanoparticles with a frequency locked whispering gallery mode microresonator. *Appl. Phys. Lett.* **2013**, *102*, 183106. [CrossRef]
29. Kim, K.W.; Song, J.; Kee, J.S.; Liu, Q.; Lo, G.-Q.; Park, M.K. Label-free biosensor based on an electrical tracing-assisted silicon microring resonator with a low-cost broadband source. *Biosens. Bioelectron.* **2013**, *46*, 15–21. [CrossRef] [PubMed]
30. Kirk, J.T.; Brault, N.D.; Baehr-Jones, T.; Hochberg, M.; Jiang, S.; Ratner, D.M. Zwitterionic polymer-modified silicon microring resonators for label-free biosensing in undiluted humanplasma. *Biosens. Bioelectron.* **2013**, *42*, 100–105. [CrossRef] [PubMed]
31. Knittel, J.; Chow, J.H.; Gray, M.B.; Taylor, M.A.; Bowen, W.P. Ultrasensitive real-time measurement of dissipation and dispersion in a whispering-gallery mode microresonator. *Opt. Lett.* **2013**, *38*, 1915–1917. [CrossRef] [PubMed]
32. Arnold, S.; Khoshsima, M.; Teraoka, I.; Holler, S.; Vollmer, F. Shift of whispering-gallery modes in microspheres by protein adsorption. *Opt. Lett.* **2003**, *28*, 272–274. [CrossRef] [PubMed]
33. Vollmer, F.; Arnold, S.; Braun, D.; Teraoka, I.; Libchaber, A. Multiplexed DNA quantification by spectroscopic shift of two microsphere cavities. *Biophys. J.* **2003**, *85*, 1974–1979. [CrossRef]
34. Dantham, V.R.; Holler, S.; Barbre, C.; Keng, D.; Kolchenko, V.; Arnold, S. Label-free detection of single protein using a nanoplasmonic-photonic hybrid microcavity. *Nano Lett.* **2013**, *13*, 3347–3351. [CrossRef] [PubMed]
35. Yano, K.; Karube, I. Molecularly imprinted polymers for biosensor applications. *TrAC Trends Anal. Chem.* **1999**, *18*, 199–204. [CrossRef]

36. Li, S.; Ge, Y.; Piletsky, S.A.; Lunec, J. *Molecularly Imprinted Sensors: Overview and Applications*; Elsevier: Amsterdam, The Netherlands, 2012; p. 390.
37. Cheng, Z.; Wang, E.; Yang, X. Capacitive detection of glucose using molecularly imprinted polymers. *Biosens. Bioelectron.* **2001**, *16*, 179–185. [CrossRef]
38. Mayes, A.; Whitcombe, M. Synthetic strategies for the generation of molecularly imprinted organic polymers. *Adv. Drug Deliv. Rev.* **2005**, *57*, 1742–1778. [CrossRef] [PubMed]
39. Kryscio, D.R.; Peppas, N.A. Critical review and perspective of macromolecularly imprinted polymers. *Acta Biomater.* **2012**, *8*, 461–473. [CrossRef] [PubMed]
40. Koshland, D.E. The key–lock theory and the induced fit theory. *Angew. Chem. Int. Ed. Engl.* **1995**, *33*, 2375–2378. [CrossRef]
41. Pauling, L. A theory of the structure and process of formation of antibodies. *J. Am. Chem. Soc.* **1940**, *62*, 2643–2657. [CrossRef]
42. Takeuchi, T.; Haginaka, J. Separation and sensing based on molecular recognition using molecularly imprinted polymers. *J. Chromatogr. B Biomed. Sci. Appl.* **1999**, *728*, 1–20. [CrossRef]
43. Owens, P.K.; Karlsson, L.; Lutz, E.S.M.; Andersson, L.I. Molecular imprinting for bio- and pharmaceutical analysis. *TrAC Trends Anal. Chem.* **1999**, *18*, 146–154. [CrossRef]
44. Wei, S.; Mizaikoff, B. Recent advances on noncovalent molecular imprints for affinity separations. *J. Sep. Sci.* **2007**, *30*, 1794–1805. [CrossRef] [PubMed]
45. Vasapollo, G.; Sole, R.D.; Mergola, L.; Lazzoi, M.R.; Scardino, A.; Scorrano, S.; Mele, G. Molecularly imprinted polymers: Present and future prospective. *Int. J. Mol. Sci.* **2011**, *12*, 5908–5945. [CrossRef] [PubMed]
46. Ulbricht, M. Molecularly imprinted polymer films and membranes. In *Molecularly Imprinted Materials*; Yan, M., Ramström, O., Eds.; CRC Press: Boca Raton, FL, USA, 2004; pp. 455–490.
47. Schneider, F.; Piletsky, S.; Piletska, E.; Guerreiro, A.; Ulbricht, M. Comparison of thin-layer and bulk mips synthesized by photoinitiated *in situ* crosslinking polymerization from the same reaction mixtures. *J. Appl. Polym. Sci.* **2005**, *98*, 362–372. [CrossRef]
48. Poma, A.; Turner, A.P.F.; Piletsky, S.A. Advances in the manufacture of mip nanoparticles. *Trends Biotechnol.* **2010**, *28*, 629–637. [CrossRef] [PubMed]
49. Chen, Q.; Ritt, M.; Sivaramakrishnan, S.; Sun, Y.; Fan, X. Optofluidic lasers with a single molecular layer of gain. *Lab Chip* **2014**, *14*, 4590–4595. [CrossRef] [PubMed]
50. Wienhold, T.; Kraemmer, S.; Bacher, A.; Kalt, H.; Koos, C.; Koeber, S.; Mappes, T. Efficient free-space read-out of wgm lasers using circular micromirrors. *Opt. Express* **2015**, *23*, 1025–1034. [CrossRef] [PubMed]
51. Kim, D.C.; Armendariz, K.P.; Dunn, R.C. Integration of microsphere resonators with bioassay fluidics for whispering gallery mode imaging. *Analyst* **2013**, *138*, 3189–3195. [CrossRef] [PubMed]
52. Soteropulos, C.E.; Hunt, H.K. Attaching biological probes to silica optical biosensors using silane coupling agents. *J. Vis. Exp.* **2012**. [CrossRef] [PubMed]
53. Donskoi, A.V.; Dresvin, S.V.; Orlova, M.A.; Osovskii, B.B.; Khait, O.D.; Paushkin, E.V. Plasma polishing of surface of wares made of silicate glass of any composition. *Glass Ceram.* **1976**, *33*, 162–165. [CrossRef]
54. Ljungberg, K.; Jansson, U.; Bengtsson, S.; Söderbärg, A. Modification of silicon surfaces with H_2SO_4:H_2O_2:HF and HNO_3:HF for wafer bonding applications. *J. Electrochem. Soc.* **1996**, *143*, 1709–1714. [CrossRef]
55. Chandekar, A.; Sengupta, S.K.; Whitten, J.E. Thermal stability of thiol and silane monolayers: A comparative study. *Appl. Surf. Sci.* **2010**, *256*, 2742–2749. [CrossRef]
56. Wang, F.; Anderson, M.; Bernards, M.; Hunt, H. Peg functionalization of whispering gallery mode optical microresonator biosensors to minimize non-specific adsorption during targeted, label-free sensing. *Sensors* **2015**, *15*, 18040–18060. [CrossRef] [PubMed]
57. Zhu, H.; Suter, J.D.; White, I.M.; Fan, X. Aptamer based microsphere biosensor for thrombin detection. *Sensors* **2006**, *6*, 785–795. [CrossRef]
58. Stringer, R.C.; Gangopadhyay, S.; Grant, S.A. Detection of nitroaromatic explosives using a fluorescent-labeled imprinted polymer. *Anal. Chem.* **2010**, *82*, 4015–4019. [CrossRef] [PubMed]
59. Stringer, R.C.; Gangopadhyay, S.; Grant, S.A. Comparison of molecular imprinted particles prepared using precipitation polymerization in water and chloroform for fluorescent detection of nitroaromatics. *Anal. Chim. Acta* **2011**, *703*, 239–244. [CrossRef] [PubMed]
60. Hunt, H.K.; Armani, A.M. Recycling microcavity optical biosensors. *Opt. Lett.* **2011**, *36*, 1092–1094. [CrossRef] [PubMed]

61. Rahachou, A.I.; Zozoulenko, I.V. Effects of boundary roughness on a Q-factor of whispering-gallery-mode lasing microdisk cavities. *J. Appl. Phys.* **2003**, *94*, 7929–7933. [CrossRef]
62. Freeman, L.M.; Li, S.; Dayani, Y.; Choi, H.-S.; Malmstadt, N.; Armani, A.M. Excitation of Cy5 in self-assembled lipid bilayers using optical microresonators. *Appl. Phys. Lett.* **2011**, *98*, 143703. [CrossRef] [PubMed]
63. Hunt, H.K.; Soteropulos, C.; Armani, A.M. Bioconjugation strategies for microtoroidal optical resonators. *Sensors* **2010**, *10*, 9317–9336. [CrossRef] [PubMed]

11

Electronic Biosensing with Functionalized rGO FETs

Ciril Reiner-Rozman [1,2,†], Caroline Kotlowski [1,2,†] and Wolfgang Knoll [1,2,*]

1 Center for Electrochemical Surface Technology (CEST), Wiener Neustadt 2700, Austria; rozman.ciril.fl@ait.ac.at (C.R.-R.); caroline.kotlowski@boku.ac.at (C.K.)
2 AIT Austrian Institute of Technology, Wien 1220, Austria
* Correspondence: wolfgang.knoll@ait.ac.at
† These authors contributed equally to this work.

Academic Editors: Mark A. Reed and Mathias Wipf

Abstract: In the following we give a short summary of examples for biosensor concepts in areas in which reduced graphene oxide-based electronic devices can be developed into new classes of biosensors, which are highly sensitive, label-free, disposable and cheap, with electronic signals that are easy to analyze and interpret, suitable for multiplexed operation and for remote control, compatible with NFC technology, *etc.*, and in many cases a clear and promising alternative to optical sensors. The presented areas concern sensing challenges in medical diagnostics with an example for detecting general antibody-antigen interactions, for the monitoring of toxins and pathogens in food and feed stuff, exemplified by the detection of aflatoxins, and the area of smell sensors, which are certainly the most exciting development as there are very few existing examples in which the typically small and hydrophobic odorant molecules can be detected by other means. The example given here concerns the recording of a honey flavor (and a cancer marker for neuroblastoma), homovanillic acid, by the odorant binding protein OBP 14 from the honey bee, immobilized on the reduced graphene oxide gate of an FET sensor.

Keywords: reduced graphene oxide (rGO graphene); FET; liquid-gate; biosensing; receptor immobilization; antigen-antibody interaction; food toxins; aflatoxins; odorant-binding proteins; olfaction; smell sensor

---

1. Introduction

The detection and quantitative monitoring of biomolecules in air, in water, in complex liquids like bodily fluids or similar is still a challenge, both from a fundamental point of view as well as in the context of practical applications. Whether it is the need for sensors in general air management scenarios—e.g., to detect air pollutants (including explosives), to sense crop disease markers, in food quality management for the identification of toxins, or in medical applications like breath analysis—Or for the detection of certain markers in blood, plasma, saliva, urine, wound liquids, *etc.*, that report a patient's health and/or disease status, in all cases we are dealing with three major problems; (i) the sensitivity of the technical device for the quantification of a particular molecule of interest; (ii) the selectivity needed to differentiate between similar molecules; and (iii) the suppression of non-specific interactions with and binding to the sensor surface by other components in the sample volume, typically in excess to the actually targeted molecule.

Numerous concepts and formats for sensors based on optical transduction principles have been reported in the literature, some of which even made it to the market place and are commercialized [1]. Not so widespread are sensors based on electrical, electrochemical or electronic transduction principles [2]. The latter category, in particular, is the youngest member of the huge family of current-based bio-sensors; typical examples are CMOS-transistor-based devices that have been used to monitor action potentials of excited neurons [3] or cardiomyocytes [4] grown on the gate surface of the device, Si-nanowire based transistor read-out of protein and DNA binding [5], or the promising use of organic ("plastic") electronics for the development of cheap and, hence, disposable sensors [6,7]. The most recent development in this area, the use of the novel carbon materials, *i.e.*, carbon nanotubes or graphene, opens a totally new but very promising range of options for biosensors based on electronic devices made from these highly interesting materials [8].

In this short summary, we will report some of our own efforts in designing, fabricating, bio-functionalizing and characterizing biosensors based on reduced graphene oxide as the gate material. We will give a very brief overview of the basic preparation protocols, and describe the electronic performance of the devices as transistors [9]. The practical examples given are (i) the detection of a standard biomolecule, bovine serum albumin (BSA), binding from solution to its antibody, immobilized on the sensor surface; (ii) the detection and quantification of food toxins (mycotoxins) binding to their antibodies; and (iii) the monitoring of an odorant molecule (dissolved in an aqueous solution) to the surface-bound odorant binding protein from an insect, the honey bee *Apis mellifera* [10].

2. Preparation and General Electronic Performance of rGO-FET Biosensors

Reduced graphene oxide field-effect transistor (rGO-FET) devices were fabricated with a typical channel width of 40 μm. Figure 1A briefly summarizes the individual preparation steps for the devices [10]. Silicon wafers with a 300 nm oxide layer were chosen as base substrates. They were cleaned following a standard RCA cleaning procedure and then submerged in a 1%–2% 3-amino-propyl-triethoxy-silane-(APTES) solution in ethanol for 1 h, with APTES forming a monolayer on the substrate that increases the adhesion of graphene (reduced graphene oxide).

Graphene oxide sheets were prepared using a variation of Hummers method [11,12]. The obtained graphene oxide flakes were deposited onto Si-wafers via spin coating. A scanning electron microscopic image of the GO flakes on the substrate before reduction of rGO and before the evaporation of the Au electrodes for the transistor are shown in Figure 1B. After rinsing with ethanol, the substrates were heated to 120 °C for two hours and then cooled to room temperature. They were then treated overnight in hermetically sealed glass petri dishes with hydrazine at 70 °C in order to reduce the graphene oxide, forming the graphene structure consisting of sp^2-hybrid bonds.

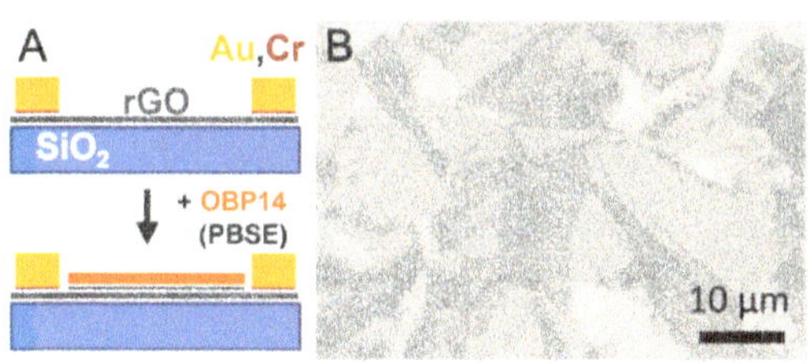

Figure 1. (**A**) Schematic illustration of the individual fabrication steps of the graphene biosensor device: After the reduction of the GO flakes to rGO, source and drain Au electrodes were evaporated (with a thin layer of Cr as an adhesion promotor), then coated (via self-assembly) by a linker, PBSE, and finally functionalized by the attachment of antibodies or by odorant binding proteins, here OBP 14 from the honey bee; (**B**) Scanning electron microscopic image of the GO flakes on the chip substrate (before reduction to rGO and before being coated with the electrodes).

For the attachment of the antibodies (here, antibodies against bovine serum albumin, BSA, and aflatoxin B1, respectively) to the sensing area, the graphene surface was chemically modified by a bi-functional linker, 1-pyrenebutanoic acid succinimidyl ester (PBSE). One end the linker firmly attaches to the graphene surface through π-π interactions with the pyrene group while the other hand covalently reacts with one of the amino group of the protein to form an amide bond. All reagents were purchased from Sigma-Aldrich unless otherwise indicated and used without further purifications.

For the detection of different odorants, the biosensors were functionalized with an odorant binding protein 14 (OBP 14) from the honey Bee, *Apis mellifera*. The protein was expressed in bacterial systems using established protocols [13,14]. Purification of the proteins was accomplished using a combination of conventional chromatographic techniques followed by a final gel filtration step on Superose-12 (GE-Healthcare) as previously described in standard protocols [14].

The chip was then mounted into a flow cell for *in situ* real-time kinetic measurements (in order to quantify the association, k_{on}, and dissociation rate constants, k_{off}, respectively) as well as for titration experiments for the determination of affinity, K_A, and dissociation constants, K_d, respectively. An artist's sketch of the FET setup and the immobilized OBP interacting with the odorant ligand, together with a photograph of the whole flow cell, are given in Figure 2.

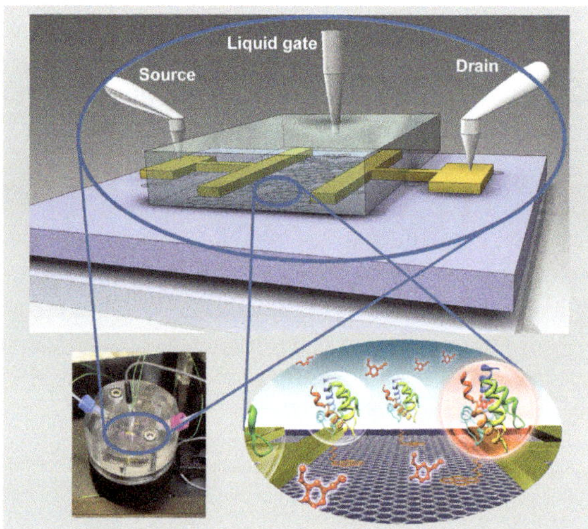

Figure 2. Schematics of the set-up and the device configuration consisting of a liquid gate electrode, source and drain electrodes, evaporated onto the reduced graphene oxide flakes on a solid Si/SiO_2 substrate, functionalized by OBPs that are covalently coupled via a linker molecule. In the lower left corner is a photograph of the mounted flow cell.

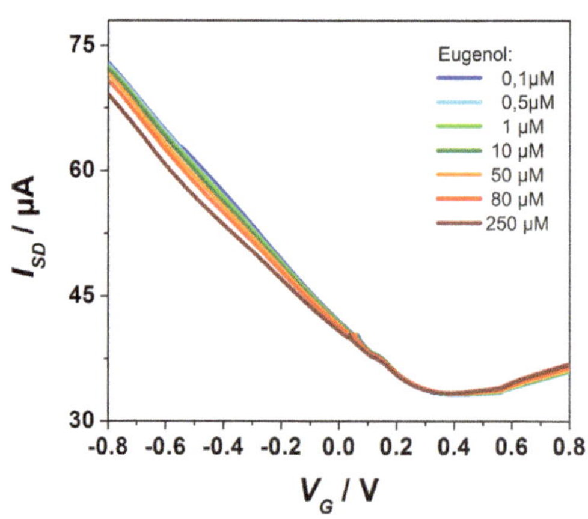

Figure 3. Source-drain current I_{SD}-vs-gate voltage V_G characteristics of the OBP14 functionalized rGO FET-biosensor device at different Eugenol concentrations (as indicated) flowing through the cell.

The electrical properties of the FET devices were tested as described before [15]. Electrical measurements were performed using a Keithley 4200 semiconductor characterization system.

An Ag/AgCl reference electrode (Flexref, World Precision Instruments) was used to operate the FET device in a liquid gate configuration with a constant source-drain bias of V_{SD} = 50 mV. The cathodic branches of the I_{SD}-vs-V_G scans (*cf.* Figure 3) are dominated by the hole mobility [9]. The Dirac voltage is seen at ca. V_G = 0.4 V. Recording these I_{SD}-vs-V_G scans at different bulk solution conditions, in particular in aqueous solutions of different ligand concentrations, results in a distinct shift of the cathodic branch which we attribute to a slight modification of the dipolar layer with the OBP protein monolayer immobilized on the graphene gate surface upon partial binding of the ligands to the free binding sites in the OBP acting as receptors.

3. Antigen–Antibody Interaction and the Limit of Detection

The first example that we describe for the use of these rGO-FETs as biosensors concerns the "classical" system, *i.e.*, the binding of the protein bovine serum albumin, BSA, as antigen to its FET-immobilized antibody. The global analysis protocol, *i.e.*, the stepwise increase of the bulk analyte concentration while simultaneously recoding the time-dependent change of the source-drain current, ΔI_{SD}, is given in Figure 4. One can see that the current decreased each time the bulk concentration was increased from an initial concentration c_0 = 100 nM, until it gradually reached a saturation level for a bulk concentration near c_0 = 25 μM. The current decrease following each concentration change contains kinetic information (*cf.* the red curves that fit the current traces) occurs by a single exponential giving a time constant, k, that is concentration dependent (increases with bulk concentration). This is in agreement with the Langmuir model for this 1:1 complex between the analyte (the antigen) from solution and the surface–immobilized receptor (the antibody). Upon rinsing with pure buffer, the current returns to its original baseline level with a single exponential (*cf.* the blue fit curve) indicating the full reversibility of the binding event (a prerequisite for any analysis according the Langmuir model). The fit to this dissociation process results in a quantitative measure of the dissociation rate constant, k_{off}. From the slope of the plot of all the rate constants determined as a function of the bulk concentration, one obtains the association rate constant, k_{on}, which together with k_{off} gives the affinity constant, K_A. This has been documented recently and reported to result in an affinity constant for the binding of BSA to this antibody of $K_A = 1.6 \times 10^5\ M^{-1}$ [9], corresponding to a dissociation constant of K_d = 6.2 μM.

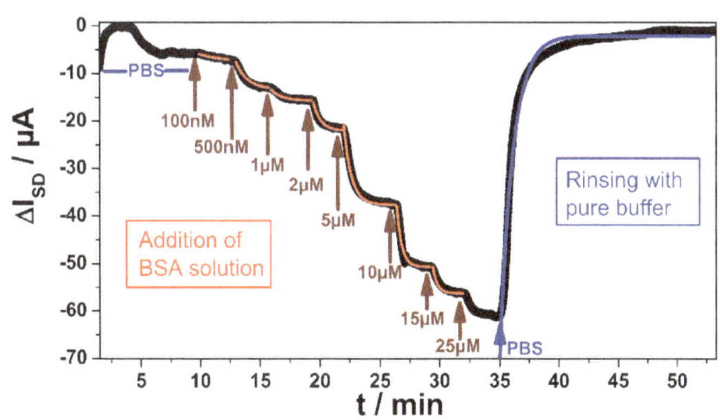

Figure 4. Global analysis of BSA binding from solution to surface-immobilized anti-BSA antibody; solutions with concentrations from 100 nM to (near) saturation at 25 μM (as indicated in red) were rinsed through the flow cell. The first few minutes show a drift due to the graphene charging behavior, which stabilizes after 7 min.

Figure 5 summarizes the results taken from Figure 4, focusing here on the titration of the equilibrium surface coverage (*i.e.*, the new source-drain current that one reads after the new equilibrium has been established) as a function of the bulk analyte concentration in solution, *i.e.*, the Langmuir isotherm. By plotting the surface coverage, Θ, *i.e.*, the source-drain current at a given concentration,

I_{SD} (c_0), divided by I_{SD} (c_∞), the source drain current at infinite bulk analyte concentration, one obtains the affinity constant, K_A:

$$\Theta = I_{SD}(c_0)/I_{SD}(c_\infty) = K_A c_0/(1 + K_A c_0) \quad (1)$$

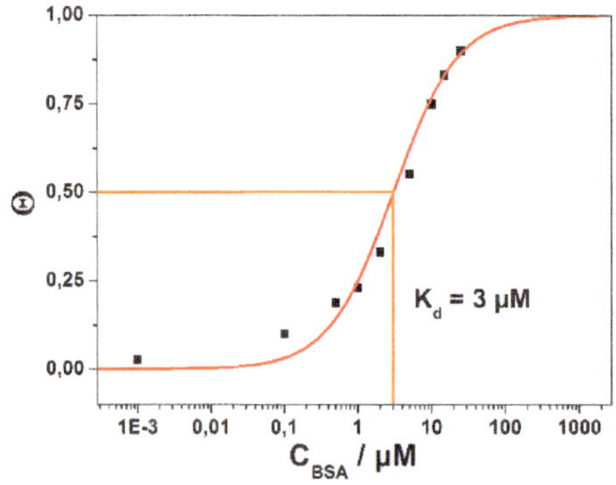

Figure 5. Langmuir adsorption isotherm obtained by plotting the (negative) change in the source-drain current, ΔI_{SD}, as obtained from Figure 4 from the new stationary current after changing the concentration in the bulk solution to a new value. The red curve is a fit to the data according to the Langmuir model, resulting in a dissociation constant (half saturation concentration) K_d = 3 μM.

In Figure 5, we have plotted the surface coverage as a function of the (logarithm of the) bulk analyte concentration, and obtain the expected S-shaped curve. The corresponding fit to the data (full red curve in Figure 5) results in an affinity constant $K_A = 3.3 \times 10^5$ M^{-1}, corresponding to a dissociation constant, *i.e.*, a half-saturation constant, K_d = 3 μM. Compared to the value obtained from the kinetic measurements (K_d = 6.2 μM) this can be considered as an excellent confirmation of the applicability of the Langmuir model to the quantitative description of the binding assay of BSA to its surface-immobilized antibody. Furthermore, it confirms that the electronic read-out of this model binding reaction can be considered as a quantitative method for general biosensing purposes.

The next question that naturally comes up is that of the limit of detection of this electronic monitoring of antigen-antibody interactions. To this end, we show in Figure 6 the kinetic recording of the current change upon switching the solution that was running through the flow cell from pure PBS buffer to a 1 nM BSA solution and then again back to pure buffer. As one can see, ΔI_{SD} can still be monitored with a superb signal-to-noise ratio. Based on this measurement, the LOD could be estimated to be in the 100 pM analyte concentration range.

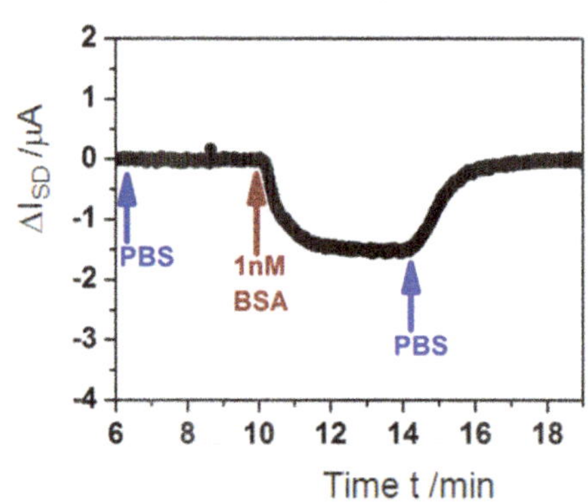

Figure 6. Single kinetic run, *i.e.*, recording of the change in the source-drain current, ΔI_{SD}, after switching in the flow cell from pure PBS buffer (blue arrow) to a 1 nM BSA solution (brown arrow) in order to monitor the association rate constant, and back to pure buffer again (blue arrow), in order to monitor the dissociation rate constant.

Within the Langmuir model this means that, according to Equation (1) with $c_0 << 1 / K_A$, the coverage at this low concentration is given by

$$\Theta = K_A c_0 \quad (2)$$

and with $K_A = 3.3 \times 10^5\ M^{-1}$, and $c_0 = 100$ pM, this then corresponds to a coverage of bound analyte of $\Theta = 3.3 \times 10^{-5}$. In other words, the minute change of the interfacial surface potential that is induced if only 1 out of 30,000 antibodies on the sensor surface binds an analyte molecule is enough to generate a current signal that can be quantified.

4. Food Toxin Detection, Comparison with Optical Sensing

The next example that we discuss concerns the detection of food pathogens, aflatoxins, in particular. They constitute a class of mycotoxins produced mainly by *Aspergillus flavus* and *Aspergillus parasiticus* which grow in a number of agricultural products. Aflatoxin M1 (AFM1) is the hydroxylated metabolite of aflatoxin B1 (AFB1) and can be found in urine, blood, milk, and internal organs of animals that have ingested AFB1-contaminated feed [16]. Due to its hepatotoxic and carcinogenic effects [17] and the relative stability during pasteurization or other thermal treatments, control measurements were established. For instance, the European Commission stipulates a maximum level of 50 $pg \cdot ml^{-1}$ for AFM1 in milk [18].

As a reference and benchmark, we start with the presentation of an optical assay based on surface-plasmon fluorescence spectroscopy, developed in our own group, combined with an inhibition immunoassay in which a derivative of AFM1 was immobilized on the sensor surface and monoclonal anti-AFM1 antibodies from the rat were used as recognition elements [19]. In this protocol the analyte sample is first incubated with a solution of anti-AFM1 antibodies of a known concentration. Some of the antibodies bind to the free AFM1 molecules; upon rinsing this cocktail through the sensor flow cell, the remaining unoccupied antibodies can then bind to the surface-immobilized AFM1 antigens, and are detected by decoration with a secondary, fluorescently labeled goat anti-rat antibody (Cy5-GaR, approximately 10.2 dyes per antibody).

The result of a series of measurements with sample solutions of different AFM1 concentrations is presented in Figure 7. The lower the bulk aflatoxin concentration the higher is the sensor signal from the unoccupied antibodies, now being immobilized on the sensor surface. The half-saturation value as a measure of the sensitivity of the optical assay is at $c_0 = 100$ pM, with a LOD of about 0.6 $pg \cdot ml^{-1}$ at a processing time of 1 h.

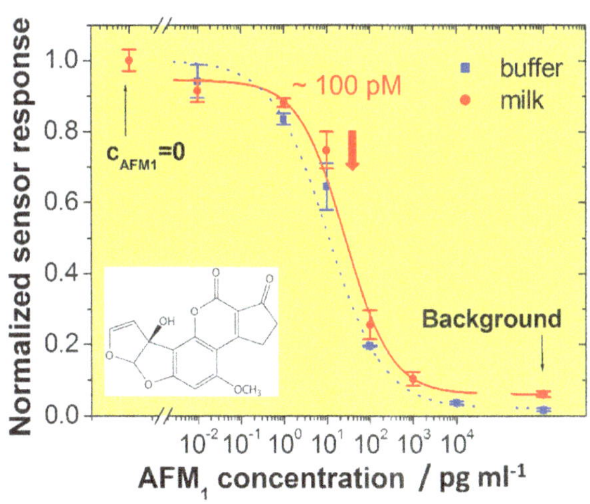

Figure 7. Normalized calibration curves for the detection of AFM1 in buffer (squares) and milk samples (circles).

In contrast to the optical reference assay, the electronic read-out has a number of advantages: (i) the sensor monitors the analyte binding in real time; hence is only diffusion limited and therefore faster; (ii) it gives direct kinetic information, *i.e.*, one also obtains association and dissociation rate constants; (iii) the assay does not use any secondary antibody, and hence requires fewer processing steps; (iv) the electronic sensing device based on "plastic electronics" is a disposable and does not need any sophisticated optical detection instrumentation, and hence is cheaper.

We first addressed the question of non-specific binding of the analyte aflatoxin to the bare rGO gate. Figure 8A demonstrates that—Not totally unexpected given the molecular structures of the analyte molecule and graphene, respectively, suggesting a significant non-specific binding by π-π-interactions—A change in the source-drain current, I_{SD}, upon the injection of a 64 nM solution of AFB1 into the flow cell, can indeed be monitored.

However, this non-specific binding can be totally suppressed for a test surface that is first functionalized by an antibody specific for a totally different analyte (BSA in this case). As can be seen in Figure 8B, even significant concentrations of AFB1 rinsed through the flow cell do not lead to any detectable change in the source-drain current, ΔI_{SD}.

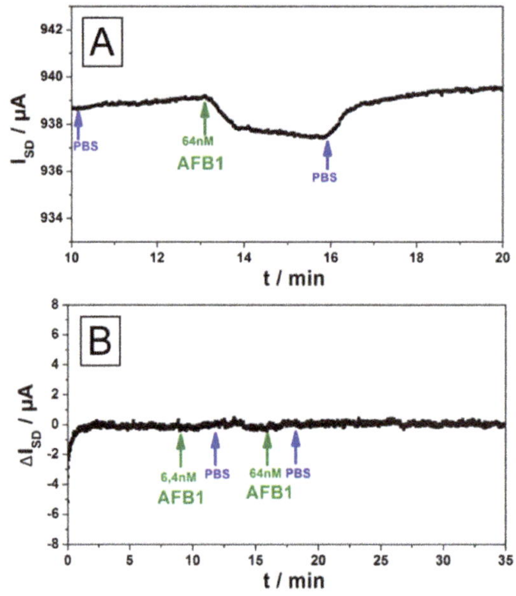

Figure 8. (**A**) Analysis of the binding of aflatoxin B1 (structure formula given in the inset of Figure 9) on a bare rGO gate surfaces using a blank FET. The signal strength for nanomolar concentrations was found to be only around 10% compared to the measurements were the target antibody was used (*cf.* Figure 9); (**B**) Unspecific responses for aflatoxin B1 were measured on graphene FET's with immobilized PBSE-linker and BSA antibodies. For all tested devices no response signal was observed, indicating that no binding of AFB1 to the linker or to a non-target antibody is occurring.

The specific binding of AFB1 to its antibody on the sensor gate surface and the sensitivity issue can be best judged by referring to the data displayed in Figure 9. Here, the antibody against AFB1, was directly immobilized on the rGO gate of the transistor. Rinsing analyte solutions of different concentrations (as indicated by the green arrows in Figure 9, alternating with pure PBS buffer, blue arrows) through the attached flow cell led to a direct sensor signal, *i.e.*, a change in the source-drain current, ΔI_{SD}, of the FET. As one can see the sensor responds with a change of its source-drain current, with a good signal-to-noise ratio, already at analyte concentrations in the several 10 pM range. This is quite comparable to the much more demanding optical approach described in Figure 7.

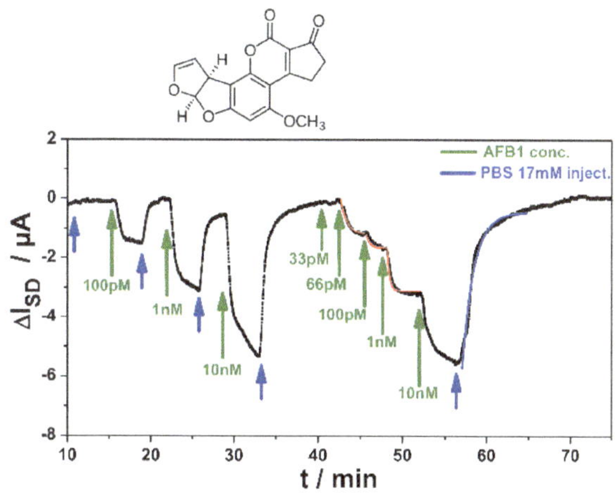

Figure 9. Real-time food pathogen sensor output, *i.e.*, ΔI_{SD}, as a function of time, while AFB1 solutions of different concentrations (green arrows), alternating with pure buffer (blue arrows) were rinsed through the sample cell.

A more comprehensive and quantitative evaluation of the kinetic and titration data of this electronic food toxin sensor is currently being performed by our group.

5. Smell Sensing

The final example that we give for the performance of the rGO FET-based biosensors concerns the development of a smell detector. Despite the enormous importance of chemical communication in nature we have essentially no technical device or sensor that could detect smells with the sensitivity and selectivity required for most applications in food quality control, for the detection of crop diseases, for medical applications like breath analysis, *etc.* Despite the fact that monitoring chemicals in chemotaxis, *i.e.*, in the search for food of many organisms or the exchange of chemicals between species as a way to communicate with each other is the oldest of our sensory repertoire, we have no sensor that offers the sensitivity and the bandwidth needed to sense and to differentiate many different odors.

The concept for a smell sensor that we are currently developing in our group is based on the functionalization of a thin film transistor with a grapheme gate by the immobilization of odorant binding proteins (OBPs) from insects as a functional element, as a bio-mimetic building block. This approach is aiming at reducing the complexity of nature to just the use of these proteins as a particularly robust element for the build-up of a first device in a bio-inspired sensor concept. OBPs from insects like those from mammals (and humans) are at the beginning of a complex amplification scheme in odorant perception that translates a first event, the binding of an odorant molecule to such an odorant binding protein, and eventually ends with the trigger of action potentials that run down the smell nerve directly into the brain.

Figure 10 gives a complete set of experimental data taken with a reduced graphene oxide (rGO) FET, functionalized with OBP14 from the honey bee (*A. mellifera*). The example concerns the monitoring of Homovanillic acid (structure formula given in Figure 10D), an odorant for bees which is also considered to be a tumor marker for neuroblastoma and malignant pheochromocytoma.

We start with the recordings of the change of the source-drain current from a transistor with an rGO gate that was coated with the linker molecule PBSE (*cf.* Section 2) but without an OBP coupled to it. As one can see form Figure 10A, this test for non-specific binding of the analyte leads to only a negligible signal which may result from residual π-stacking interactions between the odorant molecule and free sites on the reduced graphene oxide gate surface.

However, after the covalent immobilization of the receptor OBP14, the global analysis with both kinetic and titration information in one run results in a clear sensor signal with an excellent signal-to-noise ratio (Figure 10B). The different concentrations of the analyte solutions that were rinsed through the flow cell in this experiment are indicated by red arrows, and the flow of pure buffer, indicating the full reversibility of the ligand binding to the sensor-immobilized receptor is marked by a blue arrow.

The analysis of the kinetic data is given in Figure 10C. As predicted by the Langmuir model, the association process becomes faster with increasing bulk concentration, $c_{\mathbf{Homovanillic\ acid}}$. By plotting the corresponding rate constant, k, as afunction of the analyte concentration, c_0, one obtains a straight line. Also, according to $k = k_{on}c_0 - k_{off}$, the slope of this line gives $k_{on} = 1.1 \times 10^3\ M^{-1}s^{-1}$, and the intersection with the ordinate results in $k_{off} = 8 \times 10^{-3}\ s^{-1}$. This then leads to the kinetically determined affinity constant $K_A = k_{on}/k_{off} = 1.4 \times 10^5\ M^{-1}$, corresponding to a dissociation constant $K_d = 7.1\ \mu M$.

This value can be compared with the data obtained from the titration experiment displayed in Figure 10D. The fit here yields $K_A = 2.5 \times 10^5\ M^{-1}$ in excellent agreement with the kinetic determination. This confirms the applicability of the Langmuir model to this affinity binding reaction. It should be pointed out that by testing other ligands (odorants), dissociation constants ranging from a few μM to several mM were found, indicating the selectivity of this sensor concept based on an OBP receptor/FET bio-hybrid device [20].

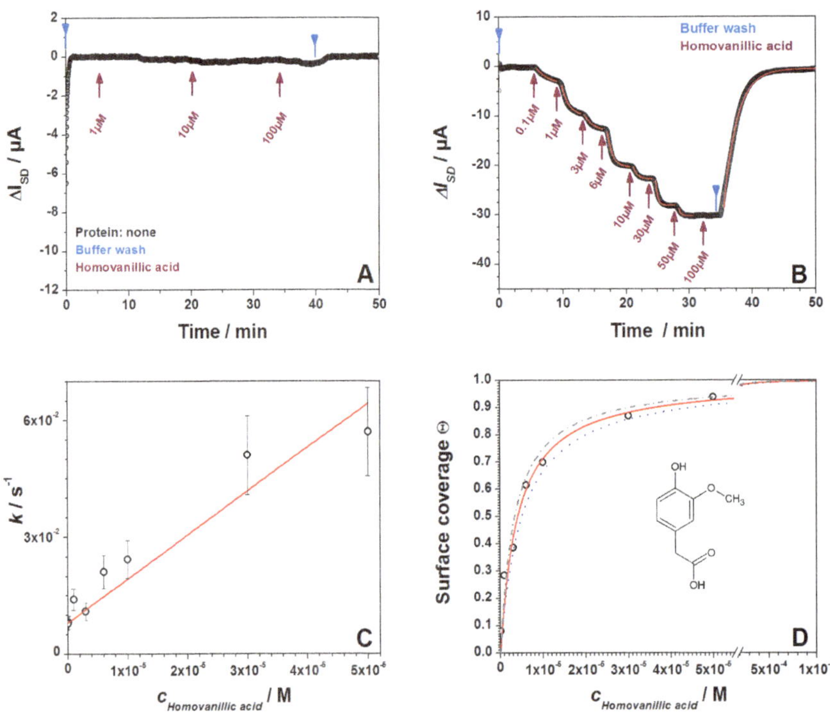

Figure 10. Full analysis of the recognition and binding of the odorant homovanillic acid to the odorant binding protein OBP14. (**A**) Taken with a sensor that was functionalized by the linker PBSE, however, had no protein coupled to it; (**B**) shows the global analysis for homovanillic acid binding to OPB 14 on the FET gate surface; (**C**) rate constants taken from the fits of (**B**), plotted as a function of the bilk concentration c_0; (**D**) Langmuir isotherm of the titration data taken from (**B**).

6. Outlook

Electronic biosensing shows great promise for complementing electrochemical detection schemes on the one hand and optical concepts for the quantitative monitoring of bioanalytes on the other. In particular, the use of graphene as the conductive gate material in the preparation of thin film transistors as the sensing device offers a tremendous advantage compared to the use of organic semiconducting materials or compared to Si-based transistors, which both require far more demanding preparation protocols.

The few examples that we presented here demonstrate the versatility of the graphene-based transistor concept for biosensing in different fields of application. It should be noted that the use of monomolecular graphene oxide flakes obtained by exfoliating graphite and their reduction to reduced graphene oxide (rGO) eventually may be replaced by higher quality graphene gate materials prepared by chemical vapor deposition (which needs to be seen, though!). The basic concept, however, of functionalizing this gate material by different types of biorecognition elements, receptors, antibodies, *etc.*, able to bind the analyte molecule of interest, has proven already to yield the sensitivity and selectivity needed for practical applications of these devices.

Some of the fundamental issues associated with rGO FET-based biosensing still need further work and clarification; e.g., the role of local pH changes, direct but also indirect modifications of the surface potential at the gate-electrolyte interface by variations of the local ionic milieu, the concentration, profile and chemical nature of ions and counter-ions associated with the biorecognition reaction, the role of dipole potentials, *etc.*, are far from being completely understood. Other than in optical biosensing, this also gives the concept of anti-fouling coatings a different meaning: it is absolutely not clear how to best minimize non-specific binding. What determines eventually the limit of detection in rGO-based electronic biosensing? What is the relationship between the gate architecture and the minimal surface coverage that is needed in order to sense an electronic signal? Would eventually a single occupied site on the biofunctionalized gate surface be enough to modify the source-drain current?

A final comment refers to the last application, *i.e.*, the sensing of smells. The example given was based on monitoring of changes induced in an odorant binding protein immobilized on the gate surface of the transistor by the binding of a ligand, an odorant, from the aqueous phase of the respective analyte solution in contact with the sensor. This format mimics to some extend the situation in the nose of vertebrates where the sensory neurons and the associated odorant binding proteins are covered and, hence, protected and hydrated by the mucosa. It also reflects properly the situation in the sensilla of the insect antennae, where the OBPs are in the lymph, *i.e.*, also in an aqueous environment. In that sense, the presented results are quite relevant also for the development of a smell sensor. In fact, a direct comparison between the sensitivity of a whole insect antenna from an insect, the red flour beetle Tribolium castaneum, responding to a certain partial pressure of an odorant in a carrier gas, with that of a rGO transistor functionalized by one of the key OBPs from this species, responding to an aqueous solution of the same odorant, gave very comparable results [21]. Of course, our final goal is to operate these devices also in air, which seems to be absolutely possible by using hydrogels as a protective coating of the device, mimicking the mucosa that keeps all the biocomponents of the sensor in a hydrated and therefore functional environment.

Acknowledgments: We would like to thank Barbara Cvak, Alois Schiessl, and Romer Labs Division Holding GmbH for their continued support. We are grateful to a number of colleagues that contributed with their advice: Jakub Dostalek, Christoph Kleber, Melanie Larisika, Rosa Mastrogiacomo, Christoph Nowak, Paolo Pelosi, and Serban F. Peteu. Partial support for this work was provided by the European Science Foundation (ESF), Grant Number: 10-EuroBioSAS-FP-005, by the European Union's Horizon 2020 program under the Sklodowska-Curie Grant Agreement No. 645686, the Austrian Science Fund (FWF) (I681-N24), the Austrian Federal Ministry for Transport, Innovation and Technology (GZ BMVIT-612.166/0001-III/I1/2010) and the Austrian Research Promotion Agency (FFG) within the COMET framework, by the Province of Lower Austria.

Author Contributions: Ciril Reiner-Rozman, Caroline Kotlowski, Wolfgang Knoll conceived and designed the experiments; Ciril Reiner-Rozman, Caroline Kotlowski performed the experiments; Ciril Reiner-Rozman,

Caroline Kotlowski, Wolfgang Knoll analyzed the data; Ciril Reiner-Rozman, Caroline Kotlowski, Wolfgang Knoll wrote the paper.

Conflicts of Interest: The authors declare no conflict of interest.

References

1. Jones, R.; Meixner, H. *Sensors, A. Comprehensive Survey, Volume 8, Micro- and Nanosensor Technology: Trends in Sensor Markets*; Jones, R., Meixner, H., Eds.; Wiley: New York, NY, USA, 2008.
2. Zhang, X.J.; Ju, H.X.; Wang, J. *Electrochemical Sensors, Biosensors and Their Biomedical Applications*; Elsevier: Amsterdam, The Netherlands, 2008.
3. Offenhäusser, A.; Maelicke, C.; Matsuzawa, M.; Knoll, W. Field-Effect Transistor Array for Monitoring Electrical Activity from Mammalian Neurons in Culture. *Biosens. Bioelectron.* **1997**, *12*, 819–826. [CrossRef]
4. Yeung, C.K.; Ingebrandt, S.; Krause, M.; Sprössler, C.; Denyer, M.; Britland, S.T.; Offenhäusser, A.; Knoll, W. The use of Field Effect Transistors (FETs) in pharmacological research. *J. Anat.* **2002**, *200*, 210.
5. Ingebrandt, S. Bioelectronics: Sensing Beyond the Limit. *Nat. Nanotechnol.* **2015**, *10*, 734–735. [CrossRef] [PubMed]
6. Khan, H.U.; Jang, J.; Kim, J.J.; Knoll, W. *In Situ* Antibody Detection and Charge Discrimination Using Aqueous Stable Pentacene Transistor Biosensors. *J. Am. Chem. Soc.* **2011**, *133*, 2170–2176. [CrossRef] [PubMed]
7. Khan, H.U.; Roberts, M.E.; Johnson, O.; Förch, R.; Knoll, W.; Bao, Z. *In Situ*, Label-Free DNA Detection Using Organic Transistor Sensors. *Adv. Mater.* **2010**, *22*, 4452–4456. [CrossRef] [PubMed]
8. Kuila, T.; Bose, S.; Khanra, P.; Mishra, A.K.; Kim, N.H.; Lee, J.H. Recent Advances in Graphene-Based Biosensors. *Biosens. Bioelectron.* **2011**, *26*, 4637–4648. [CrossRef] [PubMed]
9. Reiner-Rozman, C.; Larisika, M.; Nowak, C.; Knoll, W. Graphene-based liquid-gated field effect transistor for biosensing: Theory and experiments. *Biosens. Bioelectron.* **2015**, *70*, 21–27. [CrossRef] [PubMed]
10. Larisika, M.; Kotlowski, C.; Steininger, C.; Mastrogiacomo, R.; Pelosi, P.; Schütz, S.; Peteu, S.F.; Kleber, C.; Reiner-Rozman, C.; Nowak, C.; *et al.* Electronic Olfactory Sensor Based on *A. mellifera* Odorant Binding Protein 14 on a Reduced Graphene Oxide Field-Effect Transistor. *Angew. Chem. Int. Ed. Engl.* **2015**, *54*, 13245–13248. [CrossRef] [PubMed]
11. Larisika, M.; Huang, J.F.; Tok, A.; Knoll, W.; Nowak, C. An Improved Synthesis Route to Graphene for Molecular Sensor Applications. *Mater. Chem. Phys.* **2012**, *136*, 304–308. [CrossRef]
12. Stankovich, S.; Dikin, D.A.; Piner, R.D.; Kohlhaas, K.A.; Kleinhammes, A.; Jia, Y.; Wu, Y.; Nguyen, S.B.T.; Ruoff, R.S. Synthesis of Graphene-Based Nanosheets via Chemical Reduction of Exfoliated Graphite Oxide. *Carbon* **2007**, *45*, 1558–1565. [CrossRef]
13. Dani, F.R.; Iovinella, I.; Felicioli, A.; Niccolini, A.; Calvello, M.A.; Carucci, M.G.; Qiao, H.; Pieraccini, G.; Turillazzi, S.; Moneti, G.; *et al.* Mapping the Expression of Soluble Olfactory Proteins in the Honeybee. *J. Proteome Res.* **2010**, *9*, 1822–1833. [CrossRef] [PubMed]
14. Iovinella, I.; Dani, F.R.; Niccolini, A.; Sagona, S.; Michelucci, E.; Gazzano, A.; Turillazzi, S.; Felicioli, A.; Pelosi, P. Differential Expression of Odorant-Binding Proteins in the Mandibular Glands of the Honey Bee According to Caste and Age. *J. Proteome Res.* **2011**, *10*, 3439–3449. [CrossRef] [PubMed]
15. Ban, L.P.; Zhang, L.; Yan, Y.H.; Pelosi, P. Binding Properties of a Locust's Chemosensory Protein. *Biochem. Biophys. Res. Commun.* **2002**, *293*, 50–54. [CrossRef]
16. Shreeve, B.J.; Patterson, D.S.P.; Roberts, B.A. Mycotoxins and Their Metabolites in Humans and Animals. *Food Cosmet. Toxicol.* **1979**, *17*, 151–152. [CrossRef]
17. Paniel, N.; Radoi, A.; Marty, J.L. Development of an electrochemical biosensor for the detection of aflatoxin M1 in milk. *Sensors* **2010**, *10*, 9439–9448. [CrossRef] [PubMed]
18. Commission Regulation (EC) No. 466/2001. Available online: http://ec.europa.eu/food/fs/sfp/fcr/fcr02_en.pdf (accessed on 12 April 2016).
19. Wang, Y.; Dostalek, J.; Knoll, W. Long Range Surface Plasmon-enhanced Fluorescence Spectroscopy for the Detection of Aflatoxin M-1 in milk. *Biosens. Bioelectron.* **2009**, *24*, 2264–2267. [CrossRef] [PubMed]

20. Kotlowski, C.; Larisika, M.; Guerin, P.; Kleber, C.; Kröber, T.; Mastrogiacomo, R.; Nowak, C.; Pelosi, P.; Schütz, S.; Schwaighofer, A.; *et al.* Electronic Olfactory Biosensor Based on Honeybee Odorant Binding Protein 14 on a rGO FET. In preparation.
21. Kotlowski, C.; Ramach, U.; Balakrishnan, K.; Breu, J.; Gabriel, M.; Kleber, C.; Mastrogiacomo, R.; Pelosi, P.; Schütz, S.; Knoll, W. Monitoring Crop Disease Markers by Odorant Binding Proteins of *Tribolium castaneum*—Electroantennograms *versus* Reduced Graphene-Oxide Based Electronic Biosensor. In preparation.

12

Enhanced Biosensor Platforms for Detecting the Atherosclerotic Biomarker VCAM1 Based on Bioconjugation with Uniformly Oriented VCAM1-Targeting Nanobodies

Duy Tien Ta [1,2], Wanda Guedens [1], Tom Vranken [1], Katrijn Vanschoenbeek [3], Erik Steen Redeker [4], Luc Michiels [3] and Peter Adriaensens [1,5,*]

1 Biomolecule Design Group, Institute for Materials Research (IMO), Hasselt University, Diepenbeek BE-3590, Belgium; duytien.ta@uhasselt.be or tdtien@ctuet.edu.vn (D.T.T.); wanda.guedens@uhasselt.be (W.G.); tom.vranken@uhasselt.be (T.V.)

2 Faculty of Food Technology and Biotechnology, Can Tho University of Technology, Can Tho 900000, Vietnam

3 Immunology and Biochemistry, Biomedical Research Institute (Biomed) and School of Life Sciences, Transnationale Universiteit Limburg, Hasselt University, Diepenbeek BE-3590, Belgium; katrijn.vanschoenbeek@uhasselt.be (K.V.); luc.michiels@uhasselt.be (L.M.)

4 Maastricht Science Programme, Maastricht University, Maastricht 6200 MD, The Netherlands; erik.steenredeker@maastrichtuniversity.nl

5 Applied and Analytical Chemistry, Institute for Materials Research (IMO), Hasselt University, Diepenbeek BE-3590, Belgium

* Correspondence: peter.adriaensens@uhasselt.be

Academic Editor: Jeff D. Newman

Abstract: Surface bioconjugation of biomolecules has gained enormous attention for developing advanced biomaterials including biosensors. While conventional immobilization (by physisorption or covalent couplings using the functional groups of the endogenous amino acids) usually results in surfaces with low activity, reproducibility and reusability, the application of methods that allow for a covalent and uniformly oriented coupling can circumvent these limitations. In this study, the nanobody targeting Vascular Cell Adhesion Molecule-1 (NbVCAM1), an atherosclerotic biomarker, is engineered with a C-terminal alkyne function via Expressed Protein Ligation (EPL). Conjugation of this nanobody to azidified silicon wafers and Biacore™ C1 sensor chips is achieved via Copper(I)-catalyzed azide-alkyne cycloaddition (CuAAC) "click" chemistry to detect VCAM1 binding via ellipsometry and surface plasmon resonance (SPR), respectively. The resulting surfaces, covered with uniformly oriented nanobodies, clearly show an increased antigen binding affinity, sensitivity, detection limit, quantitation limit and reusability as compared to surfaces prepared by random conjugation. These findings demonstrate the added value of a combined EPL and CuAAC approach as it results in strong control over the surface orientation of the nanobodies and an improved detecting power of their targets—a must for the development of advanced miniaturized, multi-biomarker biosensor platforms.

Keywords: uniformly oriented bioconjugation; biosensor; CuAAC; expressed protein ligation; VCAM1-targeting nanobody

1. Introduction

In the recent years, innovative biosensor developments have made several applications with rapid detection and high accuracy possible for real-time environmental monitoring, disease diagnostics and therapy [1–7]. During the last decade, protein-based—or more particularly antibody-based—biosensors are considered as the most commonly developed platforms [8,9]. Regarding the implementation of antibody candidates in biosensor design, the variable domain of the heavy chain of the single-domain antibody (VHH)—or nanobody—found in camelidae has dedicated a great potential due to numerous advantages over the conventional antibodies [10]: small nanometer size, ease of genetic manipulation and expression in *Escherichia coli*, high stability and antigen-binding capacity as compared to full-length antibodies [11].

Many of the available surface bioconjugation methods rely on physico-chemical adsorption of the detecting proteins (also called ligands) onto the surface of the particular solid support [12–15] due to its simplicity and low cost. However, this approach most frequently results in a weak interaction and non-uniformly oriented (random) deposition of the proteins on the surface [16–19], leading to rather poor sensitivity, specificity and reproducibility of the application [15,17,20]. The main problems can be found in the limited number of available binding sites due to the heterogeneous orientation of the proteins on the surface, in addition to the leaching out/washing away during the binding and detection phases. Approaches to create more stable protein-conjugated surfaces frequently make use of strong and covalent couplings between functional groups of the endogenous amino acids, e.g., the thiol group of cysteine or the amine group of lysine, and reactive groups on the surface [13,17,19,21,22]. Although being covalently and so stably coupled, the orientation of proteins immobilized in such a way is still heterogeneous since, in most cases, multiple copies of these endogenous functional groups appear in a protein [17,20]. Alternatively, linkages between the protein and the surface can be established in a more controllable way by fusing the protein of interest with an affinity tag, e.g., a polyhistidine by which an interaction with Ni^{2+}, Cu^{2+} or Co^{2+} cations can be established [18]. A number of studies have reported the use of Cu(II)-complexing layers deposited on gold electrodes to obtain a uniformly oriented conjugation of His_6-tagged proteins, e.g., a dipyrromethene-Cu(II) layer and Receptor domains for advanced glycation end products (RAGE) [23,24], a dipyrromethene-Cu(II) layer and antibodies against H5N1 influenza virus [25], a pentetic acid-Cu(II) layer and JAK2 kinase [26], an iminodiacetic acid-like-Cu(II) layer and RIO1 kinase [27]. The thiol derivatives of these complexing reagents are firstly linked to the gold surfaces to form the layers, followed by Cu(II) complexation and His_6-tagged protein immobilization. Since the detecting method relies on changes in electrochemical properties of the Cu(II) redox centers upon binding of the analytes to the His_6-tagged proteins, the copper-complexing layers play the role of both an immobilizing mediator and a signal transducer, which is a big advantage in biosensor design. These studies reported a rather generic method for fabrication of electrochemical biosensors. However, the linkage between the His_6-tag and the transition metal cations can still be disturbed by pH change or competitive presence of imidazole, thus probably resulting in a loss of activity and reproducibility in such cases. Therefore, to combine the best of both worlds, the investigation of a stable uniformly oriented and covalent immobilization strategy is of utmost importance [10].

An alternative promising approach for controlled immobilization can be found in the site-specific introduction of a bio-orthogonal functional group in the protein. By this, a stable covalent and homogenously oriented linkage can be established between the protein and a complementary functionalized substrate surface. Such highly selective couplings can be achieved by means of "click" chemistry reactions like the copper(I)-catalyzed Huisgen 1,3-dipolar azide-alkyne cycloaddition (CuAAC) [28–30]. This reaction specifically occurs between an azide and an alkyne moiety to form a stable 5-membered 1,2,3-triazole ring under Cu(I) catalysis and mild reaction conditions. Following such strategies, a protein can be coupled not only stably but also with a uniform orientation to a solid substrate, resulting in highly functional and homogeneously covered surfaces. To site-specifically introduce a bio-orthogonal group such as alkyne or azide in a protein, the Expressed Protein Ligation (EPL) technique—first described by Muir et al. [31]—has recently (re)gained significant interest as a promising strategy [19,32–36]. Whereas EPL on the one hand has been employed for the site-specific alkynation of nanobodies and "click" chemistry and on the other hand for the selective coupling of proteins to micelles and polymersomes [37–42], studies on using the combined EPL and "click" chemistry approach to create nanobody-based biosensor platforms for detecting atherosclerosis have not been reported.

Recently, we developed an efficient protocol to functionalize nanobodies targeting the Vascular Cell Adhesion Molecule-1 (abbreviated as NbVCAM1) at the *C*-terminus with an alkyne function in order to be coupled to azide-functionalized supports with a uniform orientation via CuAAC chemistry [43]. VCAM1 is one of the inducible adhesion molecules that play a role in mediating the recruitment and attachment of leukocytes to the vascular endothelium [44] as well as further migration into the subendothelial spaces [45]. These are the major processes in the development of atherosclerotic plaques [46]. The protein is also unraveled to be associated with other diseases including rheumatoid arthritis [47], inflammatory bowel disease [48], multiple sclerosis [49], renal cell carcinoma [50], renal tumors [51] and colorectal cancer [52,53]. Therefore, VCAM1 might be considered as a pre-diagnostic marker and promising drug target for cardiovascular diseases and cancer diagnosis/therapy follow-up [54]. This explains the selection of the NbVCAM1 to demonstrate the proof of principle of the proposed conjugation strategy for the development of improved label-free optical biosensors. In particular, the *C*-terminally alkynated nanobodies are conjugated by CuAAC "click" chemistry to diverse azide-functionalized solid surfaces, including silicon wafers and gold-coated Biacore™ sensor chips, for VCAM1 antigen binding detection via ellipsometry or SPR, respectively. The resulting nanobody-conjugated surfaces display significant improvements in antigen binding capacity/affinity, sensitivity, detection limit, quantitation limit and reusability as compared to those produced via random coupling methods. Furthermore, the approach is generic and can be easily translated to other proteins.

2. Materials and Methods

All chemicals and reagents were purchased from Sigma unless stated otherwise. The PCR reagents, restriction enzymes and B-PER reagent were obtained from Thermo Scientific. The cysteine-alkyne bifunctional linker (Figure S1A, Supplementary Materials) was purchased from Eurogentec, the azido-propylamine linker from Jena bioscience (Figure S1B, Supplementary Materials) and the *N*-hydroxysuccinimide (NHS) derived ester linker 2,5-dioxopyrrolidin-1-ylhex-5-ynoate (Figure S1C, Supplementary Materials) was self-synthesized according to Jagadish et al. [55]. The pMXB10 vector, *E. coli* SHuffle® T7 competent cells and chitin resin were purchased from New England Biolabs. The two recombinant human VCAM1 antigens (hVCAM1) were bought from R & D Systems (MW of 270 kDa) and Peprotech (MW of 180 kDa) while the recombinant mouse VCAM1 (mVCAM1) antigen was purchased from Bioconnect (Huissen, The Netherlands, MW of 95 kDa). The ellipsometer and silicon wafers were bought from Synapse B.V. (Maastricht, The Netherlands) and the Biacore™ (Diegem, Belgium) C1 sensor chips from GEHealthcare. The SPR experiments were performed with a Biacore™ T200 model (GE Healthcare).

2.1. Preparation of the Nanobody Variants

The NbVCAM1-LEY nanobody was expressed as a chimeric protein (fusion with an intein and a chitin binding domain) in the *E. coli* SHuffle® T7 strain and was subjected to EPL-mediated cleavage with DTT (to produce NbVCAM1-LEY) or with the cysteine-alkyne linker to produce the *C*-terminally alkynated NbVCAM1-LEY, i.e., NbVCAM1-LEY-alkyne, as previously described [13]. The non-VCAM1-targeting NbBcII-10-LEY-alkyne (an anti-bacterial β-lactamase nanobody) was produced using the same protocol and used as a non-binding reference (negative control) in ELISA and SPR experiments. Details of expression and purification of these nanobodies are provided in the Supplementary Materials. The NbVCAM1-His_6 was produced as described by Saerens et al. [56] and used as an antigen-binding reference (a positive control in ELISA and a randomly conjugated reference via EDC/NHS chemistry in SPR). Random alkynation of the NbVCAM1-His_6 was performed for 3 h in 100 μL PBS buffer (137 mM NaCl, 2.7 mM KCl, 10 mM Na_2HPO_4 and 2 mM KH_2PO_4 at pH 7.4) containing 20 μM nanobody and a 10-fold molar excess of the *N*-hydroxysuccinimide (NHS) derived ester linker 2,5-dioxopyrrolidin-1-ylhex-5-ynoate. This linker carries a terminal alkyne function and its coupling to the nanobody can be accomplished via the reaction between the free and accessible amino groups of the protein (*N*-terminal NH_2 and lysine ε-NH_2) and the linker's carbonyl carbon, resulting in a stable amide bond. The resulting protein isomer mixture (designated as rNbVCAM1-His_6-alkyne with "r" denoting "randomly") was then immediately filtered through a Zeba™ Spin Desalting Column, 7K MWCO (Thermo Scientific, Aalst, Belgium) and used as a reference for random coupling in the ellipsometry and SPR experiments. Protein concentrations were determined with the BCA Protein Assay kit (Thermo Scientific).

2.2. *Characterization of the NbVCAM1-LEY-alkyne by Mass Spectrometry, Western Blotting and ELISA*

To test the: (i) purity; (ii) level of C-terminal alkynation; and (iii) "clickability" of the NbVCAM1-LEY-alkyne before use in subsequent coupling experiments, the NbVCAM1-LEY-alkyne was subjected to ElectroSpray Ionization-Fourier Transform Mass Spectrometry (ESI-FTMS), CuAAC-mediated biotinylation and ELISA, as described in the Supplementary Materials.

2.3. *Azidification of the Support Surfaces for Ellipsometry and SPR*

For ellipsometry, finely cut silicon wafers (0.3 × 3.2 cm) were first cleaned in a 3:1 mixture (*v*/*v*) of H_2SO_4:H_2O_2 for 5 min, followed by treatment with 6% (*v*/*v*) HF for a few seconds to create a hydrophobic surface. The slides were then oxidized with chromic acid (8% potassium dichromate (*w*/*v*) in 25% H_2SO_4 (*v*/*v*)) at 80 °C for 1 h to make them hydrophilic. The oxidized slides were washed with MilliQ water and ethanol before silanization with a solution of 15% *N*-(trimethoxysilylpropyl)ethylenediamine-triacetic acid-trisodium salt in 0.2 M acetate buffer for 1 h at 100 °C. In this way, the slides were carboxylated and after washing with MilliQ water and ethanol, the slides were azidified by submerging in a functionalization solution for 3 h at room temperature in the dark. The functionalization solution is composed of 0.4 M *N*-(3-dimethylaminopropyl)-*N*′-ethylcarbodiimide hydrochloride (EDC), 0.3 M *N*-hydroxysuccinimide (NHS) and 1 mM azido-propylamine in 220 mM HEPES buffer pH 6.8. The slides were then blocked in 1 M aminoethoxyethanol pH 7.8 for 45 min before washing with MilliQ and ethanol. The functionalized slides were N_2-dried and kept in the dark at room temperature if not used immediately.

For SPR, the commercial Biacore™ Series S carboxymethylated C1 chips were washed five times with PBS running buffer (10 μL/min) before azidification. All stock solutions were prepared in Biacore compatible plastic vials according to the manufacturer instructions (e.g., 75 mg/mL EDC, 11.5 mg/mL NHS and 15 mM azido-propylamine). The functionalization process was performed automatically according the preset EDC/NHS coupling protocol of the T200 Biacore™ Control software. The first three flow cells (Fc) of the chip were functionalized with the azido-propylamine linker (for coupling to alkynated nanobodies later via CuAAC chemistry), whereas Fc4 was directly conjugated with NbVCAM1-His_6 (10 μM) via a peptide bond between the COOH groups of the chip and an NH_2 group of the nanobody. The chips were than washed 5 times with PBS and blocked by flushing with 1 M aminoethoxyethanol pH 7.8 at a flow-rate of 10 μL/min for 10 min. The azidified chips (except for Fc4) were then washed 5 times with PBS and stored in PBS at 4 °C if not used immediately.

2.4. *Ellipsometry*

pH optimization for CuAAC-mediated conjugation. Ellipsometry was performed in null-mode [57] on a semi-automatic ellipsometer with a built-in control software and the following settings: filter 16; offset 0; gain 1; polarizer sweep angle 140° and analyzer sweep angle 175°. The functionalized silicon slides were assembled in a sample holder with eight positions and an area of approximately 0.09 cm^2 (0.3 × 0.3 cm) was dipped in 400 μL PBS in quartz cuvettes, followed by a baseline stabilization during 5 min. An external incubator is used for subsequent washing steps. Coupling with different nanobody variants was performed by either physisorption or CuAAC "click" chemistry. The CuAAC-mediated coupling was first carried out on azidified surfaces in different buffers (PBS and 10 mM sodium acetate at pH 4.0, 5.0 or 6.0) in order to select the most efficient pH. Hereto, the coupling cocktail was prepared in a quartz cuvette containing 400 μL mixture of 1 μM nanobody (NbVCAM1-LEY, NbVACM1-LEY-alkyne, rNbVCAM1-His$_6$-alkyne or NbVCAM1-His$_6$), 2.5 mM sodium L-ascorbate, 1 mM THPTA (Tris(3-hydroxypropyltriazolylmethyl)amine) and 0.5 mM $CuSO_4$. To prove the selectivity of the "click" reaction, two types of silicon substrates, i.e., carboxylated and azidified slides, were evaluated in acetate buffer pH 4.0. The Cu(II) salt is reduced to the Cu(I) catalyst by sodium ascorbate as a reducing reagent. Due to its high instability, Cu(I) is stabilized by THPTA complexing ligand [25]. The CuAAC coupling reaction was performed for 30 min at room temperature followed by consecutive washing steps with washing buffer (WB) (200 mM dihydrogen sodium phosphate, 200 mM sodium chloride, 150 mM ethylenediaminetetraacetic acid, and 50 mM ethanolamine at pH 7.5); 0.5% (*w*/*v*) SDS; PBS; 0.7 M β-mercaptoethanol (BME); and PBS (5 min for each washing step). For all nanobody conjugation experiments, the amount of surface coverage was quantified during the first PBS washing step on the basis of the sweep angle shift of the polarizer ΔP to maintain the nullified status of the reflected light on the silicon surfaces. This angle shift is proportional to the difference in surface mass density before conjugation (baseline) and during the first PBS washing. The surface mass density (Γ, ng protein/cm^2) can be calculated using the simplified Lorentz–Lorenz relation $\Gamma = 85 \times \Delta P$ [58,59]. The reported results represent the average of four measurements.

Nanobody conjugation and antigen binding. The NbVCAM1-LEY-alkyne and rNbVCAM1-His$_6$-alkyne were conjugated to the azidified slides by CuAAC as described above. A random physisorption reference was performed with non-alkynated NbVCAM1-LEY on a carboxylated slide. For this, the slide was incubated for 30 min with 1 μM nanobody in 400 μL TBS buffer pH 7.5 (50 mM Tris and 0.1 M NaCl), followed by washing with PBS to remove only the unbound proteins but not the adsorbed nanobodies. The recombinant hVCAM1 antigen (R & D Systems) was prepared in PBS at a stock concentration of 100 μg/mL (0.37 μM). In order to compare the maximal antigen binding capacity of the nanobody conjugated silicon wafers, the stock solution was only diluted to a final concentration of 5 μg/mL in 400 μL PBS and added to the cuvettes containing the slides conjugated with NbVCAM1-LEY-alkyne or rNbVCAM1-His$_6$-alkyne (via CuAAC), or NbVCAM1-LEY (by physisorption). The antigen–nanobody association was performed for 30–50 min under stirring until saturation was reached. The slides were then consecutively washed with WB, glycine-HCl buffer (0.1 M glycine-HCl and 0.2 M NaCl at pH 2.5), SDS and PBS. The ΔP and Γ values were determined by averaging the data points measured during the washing with WB. To test the reusability of the nanobody-conjugated surfaces, the slides were subjected to a second antigen binding following the same binding protocol as described above. All antigen binding measurements were performed in duplicate.

Determination of the dissociation constant (K_D) of the antigen binding. The hVCAM1 binding to surfaces conjugated with NbVCAM1-LEY-alkyne or rNbVCAM1-His$_6$-alkyne was evaluated for increasing initial antigen concentrations (0, 1.25, 2.5, 3.75 and 5 μg/mL in PBS) until saturation was achieved. The surfaces were then washed with WB and PBS. The affinity constant is determined using the Scatchard equation:

$$\frac{[\mathrm{hVCAM1_{bound}}]}{[\mathrm{hVCAM1_{free}}]} = \mathrm{n} \times \mathrm{C} \times \frac{1}{\mathrm{K_D}} - [\mathrm{hVCAM1_{bound}}] \times \frac{1}{\mathrm{K_D}} \tag{1}$$

in which [hVCAM1$_{bound}$] is the concentration (nM) of bound hVCAM1 at equilibrium as determined during the PBS washing, n is the number of binding sites per molecule (assumed to be 1 if monovalent), and C is the total amount of binding sites available. The [hVCAM1$_{bound}$] is proportional to the increase of the surface mass density increase (Γ) at equilibrium and the contact surface area (0.09 cm^2), and inversely proportional to the reaction volume (V, 400 μL or 4×10^{-4} L), and the MW (270,000 Da) of the hVCAM1 (R & D Systems), and can be calculated as:

$$[\mathrm{hVCAM1_{bound}}] = \frac{\Gamma \times 0.09}{270,000 \times 4 \times 4^{-4}} \tag{2}$$

For each initial antigen concentration [hVCAM1$_0$], the free hVCAM1 concentration can be determined according to:

$$[\text{hVCAM1}_{\text{free}}] = [\text{hVCAM1}_0] - [\text{hVCAM1}_{\text{bound}}] \tag{3}$$

The Scatchard plots were made using the data obtained from Equations (1)–(3) and a linear regression of the [hVCAM1$_{\text{bound}}$]/[hVCAM1$_{\text{free}}$] ratio as a function of the [hVCAM1$_{\text{bound}}$] was performed in order to derive the K_D (nM).

Determination of antigen binding sensitivity. For increasing [hVCAM1$_0$], the equilibrium amount of hVCAM1 bound to the surface conjugated with NbVCAM1-LEY-alkyne or rNbVCAM1-His$_6$-alkyne was used to construct the dose–response curves. Hereto, the surface mass densities were plotted against the corresponding antigen concentrations and a linear least squares fit (95% confidence level) was carried out using GraphPad Prism 5.0 software. The slopes of the curves were also used as a criterion to compare the antigen detection sensitivity according to Thevenot et al. [60].

Determination of detection limit (DL) and quantitation limit (QL). DL is defined as the lowest concentration of an analyte in a sample that can be detected. It can be determined as DL = 3.3 × σ/S where S and σ are the slope and the standard deviation of the intercept, both of which are obtained from the dose–response curve. QL is defined as the lowest concentration of an analyte in a sample that can be quantitated and can be determined as QL = 10 × σ/S [61].

2.5. Surface Plasmon Resonance

Nanobody conjugation. The azidified C1 chip (described before) was first washed five times with PBS to obtain a stable baseline. The first three flow cells were then conjugated via CuAAC with 10 μM of NbBcII-10-LEY-alkyne (Fc1), NbVCAM1-LEY-alkyne (Fc2), and rNbVCAM1-His$_6$-alkyne (Fc3) using the "click" cocktail in acetate buffer pH 4.0 as described for ellipsometry earlier (the Fc4 was already conjugated with 10 μM NbVCAM1-His$_6$ via EDC/NHS coupling). The "click" cocktail was injected at a flow-rate of 10 μL/min for 30 min. After that, the chip was washed five times and stored in PBS at 4 °C if not used immediately. The immobilization levels, expressed in Response Units (RU), were determined 10 s before the end of the PBS washing step (Figure S2, Supplementary Materials).

Analysis of the binding kinetics. Three antigens were employed in this study: two hVCAM1 antigens (270 kDa and 180 kDa from R & D Systems and Peprotech, respectively), and mVCAM1 (95 kDa from Bioconnect). The antigens were injected using a default single-cycle kinetics protocol [62], i.e., a series of initial PBS injections without antigen, followed by a continuous injection of antigen at increasing concentration between 0–1000 ng/mL in PBS. For each concentration, the association and dissociation steps were carried out during respectively 10 min (30 μL/min) and 2 min (30 μL/min), after which a final dissociation step of 10 min (30 μL/min) was accomplished. The sensorgrams of Fc2, 3 and 4 were double referenced. This includes subtraction of blanks (PBS only) in addition to the contributions of the reference Fc1 (i.e., $[\text{FcX} - \text{Fc1}]_{\text{antigen}} - [\text{FcX} - \text{Fc1}]_{\text{PBS}}$ where X is 2, 3, 4). The binding kinetic parameters (k_a and k_d) and the dissociation constant (K_D) were determined from fits using the 1:1 binding model implemented in the T200 BIAevaluation software. Regeneration of the chip was performed by injecting 10 mM NaOH (Table S4, Supplementary Materials) at a flow-rate of 100 μL/min for 1 min before starting the next kinetic binding run.

Determination of antigen binding sensitivity, detection limit and quantitation limit. The dose–response curves for hVCAM1 binding to the conjugated nanobodies on Fc2, 3 and 4 for different hVCAM1 concentrations were constructed by the BIAevaluation software. The sensitivity of antigen detection was calculated based on the slopes of the linear curves. The DL and QL are determined as described for ellipsometry.

3. Results and Discussions

3.1. *Expression and EPL-Mediated Alkynation of NbVCAM1-LEY*

In this study, non-alkynated nanobodies (NbVCAM1-LEY) and *C*-terminally alkynated nanobodies (NbVCAM1-LEY-alkyne) were produced, purified and desalted according to a previously optimized EPL-assisted protocol [38] (see Supplementary Materials for more details). The NbVCAM1-LEY-alkyne was obtained in good yield (~20 mg per liter of culture) and high purity (Figure 1A). Characterization of these nanobodies was performed with ESI-FTMS. The non-alkynated protein fraction (resulting from the intein cleavage with dithiothreitol (DTT)-containing buffer during EPL process) shows two masses: one of NbVCAM1-LEY-DTT and one of the hydrolyzed NbVCAM1-LEY (Figure 1B). This fraction was referred to as "NbVCAM1-LEY" in further experiments. The mass spectrum of the NbVCAM1-LEY-alkyne is shown in Figure 1C and the presence of an alkyne "click" function was confirmed by a successful coupling to an azido-biotin derivative (Figure S1D, Supplementary Materials) followed by Western blotting (Figure 1D). The *C*-terminally alkynated nanobody retained a similar binding capacity towards the hVCAM1 antigen as the reference non-alkynated NbVCAM1-His$_6$ in an ELISA test (Figure 1E). This procedure allows a generic preparation of *C*-terminally alkynated nanobodies as starting materials for CuAAC-mediated bioconjugation.

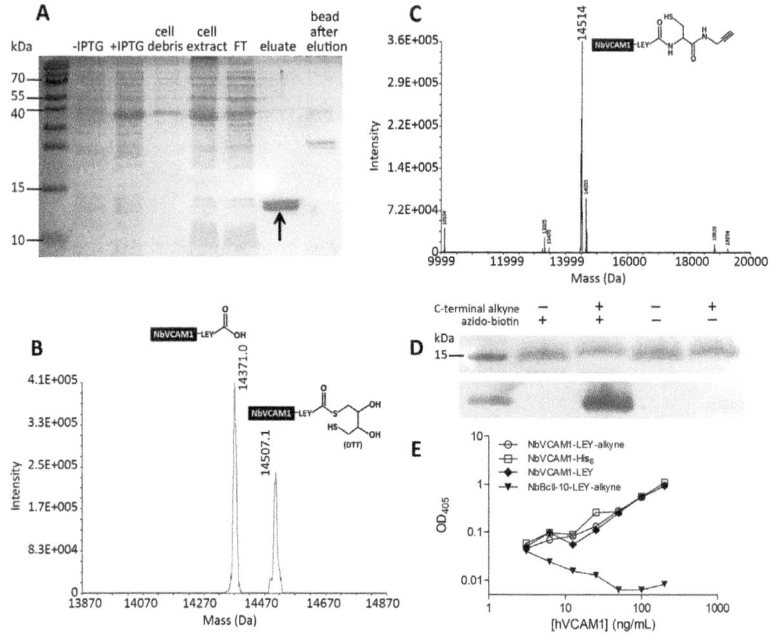

Figure 1. (**A**) SDS-PAGE of cytoplasmic expression and purification steps of NbVCAM1-LEY-alkyne during the EPL process. From left to right: non-induced and Isopropyl β-D-1-thiogalactopyranoside–induced total cell proteins, the cell debris and lysate, the proteins not bounded to the chitin column (FT: flow through), the eluted fraction (alkynated NbVCAM1-LEY) (arrow) and the extract of the beads after EPL; (**B**,**C**) Mass spectra of the purified NbVCAM1-LEY and NbVCAM1-LEY-alkyne fractions, respectively, with their structures; (**D**) CuAAC-mediated biotinylation of NbVCAM1-LEY-alkyne and analysis by SDS-PAGE (top) and Western blot (bottom), demonstrating the presence of the alkyne "click" function; (**E**) Sandwich ELISA to show the hVCAM1 antigen binding capacity of different nanobody variants. The experiment was performed in triplicate and the data are plotted on a log-log scale. The non-alkynated, fully active NbVCAM1-His$_6$ and the NbBcII-10-LEY-alkyne (will not bind VCAM1—see Supplementary Materials for more details about the production of these nanobodies) are used as positive and negative controls, respectively.

3.2. *Buffer Selection for Optimal CuAAC-Mediated Surface Conjugation*

The efficiency of the CuAAC-mediated coupling of monoalkynated NbVCAM1-LEY to azidified silicon wafers was evaluated for different buffers. As monitored by ellipsometry, the highest amount of nanobody conjugation was found for acetate buffer pH 4.0 (Table S1, Supplementary Materials). Therefore, this buffer was selected for all further CuAAC-mediated couplings of alkynated nanobodies to the silicon surfaces and the Biacore™ C1 sensor chips.

Figure 2A,B present ellipsometric data that clearly demonstrate the covalent clicking of the alkynated nanobodies to the azidified silicon slides but not to the carboxylated slides for which all nanobodies were removed by washing with washing buffer (WB) and SDS solution. Coupling of rNbVCAM1-His$_6$-alkyne (also known as randomly alkynated nanobody variant, see experimental section for synthesis details) and NbVCAM1-LEY-alkyne to azidified slides on the other hand results in an increase of the average surface mass density by respectively 267 and 291 ng protein/cm^2 (Figure 2B). This is in contrast to non-alkynated nanobodies (NbVCAM1-His$_6$ and NbVCAM1-LEY), which were washed away by the WB and SDS solution (Figure 2B).

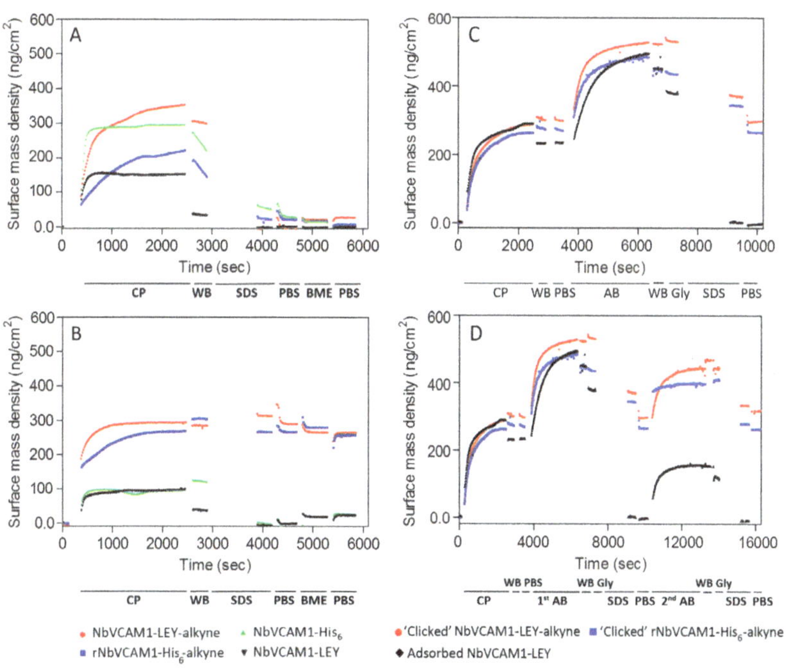

Figure 2. Ellipsometric results for the CuAAC-mediated coupling of different NbVCAM1 variants in acetate buffer pH 4.0 to: (**A**) carboxylated; and (**B**) azidified silicon wafers. The coupling process (CP) was followed by consecutive washing steps with washing buffer (WB), SDS, phosphate buffer saline (PBS), BME and PBS. Data were recorded in real-time and in quadruplicate and one representative curve is presented; (**C**) A one-cycle human VCAM1 antigen (R & D Systems) binding (A,B) on different nanobody-conjugated silicon surfaces. The nanobodies were immobilized using either CuAAC (for the rNbVCAM1-His$_6$-alkyne and NbVCAM1-LEY-alkyne) or physisorption (for the NbVCAM1-LEY). Binding was followed by consecutive washing steps with WB, Glycine-HCl, SDS and PBS; (**D**) A two-cycle AB binding process on similar slides. Measurements were carried out in duplicate and one representative curve is shown.

3.3. *Study of the Antigen Binding by Ellipsometry*

The antigen binding capacity of various nanobody-conjugated silicon wafers was examined by adding an excess of hVCAM1 antigen (5 µg/mL) in order to allow a maximum, saturating antigen binding (Figure 2C). Since the NbVCAM1-His_6 contains five amine groups (4 lysine ε-NH_2 and 1 α-NH_2) that can react with the NHS-alkyne linker (see Experimental Section and Supplementary Materials for more details), the resulting rNbVCAM1-His_6-alkyne can theoretically be coupled to the azidified surface in five different orientations. Likewise, the physically adsorbed NbVCAM1-LEY is also coupled to the surface with random orientations. In contrast, the NbVCAM1-LEY-alkyne is covalently coupled with a unique orientation to the azidified surface and shows a larger surface density increase as compared to the others. This demonstrates that more binding sites are available for the target if the surface is conjugated with uniformly oriented nanobodies. Moreover, because the *N*-terminus of the nanobody is importantly involved in antigen recognition [63–66], coupling via the *N*-terminal amine function will for sure be harmful for the activity. If the nanobodies are covalently coupled via the alkynated C-terminus on the other hand, all will have their active sites available for the antigen binding.

In order to explore the repeatability of the antigen binding for recycling the biosensing platforms, the antigen-loaded surfaces were washed thoroughly (successively with WB, Glycine-HCl, SDS, and PBS) to remove all bound antigen, after which the slides were subjected to a second cycle of antigen binding (Figure 2D). For the CuAAC conjugated surfaces, there was no significant difference in surface mass density after these washing steps as compared to the situation before the first antigen binding cycle, indicating that the covalent linkage between the alkynated nanobodies and the azidified surfaces is stable and can resist the regeneration process. In case of physically adsorbed nanobodies on the other hand, both the antigens and the nanobodies were washed away during the SDS washing. This nicely demonstrates the improvement in stability of the NbVCAM1-LEY-alkyne conjugated via CuAAC as compared to physisorption. It is remarked that the antigen binding capacity was slightly lower in the second binding cycle, probably due to partial nanobody denaturation by the SDS washing step at the end of the first cycle (Table S2, Supplementary Materials). In spite of this, the second binding cycle confirms the improved antigen binding capacity of the site-specifically conjugated NbVCAM1-LEY-alkyne.

The dissociation constant of the antigen binding can be determined from the ellipsometric binding curves (Figure 3A,B). There was a faster hVCAM1 binding of the conjugated NbVCAM1-LEY-alkyne, representing a larger association constant (k_a), as compared to the conjugated rNbVCAM1-His_6-alkyne, i.e., 25 vs. 50 min, respectively (after baseline stabilization) to reach saturation. Based on the surface mass density at equilibrium, the Scatchard plots (Figure 3C,D) were constructed from which a K_D value of 7.7 nM was determined for the NbVCAM1-LEY-alkyne-conjugated surface. The antigen binding at low concentration of the rNbVCAM1-His_6-alkyne-conjugated surface is so poor that a very large but unreliable K_D is resulted from the Scatchard plot. However, it confirms the increase in binding affinity of the site-specifically alkynated nanobody after surface conjugation. These results indicate that there are not only more binding sites available on the surfaces conjugated with the oriented NbVCAM1-LEY-alkyne, but also that these sites have an equal binding affinity towards the hVCAM1 antigen. In contrast, a rNbVCAM1-His_6-alkyne-conjugated surface has less binding sites and some of them bind the antigen with less affinity due to a conformational change resulting from conjugating via an alkyne which is localized within or close to the binding pocket.

Additionally, the dose–response curves, representing a linear correlation between the surface mass density and the antigen concentration (Figure 4), can be used for comparing antigen binding sensitivity. The slopes of the curves indicate that the sensitivity could be increased 1.82 times (38.39 vs. 21.04) by using the *C*-terminally alkynated nanobody as compared to the randomly alkynated nanobody. It is noticed that the hVCAM1 binding of the surface conjugated with the NbVCAM1-LEY-alkyne reaches saturation at 3.75 μg/mL antigen. Therefore, the dose–response curve was fitted with only the data points in the linear range. The LD and LQ of the NbVCAM1-LEY-alkyne conjugated surfaces are, respectively, 0.51 and 1.54 μg/mL, and so slightly lower than the values of 0.62 and 1.88 μg/mL found for the rNbVCAM1-His_6-alkyne conjugated surfaces. It further is experimentally observed that hVCAM1 concentrations below 1.25 μg/mL indeed become difficult to quantify with ellipsometry.

In an attempt to achieve a higher sensitivity (i.e., a lower detection limit) for biosensing applications, surface plasmon resonance (SPR) was employed using a Biacore™ T200 workstation.

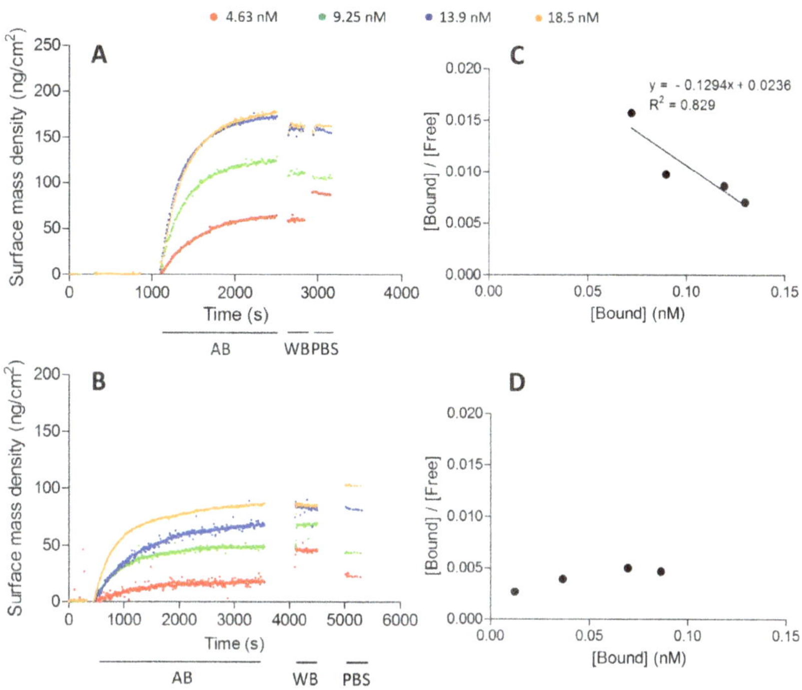

Figure 3. Antigen binding curves of azidified silicon wafers conjugated by CuAAC with: NbVCAM1-LEY-alkyne (**A**); and rNbVCAM1-His$_6$-alkyne (**B**) for different hVCAM1 antigen concentrations as detected by ellipsometry. The association process was followed by washing with washing buffer and PBS, after which the surface mass density was determined. (**C**,**D**) The corresponding Scatchard plots. The dissociation constants K_D were derived from the inverse of the slopes of the linear regression equations.

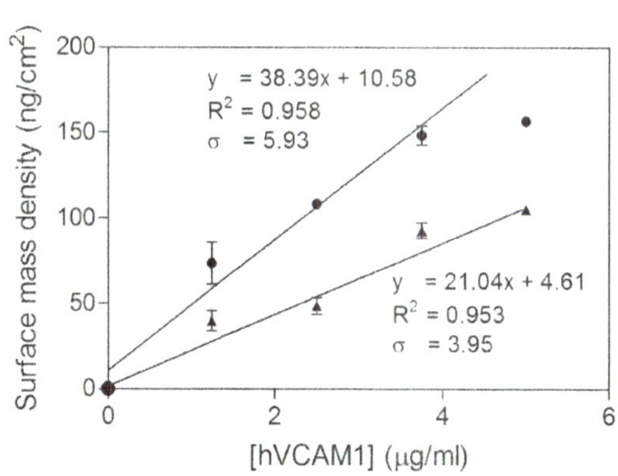

Figure 4. Dose–response curves for the hVCAM1 (R & D Systems) binding to NbVCAM1-LEY-alkyne (●) and rNbVCAM1-His$_6$-alkyne (▲) conjugated silicon slides obtained by ellipsometry. The data were analyzed by means of a linear least squares fitting (95% confidence level; note that only the non-saturating antigen concentrations (0–3.75 μg/mL) were taken into account for NbVCAM1-LEY-alkyne conjugated surfaces).

3.4. Study of the Antigen Binding by Surface Plasmon Resonance

Compared to ellipsometry, SPR is a more advanced label-free technique to study biomolecular interactions due to its higher degree of automation and sensitivity in addition to limited sample preparation. In a previous study on hVCAM1 antigen binding using SPR, Broisat et al. [63] reported a dissociation constant in the nanomolar range for NbVCAM1-His$_6$. However, these authors immobilized the antigen as the "ligand" and used the nanobody as the "analyte", a set-up not aimed for bio-sensing applications. In this study, we construct Biacore™ C1 chip surfaces conjugated with nanobodies that are not only bound covalently but also with a uniformly orientation, and therefore exhibit an improved binding sensitivity as compared to randomly bound nanobodies.

The improvement in binding sensitivity of conjugated NbVCAM1-LEY-alkyne (as compared to rNbVCAM1-His$_6$-alkyne conjugated via CuAAC and NbVCAM1-His$_6$ coupled via EDC/NHS chemistry) can be observed for two different hVCAM1 antigens by comparing the slopes of the dose–response curves (Figure 5A,B and Table 1). For the hVCAM1 of R & D Systems, the sensitivity was increased 6.7 times and 53.9 times, respectively. For the hVCAM1 from Peprotech, the sensitivity was increased 1.6 times and 4.1 times, respectively. Improvements in detection and quantitation limit were also observed for the binding of both hVCAM1 antigens to NbVCAM1-LEY-alkyne as compared to the other nanobody variants (Table 1). In addition, and this for ellipsometry as well as for SPR, the antigen binding experiments were performed on three independent surfaces (three replicates) and the resulting measurements show small relative standard deviations and high correlation coefficients (Figure 5), indicative for a good reproducibility.

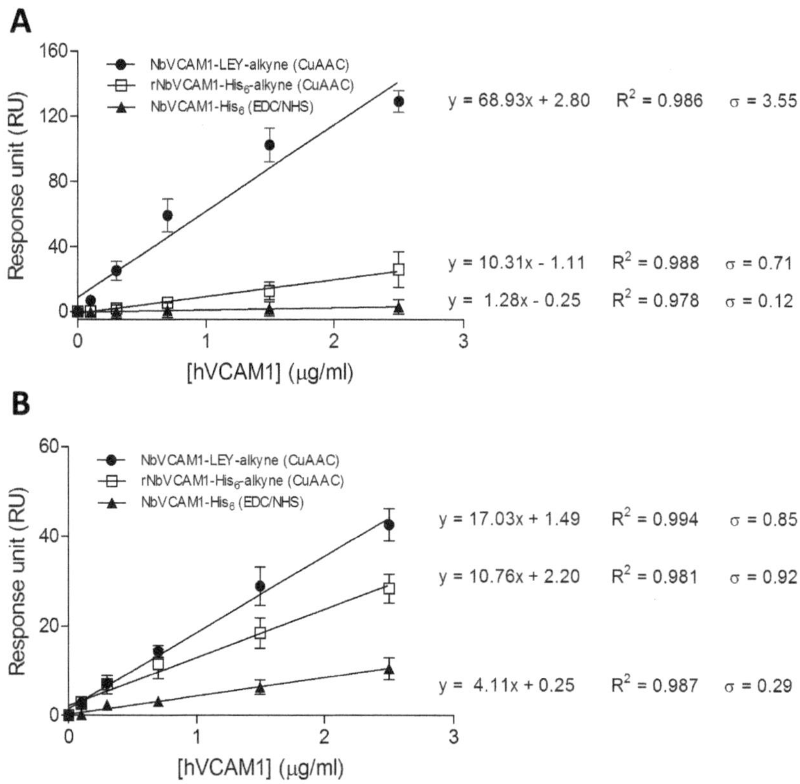

Figure 5. Dose–response curves for the binding of hVCAM1 from: R & D Systems (**A**); and Peprotech (**B**) to VCAM1-targeting nanobodies that are conjugated to different flow cells of the C1 chips via different chemistries.

Table 1. The sensitivity (S), detection limit (DL) and quantitation limit (QL), all displayed in μg/mL, for the binding of recombinant human VCAM1 antigens to the nanobody-conjugated flow cells prepared by the different coupling methods.

	hVCAM1 (R & D System)			hVCAM1 (Peprotech)		
	S	DL	QL	S	DL	QL
NbVCAM1-LEY-alkyne (CuAAC chemistry)	68.93	0.17	0.51	17.03	0.16	0.50
rNbVCAM1-His$_6$-alkyne (CuAAC chemistry)	10.31	0.23	0.69	10.76	0.28	0.86
NbVCAM1-His$_6$ (EDC/NHS chemistry)	1.28	0.31	0.94	4.11	0.23	0.71

As shown in Table 2, the binding kinetics and affinity of VCAM1 for the nanobody-conjugated surfaces was further evaluated on the basis of the K_D constants. The association constant (k_a) and dissociation constant (k_d) are shown in Table S3 (Supplementary Materials). It is firstly noticed that the NbVCAM1-LEY-alkyne conjugated flow cell (Fc) is able to bind both human and mouse VCAM1 antigens with nanomolar affinities, which is in accordance with the findings of Broisat et al. [63]. Moreover, the site-specifically conjugated NbVCAM1-LEY-alkyne shows a significant increase in binding affinity for the two hVCAM1 antigens, i.e., with a factor of 6–14 as compared to rNbVCAM1-His$_6$-alkyne and even a factor of 138 as compared to NbVCAM1-His$_6$ coupled via EDC/NHS chemistry (Table 2). These data are in accordance with the ellipsometry results, supporting the hypothesis that random conjugation via the lysines (or alkynated lysines) disturbs the conformation of the nanobody's binding domains if the anchoring amine is directly involved in the antigen binding or is changing the spatial structure of the binding pocket. These results also show that SPR is more sensitive to detect the differences in binding affinity as compared to ellipsometry, mainly due to the lower detection limit (subnanomolar concentrations of antigen) and higher level of automation (limited sample preparation and handling) of the Biacore™ system.

Table 2. The dissociation constant (K_D in nM $\pm$ standard error) for the binding of the human and mouse recombinant VCAM1 antigens to the nanobody-conjugated flow cells prepared by the different coupling methods.

	hVCAM1 (R & D System)	hVCAM1 (Peprotech)	mVCAM1 (Bioconnect)
NbVCAM1-LEY-alkyne (CuAAC chemistry)	0.15 $\pm$ 0.01	1.61 $\pm$ 0.14	1.45 $\pm$ 0.55
rNbVCAM1-His$_6$-alkyne (CuAAC chemistry)	2.10 $\pm$ 0.71	8.67 $\pm$ 0.27	N/D
NbVCAM1-His$_6$ (EDC/NHS chemistry)	20.70 *	49.30 *	N/D

N/D: not determined, *: insufficient data to calculate the standard error.

In addition, the difference in K_D for the binding of the different antigens to conjugated NbVCAM1-LEY-alkyne (Table 2) can be explained by the structural differences between these antigens. The single domain hVCAM1 (from Peprotech) and mVCAM1 (from Bioconnect) bind with similar affinity constants, whereas the heterodimeric hVCAM1 (from R & D Systems) exhibits a smaller K_D, i.e., a higher affinity. Since this antigen contains a VCAM1 and a partial IgG1 domain, both of which belong to the immunoglobulin superclass, they might share some structural similarities which probably enables occasional binding to the nanobody with the IgG1 domain (although with much less affinity as compared to the VCAM1 domain). It therefore has to be noted that the results calculated for the binding of the chimeric hVCAM1 antigen by means of the monovalent binding model have to be considered as useful approximations.

After regeneration of the nanobody-conjugated sensor chips, it was shown that 70% of the binding activity was retained for the NbVCAM1-LEY-alkyne based sensor (Table S4, Supplementary Materials), whereas more than 50% was lost for the rNbVCAM1-His$_6$-alkyne and the NbVCAM1-His$_6$ based reference sensors (data not shown). It again indicates that nanobodies that are conjugated via the

C-terminally alkyne to the azidified surfaces resist the regeneration conditions better, and are thus more stable, than the nanobodies on the reference sensors. It should be noted that the reusability of all above platforms might be improved upon applying different regeneration protocols.

All the results presented above show that: (i) the EPL technique is an efficient tool to site-specifically append a bio-orthogonal functional group to a nanobody for (ii) site-specific coupling to surfaces for advanced biosensing. As reported before, our adapted EPL protocol allows a one-step synthesis and purification of C-terminally alkynated nanobodies in high yield for subsequent CuAAC-mediated coupling [43]. This is highly advantageous as compared to the two-step procedure (purification of NbVCAM1-His_6 and its random alkynation separately) used to prepare the randomly alkynated nanobodies. However, more importantly, our findings additionally demonstrate that the combined use of EPL and CuAAC chemistry allows to uniformly conjugate solid supports with nanobodies, resulting in higher binding affinities and sensitivities as well as improved detection limit, quantitation limit and repeatability as compared to non-oriented (random) approaches. More specifically for the NbVCAM1-LEY-alkyne nanobody, a SPR-based VCAM1 biosensor would allow to detect human and mouse VCAM1 antigens at (sub)nanomolar concentrations in atherosclerotic serum.

4. Conclusions

The combined use of EPL and highly selective CuAAC "click" chemistry is reported in this study in order to develop biosensor platforms for VCAM1 binding detection with significantly improved performances. The proof of principle of the approach, being generic in nature, is demonstrated in this study for a specific NbVCAM1-LEY-alkyne nanobody and SPR-based read-out platform. More specifically, the EPL principle is applied to engineer the nanobody NbVCAM1-LEY with a site-specific, i.e., C-terminal, alkynated linker molecule while maintaining full antigen binding capacity. The alkyne function of this linker allows conjugating the resulting NbVCAM1-LEY-alkyne nanobodies covalently and with a uniform orientation to azidified solid supports via a stable triazole linkage resulting from the CuAAC "click" reaction. This paper also demonstrates the potential, feasibility and benefits of this innovative strategy for biosensor development and can pave the way to further device miniaturization needed for the development of sensors for detecting multiple antigens in a single assay.

Acknowledgments: This research is funded by the FWO project G.0581.12N. The authors gratefully thank S. Muyldermans and N. Devoogdt (Vrije Universiteit Brussel, Belgium) for the vector pHEN6(c):*pelB*-NbVCAM1-His6, and J.-P. Noben and E. Rooyackers for the MS measurements. We further acknowledge the Hercules Foundation for the project "LC-MS@UHasselt: Linear Trap Quadrupole-Orbitrap mass spectrometer", and the Interreg IV-A project "BioMiMedics" which is financed by the EU and the province of Limburg (Belgium). We further thank the Interuniversity Attraction Poles program (P7/05) initiated by the Belgian Science Policy Office (BELSPO).

Author Contributions: D.T.T., E.S.R., W.G. and P.A. conceived and designed the experiments; D.T.T. performed the experiments; D.T.T., W.G. and P.A. analyzed the data; T.V. performed azidification of the silicon wafers; K.V. and L.M. helped perform the SPR; and D.T.T., W.G. and P.A. wrote the paper.

Conflicts of Interest: The authors declare no conflict of interest. The founding sponsors had no role in the design of the study; in the collection, analyses, or interpretation of data; in the writing of the manuscript, and in the decision to publish the results.

References

1. Dover, J.E.; Hwang, G.M.; Mullen, E.H.; Prorok, B.C.; Suh, S.J. Recent advances in peptide probe-based biosensors for detection of infectious agents. *J. Microbiol. Methods* **2009**, *78*, 10–19. [CrossRef] [PubMed]
2. Kang, J.; Kim, S.; Kwon, Y. Antibody-based biosensors for environmental monitoring. *J. Toxicol. Environ. Health Sci.* **2009**, *1*, 145–150. [CrossRef]

3. Kim, J.P.; Lee, B.Y.; Hong, S.; Sim, S.J. Ultrasensitive carbon nanotube-based biosensors using antibody-binding fragments. *Anal. Biochem.* **2008**, *381*, 193–198. [CrossRef] [PubMed]
4. Omidfar, K.; Khorsand, F.; Darziani Azizi, M. New analytical applications of gold nanoparticles as label in antibody based sensors. *Biosens. Bioelectron.* **2013**, *43*, 336–347. [CrossRef] [PubMed]
5. Ciani, I.; Schulze, H.; Corrigan, D.K.; Henihan, G.; Giraud, G.; Terry, J.G.; Walton, A.J.; Pethig, R.; Ghazal, P.; Crain, J.; et al. Development of immunosensors for direct detection of three wound infection biomarkers at point of care using electrochemical impedance spectroscopy. *Biosens. Bioelectron.* **2012**, *31*, 413–418. [CrossRef] [PubMed]
6. Wan, Y.; Su, Y.; Zhu, X.; Liu, G.; Fan, C. Development of electrochemical immunosensors towards point of care diagnostics. *Biosens. Bioelectron.* **2013**, *47*, 1–11. [CrossRef] [PubMed]
7. Julie-Ann, O.R.; Kara, L.M.M.; Richard, J.O.K. Antibody-based sensors for disease detection, in biosensors and their applications in healthcare. *Future Sci. Ltd.* **2013**. [CrossRef]
8. Huy, T.Q.; Hanh, N.T.; Thuy, N.T.; Chung, P.V.; Nga, P.T.; Tuan, M.A. A novel biosensor based on serum antibody immobilization for rapid detection of viral antigens. *Talanta* **2011**, *86*, 271–277. [CrossRef] [PubMed]
9. Zeng, X.; Shen, Z.; Mernaugh, R. Recombinant antibodies and their use in biosensors. *Anal. Bioanal. Chem.* **2012**, *402*, 3027–3038. [CrossRef] [PubMed]
10. Trilling, A.K.; Beekwilder, J.; Zuilhof, H. Antibody orientation on biosensor surfaces: A minireview. *Analyst* **2013**, *138*, 1619–1627. [CrossRef] [PubMed]
11. Dumoulin, M.; Conrath, K.; van Meirhaeghe, A.; Meersman, F.; Heremans, K.; Frenken, L.G.; Muyldermans, S.; Wyns, L.; Matagne, A. Single-domain antibody fragments with high conformational stability. *Protein Sci.* **2002**, *11*, 500–515. [CrossRef] [PubMed]
12. Arenkov, P.; Kukhtin, A.; Gemmell, A.; Voloshchuk, S.; Chupeeva, V.; Mirzabekov, A. Protein microchips: Use for immunoassay and enzymatic reactions. *Anal. Biochem.* **2000**, *278*, 123–131. [CrossRef] [PubMed]
13. Lee, K.B.; Park, S.J.; Mirkin, C.A.; Smith, J.C.; Mrksich, M. Protein nanoarrays generated by dip-pen nanolithography. *Science* **2002**, *295*, 1702–1705. [CrossRef] [PubMed]
14. Rusmini, F.; Zhong, Z.; Feijen, J. Protein immobilization strategies for protein biochips. *Biomacromolecules* **2007**, *8*, 1775–1789. [CrossRef] [PubMed]
15. Zhu, H.; Snyder, M. Protein chip technology. *Curr. Opin. Chem. Biol.* **2003**, *7*, 55–63. [CrossRef]
16. Huang, W.; Wang, J.; Bhattacharyya, D.; Bachas, L.G. Improving the activity of immobilized subtilisin by site-specific attachment to surfaces. *Anal. Chem.* **1997**, *69*, 4601–4607. [CrossRef] [PubMed]
17. Steen Redeker, E.; Ta, D.T.; Cortens, D.; Billen, B.; Guedens, W.; Adriaensens, P. Protein engineering for directed immobilization. *Bioconjug. Chem.* **2013**, *24*, 1761–1777. [CrossRef] [PubMed]
18. Hernandez, K.; Fernandez-Lafuente, R. Control of protein immobilization: Coupling immobilization and site-directed mutagenesis to improve biocatalyst or biosensor performance. *Enzym. Microb. Technol.* **2011**, *48*, 107–122. [CrossRef] [PubMed]
19. Camarero, J.A. New developments for the site-specific attachment of protein to surfaces. *Biophys. Rev. Lett.* **2006**, *1*, 1–28. [CrossRef]
20. Yoshimura, S.H.; Khan, S.; Ohno, S.; Yokogawa, T.; Nishikawa, K.; Hosoya, T.; Maruyama, H.; Nakayama, Y.; Takeyasu, K. Site-specific attachment of a protein to a carbon nanotube end without loss of protein function. *Bioconjug. Chem.* **2012**, *23*, 1488–1493. [CrossRef] [PubMed]
21. Liu, G.Y.; Amro, N.A. Positioning protein molecules on surfaces: A nanoengineering approach to supramolecular chemistry. *Proc. Natl. Acad. Sci. USA* **2012**, *99*, 5165–5170. [CrossRef] [PubMed]
22. Van Vught, R.; Pieters, R.J.; Breukink, E. Site-specific functionalization of proteins and their applications to therapeutic antibodies. *Comput. Struct. Biotechnol. J.* **2014**. [CrossRef] [PubMed]
23. Mikula, E.; Wysłouch-Cieszyńska, A.; Zhukova, L.; Puchalska, M.; Verwilst, P.; Dehaen, W.; Radecki, J.; Radecka, H. Voltammetric detection of S100B protein using His-tagged receptor domains for advanced glycation end products (RAGE) immobilized onto a gold electrode surface. *Sensors* **2014**, *14*, 10650–10663. [CrossRef] [PubMed]
24. Jargiło, A.; Grabowska, I.; Radecka, H.; Sulima, M.; Marszałek, I.; WysłouchCieszyńska, A.; Dehaen, W.; Radecki, J. Redox active dipyrromethene-Cu(II) monolayer for oriented immobilization of his-tagged RAGE domains—The base of electrochemical biosensor for determination of $A\beta_{16-23'}$. *Electroanalysis* **2013**, *25*, 1185–1193. [CrossRef]

25. Jarocka, U.; Sawicka, R.; Stachyra, A.; Góra-Sochacka, A.; Sirko, A.; Zagórski-Ostoja, W.; Sączyńska, V.; Porębska, A.; Dehaen, W.; Radecki, J.; et al. A biosensor based on electroactive dipyrromethene-Cu(II) layer deposited onto gold electrodes for the detection of antibodies against avian influenza virus type H5N1 in hen sera. *Anal. Bioanal. Chem.* **2015**, *407*, 7807–7814. [CrossRef] [PubMed]
26. Wojtasik, J.; Mielecki, M.; Kurzatkowska, K.; Grzelak, K.; Verwilst, P.; Dehaen, W.; Radecki, J.; Radecka, H. Pentetic acid (DPTA) Cu(II) monolayer deposited on gold electrode—The base of biosensors for electrochemical screening of kinase JAK2 and potential inhibitor interactions. *Sens. Actuators B Chem.* **2014**, *196*, 223–230. [CrossRef]
27. Mielecki, M.; Wojtasik, J.; Zborowska, M.; Kurzatkowska, K.; Grzelaka, K.; Dehaen, W.; Radecki, J.; Radecka, H. Oriented immobilization of His-tagged kinase RIO1 protein on redox active *N*-(IDA-like)-Cu(II) monolayer deposited on gold electrode—The base of electrochemical biosensor. *Electrochim. Acta* **2013**, *96*, 147–154. [CrossRef]
28. Rostovtsev, V.V.; Green, L.G.; Fokin, V.V.; Sharpless, K.B. A stepwise huisgen cycloaddition process: Copper(I)-catalyzed regioselective "Ligation" of azides and terminal alkynes. *Angew. Chem. Int. Ed. Engl.* **2002**, *41*, 2596–2599. [CrossRef]
29. Tornoe, C.W.; Christensen, C.; Meldal, M. Peptidotriazoles on solid phase: [1,2,3]-Triazoles by regiospecific copper(I)-catalyzed 1,3-dipolar cycloadditions of terminal alkynes to azides. *J. Org. Chem.* **2002**, *67*, 3057–3064. [CrossRef] [PubMed]
30. Meldal, M.; Tornoe, C.W. Cu-catalyzed azide-alkyne cycloaddition. *Chem. Rev.* **2008**, *108*, 2952–3015. [CrossRef] [PubMed]
31. Muir, T.W.; Sondhi, D.; Cole, P.A. Expressed protein ligation: A general method for protein engineering. *Proc. Natl. Acad. Sci. USA* **1998**, *95*, 6705–6710. [CrossRef] [PubMed]
32. Berrade, L.; Camarero, J.A. Expressed protein ligation: A resourceful tool to study protein structure and function. *Cell Mol. Life Sci.* **2009**, *66*, 3909–3022. [CrossRef] [PubMed]
33. Hauser, P.S.; Ryan, R.O. Expressed protein ligation using an *N*-terminal cysteine containing fragment generated in vivo from a Pelb fusion protein. *Protein Expr. Purif.* **2007**, *54*, 227–233. [CrossRef] [PubMed]
34. Hauser, P.S.; Raussens, V.; Yamamoto, T.; Abdullahi, G.E.; Weers, P.M.; Sykes, B.D.; Ryan, R.O. Semisynthesis and segmental isotope labeling of the apoe3 *N*-terminal domain using expressed protein ligation. *J. Lipid Res.* **2009**, *50*, 1548–1555. [CrossRef] [PubMed]
35. Tanaka, T.; Wagner, A.M.; Warner, J.B.; Wang, Y.J.; Petersson, E.J. Expressed protein ligation at methionine: *N*-terminal attachment of homocysteine, ligation, and masking. *Angew. Chem. Int. Ed. Engl.* **2013**, *52*, 6210–6213. [CrossRef] [PubMed]
36. Baumann, L.; Steinhagen, M.; Beck-Sickinger, A.G. Preparation of *C*-terminally modified chemokines by expressed protein ligation. *Methods Mol. Biol.* **2013**, *1047*, 103–118. [PubMed]
37. Debets, M.F.; van Berkel, S.S.; Dommerholt, J.; Dirks, A.T.; Rutjes, F.P.; Delft, F.L. Bioconjugation with strained alkenes and alkynes. *Acc. Chem. Res.* **2011**, *44*, 805–815. [CrossRef] [PubMed]
38. Reulen, S.W.; van Baal, I.; Raats, J.M.; Merkx, M. Efficient, chemoselective synthesis of immunomicelles using single-domain antibodies with a *C*-terminal thioester. *BMC Biotechnol.* **2009**. [CrossRef] [PubMed]
39. Debets, M.F.; Leenders, W.P.; Verrijp, K.; Zonjee, M.; Meeuwissen, S.A.; Otte-Holler, I.; van Hest, J.C. Nanobody-functionalized polymersomes for tumor-vessel targeting. *Macromol. Biosci.* **2013**, *13*, 938–945. [CrossRef] [PubMed]
40. Lin, P.C.; Ueng, S.H.; Tseng, M.C.; Ko, J.L.; Huang, K.T.; Yu, S.C.; Adak, A.K.; Chen, Y.J.; Lin, C.C. Site-specific protein modification through Cu(I)-catalyzed 1,2,3-triazole formation and its implementation in protein microarray fabrication. *Angew. Chem. Int. Ed. Engl.* **2006**, *45*, 4286–4290. [CrossRef] [PubMed]
41. Steinhagen, M.; Holland-Nell, K.; Meldal, M.; Beck-Sickinger, A.G. Simultaneous "One Pot" expressed protein ligation and Cui-catalyzed azide/alkyne cycloaddition for protein immobilization. *Chembiochem* **2011**, *12*, 2426–2430. [CrossRef] [PubMed]
42. Trilling, A.K.; Hesselink, T.; van Houwelingen, A.; Cordewener, J.H.; Jongsma, M.A.; Schoffelen, S.; van Hest, J.C.; Zuilhof, H.; Beekwilder, J. Orientation of llama antibodies strongly increases sensitivity of biosensors. *Biosens. Bioelectron.* **2014**, *60*, 130–136. [CrossRef] [PubMed]
43. Ta, D.T.; Steen Redeker, E.; Billen, B.; Reekmans, G.; Sikulu, J.; Noben, J.P.; Guedens, W.; Adriaensens, P. An efficient protocol towards site-specifically clickable nanobodies in high yield: Cytoplasmic expression in *Escherichia coli* combined with intein-mediated protein ligation. *Protein Eng. Des. Sel.* **2015**, *28*, 351–363. [CrossRef] [PubMed]

44. Springer, T.A. Adhesion receptors of the immune system. *Nature* **1990**, *346*, 425–434. [CrossRef] [PubMed]
45. Libby, P.; Hansson, G.K. Involvement of the immune system in human atherogenesis: Current knowledge and unanswered questions. *Lab. Investig.* **1991**, *64*, 5–15. [PubMed]
46. Hwang, S.J.; Ballantyne, C.M.; Sharrett, A.R.; Smith, L.C.; Davis, C.E.; Gotto, A.M., Jr.; Boerwinkle, E. Circulating adhesion molecules Vcam-1, Icam-1, and E-Selectin in carotid atherosclerosis and incident coronary heart disease cases: The atherosclerosis risk in communities (Aric) study. *Circulation* **1997**, *96*, 4219–4225. [CrossRef] [PubMed]
47. Navarro-Hernandez, R.E.; Oregon-Romero, E.; Vazquez-Del Mercado, M.; Rangel-Villalobos, H.; Palafox-Sanchez, C.A.; Munoz-Valle, J.F. Expression of Icam1 and Vcam1 serum levels in rheumatoid arthritis clinical activity. *Dis. Mark.* **2009**, *26*, 119–126. [CrossRef] [PubMed]
48. Jurisic, G.; Sundberg, J.P.; Bleich, A.; Leiter, E.H.; Broman, K.W.; Buechler, G.; Alley, L.; Vestweber, D.; Detmar, M. Quantitative lymphatic vessel trait analysis suggests Vcam1 as candidate modifier gene of inflammatory bowel disease. *Genes Immun.* **2010**, *11*, 219–231. [CrossRef] [PubMed]
49. Matsuda, M.; Tsukada, N.; Miyagi, K.; Yanagisawa, N. Increased levels of soluble vascular cell-adhesion molecule-1 (Vcam-1) in the cerebrospinal-fluid and sera of patients with multiple-sclerosis and human T-lymphotropic virus type-1-associated myelopathy. *J. Neuroimmunol.* **1995**, *59*, 35–40. [CrossRef]
50. Wu, T.C. The role of vascular cell adhesion molecule-1 in tumor immune evasion. *Cancer Res.* **2007**, *67*, 6003–6006. [CrossRef] [PubMed]
51. Shioi, K.; Komiya, A.; Hattori, K.; Huang, Y.; Sano, F.; Murakami, T.; Nakaigawa, N.; Kishida, T.; Kubota, Y.; Nagashima, Y.; et al. Vascular cell adhesion molecule 1 predicts cancer-free survival in clear cell renal carcinoma patients. *Clin. Cancer Res.* **2006**, *12*, 7339–7346. [CrossRef] [PubMed]
52. Touvier, M.; Fezeu, L.; Ahluwalia, N.; Julia, C.; Charnaux, N.; Sutton, A.; Mejean, C.; Latino-Martel, P.; Hercberg, S.; Galan, P.; et al. Pre-diagnostic levels of adiponectin and soluble vascular cell adhesion molecule-1 are associated with colorectal cancer risk. *World J. Gastroenterol.* **2012**, *18*, 2805–2812. [CrossRef] [PubMed]
53. Yamada, Y.; Arao, T.; Matsumoto, K.; Gupta, V.; Tan, W.; Fedynyshyn, J.; Nakajima, T.E.; Shimada, Y.; Hamaguchi, T.; Kato, K.; et al. Plasma concentrations of Vcam-1 and Pai-1: A predictive biomarker for post-operative recurrence in colorectal cancer. *Cancer Sci.* **2010**, *101*, 1886–1890. [CrossRef] [PubMed]
54. Nguyen, V.K.; Su, C.; Muyldermans, S.; van der Loo, W. Heavy-chain antibodies in camelidae; a case of evolutionary innovation. *Immunogenetics* **2002**, *54*, 39–47. [PubMed]
55. Jagadish, B.; Sankaranarayanan, R.; Xu, L.; Richards, R.; Vagner, J.; Hruby, V.J.; Gillies, R.J.; Mash, E.A. Squalene-derived flexible linkers for bioactive peptides. *Bioorg. Med. Chem. Lett.* **2007**, *17*, 3310–3313. [CrossRef] [PubMed]
56. Saerens, D.; Kinne, J.; Bosmans, E.; Wernery, U.; Muyldermans, S.; Conrath, K. Single domain antibodies derived from dromedary lymph node and peripheral blood lymphocytes sensing conformational variants of prostate-specific antigen. *J. Biol. Chem.* **2004**, *279*, 51965–51972. [CrossRef] [PubMed]
57. Damen, C.W.N.; Speijer, H.; Hermens, W.T.; Schellens, J.H.M.; Rosing, H.; Beijnen, J.H. Nanobody-based cancer therapy of solid tumors. *Anal. Biochem.* **2009**, *293*, 73–79. [CrossRef] [PubMed]
58. Giesen, P.L.; Willems, G.M.; Hemker, H.C.; Stuart, M.C.; Hermens, W.T. Monitoring of unbound protein in vesicle suspensions with off-null ellipsometry. *Biochim. Biophys. Acta* **1993**, *1147*, 125–131. [CrossRef]
59. Robers, M.; Rensink, I.J.; Hack, C.E.; Aarden, L.A.; Reutelingsperger, C.P.; Glatz, J.F.; Hermens, W.T. A new principle for rapid immunoassay of proteins based on in situ precipitate-enhanced ellipsometry. *Biophys. J.* **1999**, *76*, 2769–2776. [CrossRef]
60. Thevenot, D.R.; Toth, K.; Durst, R.A.; Wilson, G.S. Electrochemical biosensors: Recommended definitions and classification. *Biosens. Bioelectron.* **2001**, *16*, 121–131. [CrossRef] [PubMed]
61. Swartz, M.E.; Krull, I.S. Chapter 4: Method validation basics. In *Handbook of Analytical Validation*; CRC Press Taylor & Francis Group: Boca Raton, FL, USA, 2012; pp. 70–73.
62. Karlsson, R.; Katsamba, P.S.; Nordin, H.; Pol, E.; Myszka, D.G. Analyzing a kinetic titration series using affinity biosensors. *Anal. Biochem.* **2006**, *349*, 136–147. [CrossRef] [PubMed]
63. Broisat, A.; Hernot, S.; Toczek, J.; de Vos, J.; Riou, L.M.; Martin, S.; Ahmadi, M.; Thielens, N.; Wernery, U.; Caveliers, V.; et al. Nanobodies targeting mouse/human Vcam1 for the nuclear imaging of atherosclerotic lesions. *Circ. Res.* **2012**, *110*, 927–937. [CrossRef] [PubMed]

64. De Genst, E.; Saerens, D.; Muyldermans, S.; Conrath, K. Antibody repertoire development in camelids. *Dev. Comp. Immunol.* **2006**, *30*, 187–198. [CrossRef] [PubMed]
65. Muyldermans, S.; Baral, T.N.; Retamozzo, V.C.; De Baetselier, P.; de Genst, E.; Kinne, J.; Leonhardt, H.; Magez, S.; Nguyen, V.K.; Revets, H.; et al. Camelid immunoglobulins and nanobody technology. *Vet. Immunol. Immunopathol.* **2009**, *128*, 178–183. [CrossRef] [PubMed]
66. Kijanka, M.; Dorresteijn, B.; Oliveira, S.; van Bergen En Henegouwen, P.M. Nanobody-based cancer therapy of solid tumors. *Nanomedicine* **2015**, *1*, 161–174. [CrossRef] [PubMed]

13

Development of Formaldehyde Biosensor for Determination of Formalin in Fish Samples; Malabar Red Snapper (*Lutjanus malabaricus*) and Longtail Tuna (*Thunnus tonggol*)

Bohari Noor Aini, Shafiquzzaman Siddiquee * and Kamaruzaman Ampon

Biotechnology Research Institute, Universiti Malaysia Sabah, Jln UMS, 88400 Kota Kinabalu, Sabah, Malaysia; noorainibohari@gmail.com (B.N.A.); amponk@ums.edu.my or profkamaru@gmail.com (K.A.)

* Correspondence: shafiqpab@ums.edu.my or shafiqpab@hotmail.com

Academic Editor: Nastaran Hashemi

Abstract: Electrochemical biosensors are widely recognized in biosensing devices due to the fact that gives a direct, reliable, and reproducible measurement within a short period. During bio-interaction process and the generation of electrons, it produces electrochemical signals which can be measured using an electrochemical detector. A formaldehyde biosensor was successfully developed by depositing an ionic liquid (IL) (e.g., 1-ethyl-3-methylimidazolium trifluoromethanesulfonate ([EMIM][Otf])), gold nanoparticles (AuNPs), and chitosan (CHIT), onto a glassy carbon electrode (GCE). The developed formaldehyde biosensor was analyzed for sensitivity, reproducibility, storage stability, and detection limits. Methylene blue was used as a redox indicator for increasing the electron transfer in the electrochemical cell. The developed biosensor measured the NADH electron from the NAD^+ reduction at a potential of 0.4 V. Under optimal conditions, the differential pulse voltammetry (DPV) method detected a wider linear range of formaldehyde concentrations from 0.01 to 10 ppm within 5 s, with a detection limit of 0.1 ppm. The proposed method was successfully detected with the presence of formalin in fish samples, *Lutjanus malabaricus* and *Thunnus Tonggol*. The proposed method is a simple, rapid, and highly accurate, compared to the existing technique.

Keywords: formaldehyde biosensor; glassy carbon electrode; gold nanoparticles; ionic liquid; methylene blue

---

1. Introduction

The fast urbanization of society has led to an accumulation of many toxic elements, especially carcinogens in the environment. Formaldehyde is considered as a toxic element since it has been classified as Group 1 carcinogen to human beings by the International Agency for Research on Cancer (IARC). Formaldehyde accumulates in the body and adversely affects lifespan. Formaldehyde is commonly used as bath treatment in aquaculture and the preservation of any biological samples. Nowadays, the fish vendors have learned to use formaldehyde, better known as formalin (40% formaldehyde), to preserve fish, as the chemical is a renowned food preservative. This has been proven by recent news and research, claiming the use of formaldehyde in fish preservation is very popular, particularly in Asian countries [1,2].

Fish and seafood are an important part of a healthy diet and are deliberated as the largest source of protein in Malaysia. By composition, fish contains fat, free amino acids, and water, which is susceptible to spoilage by microorganisms and biochemical reactions during *post mortem* processing [3]. The flesh of fish can spoil quickly and it should be eaten on the day of capture, unless cured [4]. Microbial and enzymatic activities in fresh fish can deteriorate the fish and alter the biological compounds under normal freezing storage. Thus, fish and seafood are very perishable and can only be kept fresh in ice for 8 to 14 days, depending on the species. In order to keep the freshness of fish and seafood, fishermen and fish vendors tend to carelessly use formaldehyde as a preservation agent because formaldehyde is well-known in food preserving. However, the dose of formaldehyde used in the fish preservation activity has yet to be disclosed. Lack of knowledge on the lethal effect of formaldehyde has led to its misuse.

The formaldehyde mechanism of action for fixing lies in its ability to form cross-links between soluble and structural proteins. The resulting structure retains its cellular constituents in their in vivo relationships to each other, giving it a degree of mechanical strength which enables it to withstand subsequent processing, as reported by Environmental and Occupational Health and Safety Services, 2004 [5].

The limitation on exposure and health risk towards this hazardous substance in occupational settings has been set by the Occupational Safety and Health Administration and Environmental Protection Agency. According to the United States Environmental Protection Agency (EPA), maximum daily dose reference (RfD) for formaldehyde is 0.2 $\mu g \cdot g^{-1}$ body weight per day [6]. According to Malaysian Food Regulations 1985, Regulations 148 and 159 (2006), only smoked fish and meat are permitted to incidentally absorb formaldehyde during processing in a proportion not exceeding 5 $\mu g \cdot g^{-1}$ [7]. However, for fresh fish, the permitted amount of formaldehyde is not yet specified [8].

Standards have been fixed by the Occupational Safety and Health Administration, Malaysian Food Regulations, as well as by the EPA, to limit human exposure and health risk in occupations involving formaldehyde use. Formaldehyde levels must be accurately monitored to act in accordance with these standards. Many conventional methods are available for determination of formaldehyde concentration levels in the laboratory, such as gas chromatography-mass spectrometry (GC-MS), high-performance liquid chromatography (HPLC), fluorimetry, Nash test, gravimetric methods, and other chemical-based biosensors [8–11]. Colorimetric detection methods, such as Deniges' method, and Eegriwe's method, have been known since the beginning of the 20th century [6]. Unluckily, these methods, reagents, and reaction products are often just as harmful to human health. All of these conventional methods require similarly hazardous reagents and suffer from a number of interferences, resulting in false positives. Additionally, these methods are impracticable for real-time measurements because of the required time for apparatus setup. Recent efforts have turned toward the development of biological methods of detection combined with physical transducers, and biosensors. Electrochemical-based biosensors enable direct, reliable, and reproducible measurements. The developed formaldehyde biosensor is a simple sample preparation procedure, resulting in faster response, lower cost, zero pollution, and user friendliness.

Determination of formaldehyde in Indian mackerel (*Restrelliger kanagurta*) was previously detected with different levels of formaldehyde using electrochemical biosensors which were reported by Marzuki et al. [2], it lacks performance regarding the nanomaterials-based detection of formaldehyde in fish samples. Owing to the gap, this study is a stepping stone for the research on formaldehyde determination in fresh fish samples using nanomaterials.

For this study, the electrochemical biosensor was developed based on the gold nanoparticles (AuNPs), ionic liquid [EMIM][Otf], chitosan (nanocomposite membrane), and glassy carbon electrode for determination of formaldehyde (Schemes 1 and 2). Formaldehyde dehydrogenase used as bio-recognition receptor in the system, so any interference can be avoided (selective towards the substrate, formaldehyde). Immobilization of the enzyme is applied using chitosan, which acts as a binder. Immobilization could enhance the electro-catalytic properties of the electrode or, in other words, increase the rate of chemical reactions without being consumed in the process (decrease the fouling effects) and obtain better results.

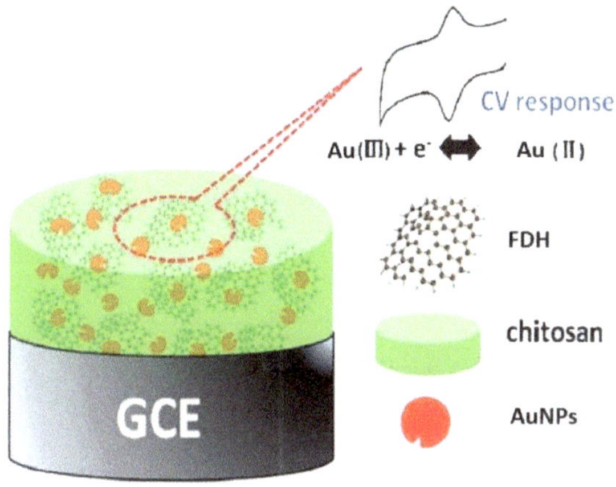

Scheme 1. The interaction of formaldehyde dehydrogenase, chitosan, and Au nanoparticles on a glassy carbon electrode.

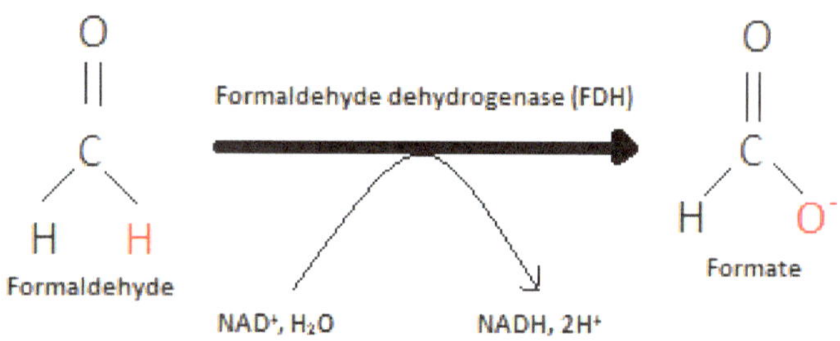

Scheme 2. Scheme of a formaldehyde biosensor. Formaldehyde is oxidized into formate and produces NADH as byproduct. The amount of NADH can be measured by the electrode.

A formaldehyde biosensor (FDH) was initially immobilized onto the surface of chitosan, which was employed to hydrolyze formaldehyde with the production of formic acid and NADH, as displayed in Equation (1). FDH immobilized onto chitosan has been investigated, with respect to the effects of response time, pH range, scan rate, and formaldehyde concentration on the hydrolysis of formaldehyde.

$$HCHO + NAD^{+} + H_2O \xrightarrow[\text{Formandehyde dehydrogenase}]{} HCOOH + NADH + H^{+} \quad (1)$$

The use of chitosan (CHIT) film for enzyme immobilization has low cost, zero toxicity [12,13], and is easily controlled by pH manipulation [14]. Nanoparticles (AuNPs) are commonly immobilized onto chitosan along with formaldehyde (FDH) enzymes to provide large surface areas for a higher electrochemical reaction rate [15]. This research has included ionic liquids in the electrochemical electrode to enhance the high sensitivity and homogenous deposition. FDH is found to be specifically reactive to formaldehyde [16], whereas the presence of a cofactor NAD^{+} will provide higher stability of the reaction.

The aim of the project was to develop an electrochemical biosensor using formaldehyde dehydrogenase (FDH) and chemically-modified electrode based on nanomaterials-coated with chitosan. Since there are a very limited number of techniques for the real-time determination of formaldehyde on the real fish sample, it is important to investigate the formaldehyde content in the fish in real-time since it is claimed to be the major contaminant in fish, in order to understand better the risks of fish consumption, to manage the risks of consumption and to provide additional information in food safety.

2. Materials and Methods

2.1. Chemical and Materials

Formaldehyde dehydrogenase (EC 1.2.1.46) collected from *Pseudomonas putida* (specific activity 1.6 U/mg) and β-nicotinamide adenine nucleotide (NAD^+) obtained from Sigma (Spruce Street, St. Louis, USA). Methylene blue (MB) was purchased from Sigma (Spruce Street, St. Louis, USA). Formaldehyde (37%) and acetic acid were purchased from Merck company. Gold nanoparticles (AuNPs) and ionic liquid [EMIM][OTF] were purchased from Sigma (Spruce Street, St. Louis, USA). All chemicals used in the experiments were analytical reagent grade. Deionized water was obtained from a Millipore Milli-Q purification system. The Malabar Red Snapper *(Lutjanus malabaricus)* and Longtail Tuna *(Thunnus Tonggol)* samples were collected from the three different local wet markets in Kota Kinabalu, Sabah, Malaysia.

2.2. Apparatus and Equipments

An electrochemical study was carried out using a Metrohm AutoLab Eco-chemie, Netherlands, with the software package NOVA 1.8. A Metrohm 3 mm glassy carbon electrode (GCE) was used as the working electrode to be coated with the enzyme and nanomaterials onto the membrane via covalent immobilization. An Ag | AgCl | KCl 3M electrode, referred as the reference electrode, and a platinum (Pt) wire were employed as a counter-electrode.

2.3. Preparation of Reagents

Stock solution of MB (1 mM) was prepared in a 50 mM Tris–HCl (pH 7.0) solution. The diluted solutions were prepared by an appropriate dilution with the Tris–HCl buffer. The FDH mixed thoroughly with chitosan, gold nanoparticles (AuNPs), and ionic liquid ([EMIM][OTF]), the mixtures were homogenized for 24 h with 3000 rpm. The pH (50 mM Tris-HCl buffer) was determined using a pH meter, model PC 2700-meter kit. Before use, the pH meter was calibrated with standard buffer solutions of pH 4, 7, and 10. The amounts of chemicals were weighed accurately by using a digital electronic balance, model GR-200. For the preparation of NAD^+ solution (0.5 mM) 2.5 μL of NAD^+ solution (5 mM) was dissolved in 25 mL of deionized water. Standard formaldehyde stock solution (100 ppm) was prepared by adding 25 mL deionized water to 6.8 μL of formaldehyde (37%) solution. Different concentrations of standard formaldehyde were prepared on the range of 0.01–10 ppm. All of the solutions were prepared fresh at the beginning of each experiment.

2.4. Preparation of the FDH/AuNPS/([EMIM][OTF])/CHIT Modified Electrode

Before modification, pre-treatment of GCE was performed according to Siddiquee et al. [17] procedure with some modifications. The glassy carbon electrode (GCE) was polished with 0.05 μm alumina slurry for 2 min on a smooth cloth in order to make sure the surface is cleaned of any foreign residues. Then, the electrode was ultrasonicated in an ultrasonic bath for 15 min and dried at room temperature. For immobilization of FDH with chitosan, FDH solution (30 mg/mL) was prepared by dissolving 6 μL of stock FDH solution (50 mg/mL) in 10 μL of 0.05 mM buffer (pH 7.0), which corresponded to the optimum pH. The FDH solution was thoroughly mixed with the chitosan in a volume ratio of 1:20 and sonicated for 15 min. Then, 10 μL of the mixture was deposited on the surface of the GCE and allowed to evaporate at room temperature. This procedure resulted in the fabrication of homogenously-dispersed FDH/CHIT immobilized on the glassy carbon electrode surface.

An appropriate amount of the AuNPs was dispersed on the CHIT. Then it was sonicated for 20 min after stirring for 8 h. The mass ratio of AuNPs: CHITwas 1:5. A 20 μL of FDH solution in a Tris-HCl (pH 7.0, 0.05 M) was added. An ionic liquid was dispersed in the AuNPs/CHIT composite, and then sonicated for 3 h to produce homogeneous suspension. The ratio of ionic liquid was fixed at 3% (v/v) in the experiments. Methylene blue (MB) was accumulated onto the membrane surface by immersing the electrode and stirred into 10 mL of MB for 2 min without applying any potential.

After accumulation of MB, the electrode was rinsed with buffer (pH 7.2, 0.5 M) for 2 min to remove any non-specifically-bound MB. It was then transferred into an analytical buffer added with substrate in an electrochemical cell for cyclic voltammetry and differential pulse voltammetry measurements.

2.5. Assembly of Electrochemical Biosensor

FDH-immobilized chitosan was deposited on the surface of a Thermo-Orion glassy carbon electrode and kept in a steady position by an O-ring. The electrode was dried at room temperature for at least 4 h. The counter and reference electrodes were immersed together into a stirred reaction media containing phosphate buffer solution. A 5 mL of substrate was injected into the reaction media and the accumulation products signal was measured and processed by the AutoLab Nova 1.8 software package. The same protocol was applied to the unmodified GCE.

2.6. Reproducibility Assay

Reproducibility was associated with precision, where the functional ability of the electrode was kept in an acceptable range, especially when the electrodes were produced in large quantity [1]. Individually, five different working electrodes were prepared and analyzed the reproducibility by using the same concentration of formaldehyde solution, five times.

2.7. Detection of Formaldehyde in Fish Samples

Fresh Malabar red snapper fish samples were collected from wet market in Kota Kinabalu, Sabah. The samples were stored at 4 ± 1 °C. Formaldehyde extraction procedure exactly followed the previously established method reported by Marzuki et al. [1]. The fish was thawed and only the flesh was taken and cut into small pieces. A 15 g of the flesh was homogenized with 30 mL of Tris–HCl (pH 7, 0.5 M) for 5 min, and the aliquots (a portion of a total amount of solution) were filtered. The filtration was done using Whatmann 1 filter paper. The sample was directly used without further extraction and treatment. Formaldehyde was determined using the modified electrode and the storage stability was measured in a real sample from 0 to 35 days at 4 °C. The experimental works were conducted with five replicates. Recovery assays were analyzed with varying storage periods.

3. Results and Discussion

3.1. Morphological Characterization of Modified GCE

3.1.1. Morphological Analysis via Scanning Electron Microscope

The surface morphological analysis of the CHIT, AuNPs/CHIT, and AuNPs/[EMIM][OTF])/CHIT were observed by scanning electron microscope (SEM). Figure 1A shows the microporous protein fiber of the chitosan membrane. Based on the results, AuNPs were well dispersed, spherical in shape on the chitosan, and appeared as white dots on the protein fiber of the chitosan. FDH attached well with the AuNPs/[EMIM][OTF] net fiber matrix as shown in Figure 1B. Additionally, the image clearly illustrated that FDH molecules were scattered on the whole surface of AuNPs/[EMIM][OTF]/CHIT. When FDH was immobilized on the membrane fibers, the rougher fibers appeared with clusters of lumps of FDH as compared to without, using FDH on chitosan. The fibers of FDH/AuNPs/[EMIM][OTF]/CHIT were found rougher than that of the FDH/CHIT. The protein fibers were covered with many small spherical nanoparticles which increased the surface area of the chitosan. In the presence of [EMIM][OTF], it appears as a smooth surface and recovers the conductivity of modified GCE [18]. Additionally, [EMIM][OTF] acts as an efficient solvent in the electrochemical sensor. [EMIM][OTF] is an important source of ion transporters to transport charges in the nanomaterials. The conductivity performance of the biosensor containing AuNPs/[EMIM][OTF]/CHIT remarkably enhanced the potential current due to the presence of nanoparticles and ionic liquid contributions. From these results, it is strongly concluded that the combination of FDH and AuNPs are successfully immobilized on the chitosan for the development of a formaldehyde biosensor. The interaction of chitosan with AuNPs leads to the formation of cross-linked chitosan and nanoparticles [19]. Thus, the FDH/AuNPs/[EMIM][OTF]/CHIT structure has provided a large effective surface area for excellent adsorption and substrate diffusion, which is a critical issue for improving the response properties of the electrochemical enzyme sensor.

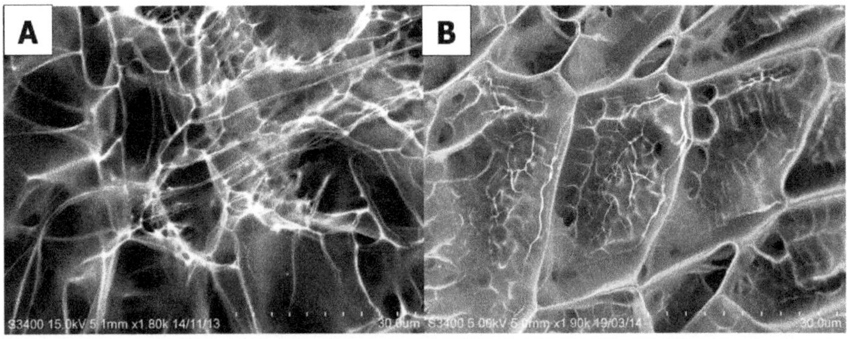

Figure 1. A scanning electron micrograph of (**A**) chitosan, CHIT; and (**B**) chitosan immobilized with Au nanoparticles and formaldehyde dehydrogenase, FDH/AuNPs/[EMIM][Otf]/CHIT/GCE.

3.1.2. Energy Dispersive Spectroscopy (EDS) Spectrum

The EDX spectrum in Figure 2 is a plot of X-ray counts vs. energy (keV). Energy peaks correspond to various elements in the modified membrane since it determines the abundance of specific elements. They are narrow and readily resolved, but many elements yield multiple peaks. The analysis indicates that the membrane has the phase structure and composition of the rutile form of FDH/NPs/([EMIM][OTF])/CHIT. Carbon (C), oxygen (O), and gold elements (Au) showed strong peaks. Elements in low abundance will generate X-rays that may not be resolvable from the background radiation. There are energy peak overlaps among different elements, particularly those corresponding to X-rays generated by emission from different energy level shells (C and O) in different elements. In the spectrum, there were closed overlaps of C or O and various lines with Au. Particularly at higher energy, individual peaks may correspond to several different elements. Therefore, there is an EDX spectrum peak of Au at 280 keV. Since lower atomic number elements have fewer filled shells, they have fewer X-ray peaks. Carbon, for example, only has one peak at 40 keV. Conversely, the higher atomic numbered elements have a greater number of X-ray peaks. While some of the high atomic numbered X-rays can be over 50 keV, a spectral range of 0–20 keV can detect all of the elements, as summarized in Table 1. From these results, it is strongly concluded that the combination of FDH and AuNPs are successfully immobilized on the chitosan for fabrication of the formaldehyde biosensor. The interaction of chitosan with AuNPs leads to the formation of cross-linked chitosan and nanoparticles as mentioned before.

Table 1. Chemical analysis of the energy-dispersive X-Ray (EDX) spectrum.

Element	Series Unn (wt.%)	C Norm. (wt.%)	C Norm. (at.%)	C Error (1 Sigma) (wt.%)
Carbon	K-series 24.90	26.64	45.49	4.92
Nitrogen	K-series 6.28	6.72	9.84	2.26
Oxygen	K-series 21.52	23.03	29.52	4.21
Fluorine	K-series 6.88	7.37	7.95	1.76
Aluminium	K-series 0.53	0.57	0.43	0.08
Sulfur	K-series 5.34	5.71	3.65	0.26
Gold	L-series 28.02	29.98	3.12	4.26
	Total	93.46	100.00	100.00

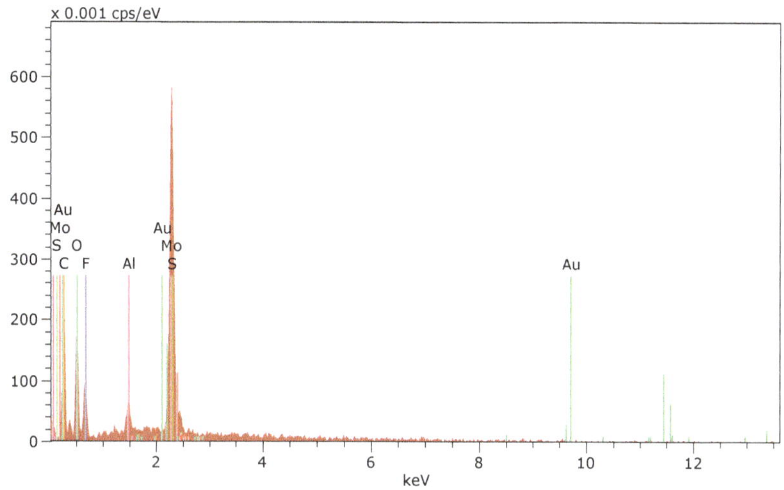

Figure 2. EDX spectrum of FDH/AuNPs/[EMIM][Otf]/CHIT.

3.2. Optimization Condition for Formaldehyde Determination

To study the effects of using a redox reaction indicator, the unmodified glassy carbon electrode was soaked in a methylene blue solution for 5 min before running the analysis with known concentrations of the formaldehyde solution. The comparison was done after running the analysis with the presence and absence of the methylene blue solution (Figure 3). The methylene blue mediator is strongly retained inside the membrane through hydrophobic interaction. The first step was conducted using an unmodified electrode for examination with the effects of using a redox indicator. Then, the unmodified electrode was applied for an examination of the scan rate, pH, and interaction time, as well as the response range of formaldehyde.

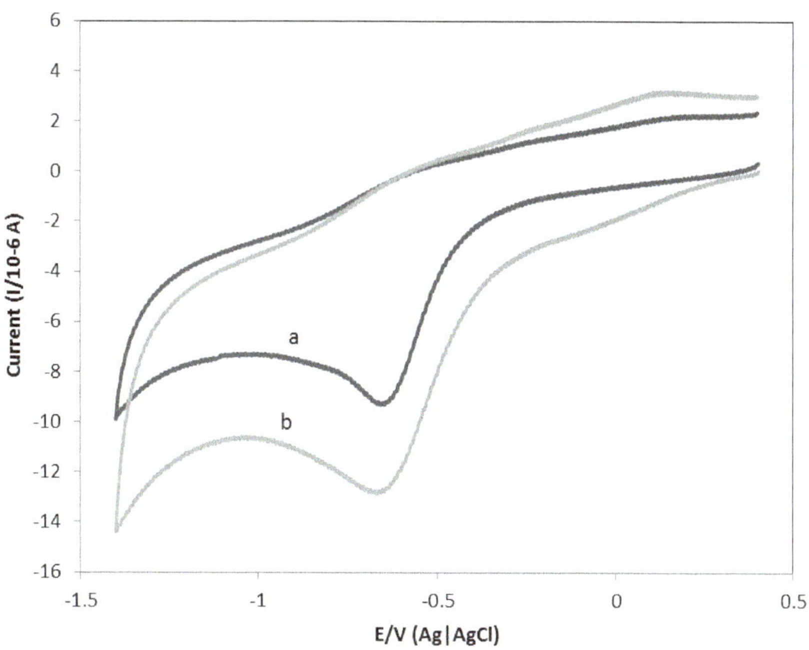

Figure 3. A cyclic voltammogram of a bare electrode (**a**) without being soaked in methylene blue; and (**b**) soaked in methylene blue (0.1 M of MB, in 10 ppm of formaldehyde).

The cathodic peak of bare GCE accumulated with 1 mM methylene blue (MB) increased, as compared to the cathodic peak currents, in the range of -9.30×10^{-7} to -12.89×10^{-7} A. 8 ppm of formaldehyde concentration was significant in the presence of MB as a remarkable marker for current signal. Determination of formaldehyde depends on the electrode modification components and the presence of mediator. Direct electron transfers between enzyme and electrode require a mediator since the transformation of electrons occur at a leisurely rate. MB is a cationic dye which has a reserved potential between 0.08 and −0.25 V in pH 2–8 solution. Hence, it is close to the potential used in this project. MB diffuses into CHIT fiber by electrostatic interaction [20]. According to Yao et al. [19], the role of the mediator is to shuttle electrons effectively between the electrolyte in the electrochemical cell and the bioactive center of the electrode.

The optimum working conditions were studied at 0.10 Vs^{-1} (voltage at which maximum current was generated) in analytical buffer, at pH 7.0. Different concentrations of formaldehyde were detected in the range of 0.01 to 10.0 ppm. The current signals of the enzyme reaction were measured using cyclic voltammetry (CV) and differential pulse voltammetry (DPV). All measurements were completed with three replications.

3.2.1. Scan Rate Effects

Useful information involving electrochemical reactions can be obtained from the relationship between the cathodic peak current and the scan rate. The kinetics of the bioactive center GCE reaction was investigated by studying the effects of the scan rate on the peak currents. The influence of scan rate on reduction of NAD^+ at the GCE surface was investigated in the range of 0.10–0.50 Vs^{-1} by cyclic voltammetry (CV) (Figure 4). The peak current increased with an increasing scan rate. As can be seen, increasing the scan rate let anodic and cathodic peak potentials shift towards the positive and negative directions, indicating a charge transfer kinetics limitation. The higher scan rate gave fragmented peaks and the potential range was shifted to the more negative region, which means it requires a larger number of voltages per second. Both the anodic and cathodic peak currents were increased linearly, proportional to the scan rate ranging from 0.04 to 0.10 Vs^{-1}. The overall redox process is focused at the electrode surface, which can be considered to be relatively fast on the voltammetry time scale, indicating a surface-confined redox process and corresponds to the rapid conversion of a surface electrode without a diffusion-controlled reaction step. Therefore, 0.1 Vs^{-1} was selected as the optimum scan rate. The reaction was stable at a low scan rate; therefore, 0.1 Vs^{-1} was chosen and applied, similarly to Marzuki et al. [4].

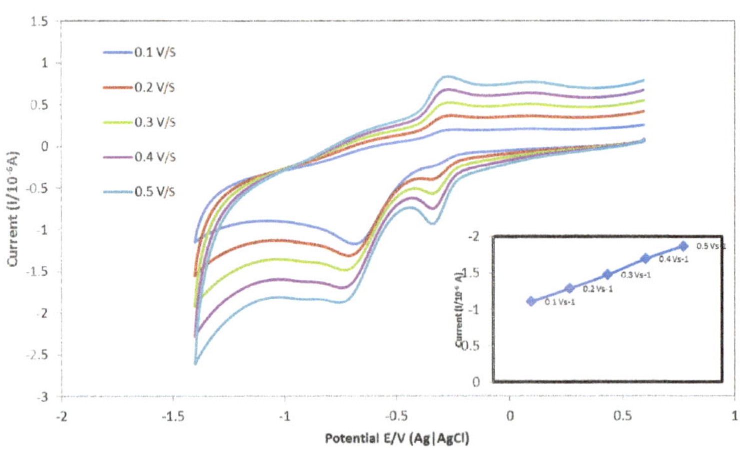

Figure 4. The cyclic voltammogram of the scan rate effects on the detection of formaldehyde. Scan rates used were 0.1, 0.2, 0.3, and 0.5 V/s. All were performed at room temperature, 25 ± 1 °C, and with the same concentration of formaldehyde, 8.0 ppm.

3.2.2. pH of Analytical Electrolyte Effects

The pH value of the electrolyte is important for the performance of the electrochemical biosensor. Therefore, the effects of the pH of the supporting electrolyte were studied from 6.0 to 8.5 at intervals of 0.5 using the Tris–HCl buffer (50 mM). The response current increased and reached a maximum at pH 6.5 and decreased obviously, as shown in Figure 5. The cathodic peak potentials seem to be intensely dependent on the pH of the electrolyte. A linear negative shift was observed in the cathodic peak current by increasing the pH value. The results showed that the oxidation of formaldehyde involves a dissimilar number of transferred H^+ or OH^- at various pH values, which led to a different response, similarly reported previously by Lei et al. [21]. The peaks drop at pH 7.0–8.0 due to deprotonation of ions occurred. The obtained results were similar to those previously reported by Qian et al. [22]. The acidic environment enhances the reaction because H^+ is needed for NAD^+ to reduce to NADH. In fact, the immobilized FDH can retain its activity under broad pH conditions, indicating that the membrane and AuNPs are provided a favorable biocompatible microenvironment for the survival of FDH. Thus, pH 6.5 was selected as the optimum pH to obtain maximum sensitivity and bioactivity and used throughout the studies.

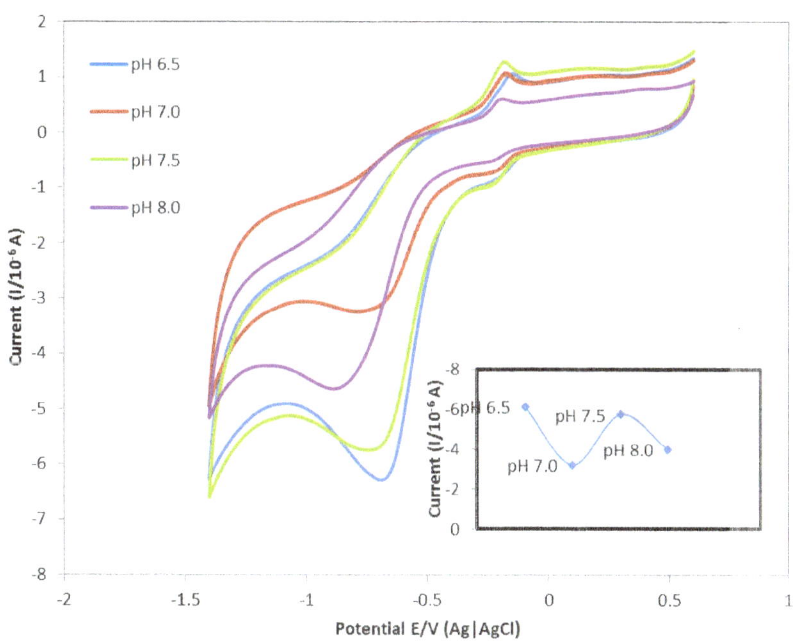

Figure 5. The cyclic voltammetry of effects of pH of the analytical buffer. The pH of the buffer used were 6.0, 6.5, 7.0, 7.5, and 8.0. All were performed at room temperature, 25 ± 1 °C, and with the same concentration of formaldehyde, 8.0 ppm.

3.2.3. Interaction Time Effects

The interaction time of formaldehyde dehydrogenase and the substrate were influenced the the performance of the GCE in the presence of MB. The electrochemical cell was obtained from about 8 ppm of standard formaldehyde with 0.05 mM Tris-HCl buffer (pH 7.0). The interaction time was from 5 to 50 s and the scan rate fixed at 0.10 Vs^{-1} (Figure 6). The maximum current response was found at 5 s, implying that the accumulation of FDH and the substrate were saturated at the surface of the bioactive center of GCE. At 5 s, a complete enzymatic reaction was reached. There was sufficient time within 5 s to transform the formaldehyde to formic acid and reduced NAD^+ to NADH. The cathodic peak value increased slowly and flattened with time; thus, 5 s was chosen as the optimum interaction time for the determination of formaldehyde.

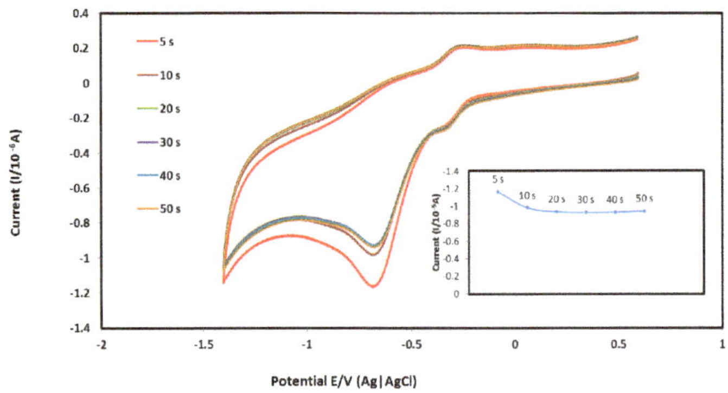

Figure 6. The cyclic voltammetry of effects of interaction time for detection of formaldehyde. The interaction times of the biosensor used were 5, 10, 20, 30, 40, 50, and 60 s. All were performed at room temperature, 25 ± 1 °C, and with the same concentration of formaldehyde, 8.0 ppm.

3.3. Formaldehyde Detection

The electrochemical behavior of the bare GCE and modified GCE were characterized by DPV using MB as an electroactive indicator (Figure 3). DPV was employed for the quantitative determination of formaldehyde, which is relatively sensitive compared to CV analysis. The shifting of the peak depended on many factors, such as scan rate, interaction time between enzyme and substrate, pH, and concentration of substrate. The developed formaldehyde biosensor was conducted using the modified FDH/AuNPs/[EMIM][Otf]/CHIT to react with different concentrations of formaldehyde as shown in Figure 7. Under optimum conditions, the DPV method was detected with different concentrations of formaldehyde in the range from 0.01 to 10 ppm, with detection limit of 0.1 ppm (n = 5). Due to the presence of AuNPs and ionic liquid ([EMIM][Otf]), large surface areas of the electrode for immobilizing homogenous formaldehyde were established. The performances of the constructed formaldehyde biosensors are compared and the results are shown in Table 2. The results indicate a good analytical performance for the development of a formaldehyde biosensor.

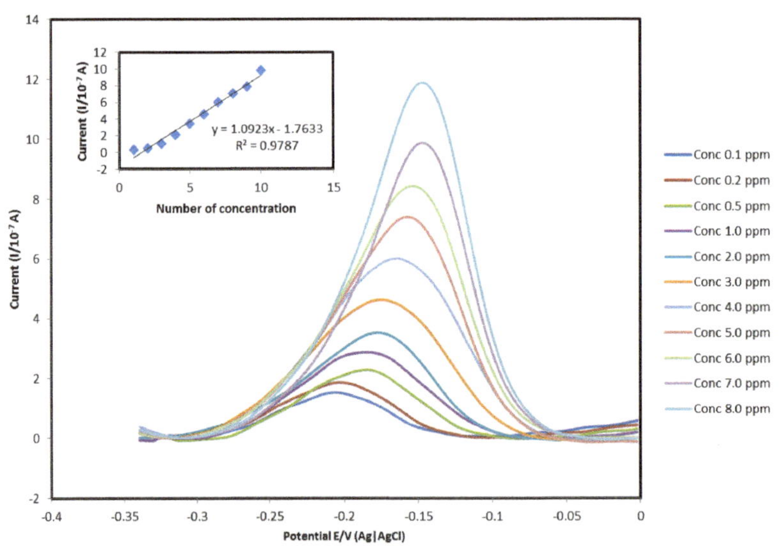

Figure 7. The diffrential pulse voltammogram of different concentrations based on FDH/AuNPs/[EMIM][Otf]/CHIT/GCE, conducted at pH 6.5 and temperature of 25 ± 1 °C. The concentrations of formaldehyde used were in between range 0.1–10 ppm.

Table 2. Comparison of analytical performance of various formaldehyde biosensors.

References	Range of Concentration	Detection Limit	Mode of Operation	Enzyme	Mediator
[20]	1.3 ppb–1.2 ppm	-	Amperometry (E_{ap} = 800 mV)	FDH	-
[23]	0.3 ppb–1.5 ppm	0.3 ppb	Amperometry (E_{ap} = 800 mV)	FDH	Os polymer
[23]	-	-	Amperometry (E_{ap} = 800 mV)	FDH	Tetrathiafulvalene
[24]	1.5–90 ppm	22.8 ppm	Amperometry (E_{ap} = 800 mV)	AOX + FDH	-
[24]	30–210.2 ppm	22.22 ppm	Amperometry (E_{ap} = 800 mV)	AOX + FDH	DCIP
[25]	9.09–120.12 ppm	8.1 ppm	Amperometry (E_{ap} = 800 mV)	AOX	-
[25]	0.1–100 μM	0.1 μM	Amperometry (E_{ap} = 300 mV, pH 7.5)	FDH	-
[26]	1.8–15.4 ppm	9 ppm	Potentiometry	AOX	-
[26]	1.8–15.4 ppm	1.8 ppm	Amperometry (E_{ap} = 100 mV, pH 7.5)	AOX	-
[4]	1–10 ppm	1 ppm	Electrochemical	FDH	-
This study	0.01–10 ppm	0.1 ppm	Electrochemical (E_{ap} = 100 mV, pH 6.5)	FDH	Methylene blue

3.4. Mechanism of the Formaldehyde Biosensor

In this reaction, formaldehyde dehydrogenase acts as the electron transfer to facilitate the addition of one hydrogen atom to NAD^+ and reduced it to NADH, whereas formaldehyde converted to formic acid. In fact, cofactor NAD^+ avoided the blocking of O_2 from electrocatalytic oxidation. The compact combination of FDH/AuNPs/([EMIM][OTF])/CHIT with the electrode surface enhanced the transfer speed of electrons and further increased the catalytic activity of formaldehyde due to AuNPs properties which have high biological compatibility, high catalytic efficiency, strong adsorption ability, a fast electron transfer rate, and easy preparation. The cathodic current of formaldehyde (started at about −0.5 V vs. Ag | AgCl) decreased with increasing formaldehyde concentration until 10 ppm, indicating that the consumption of oxygen over the course of the enzymatic reaction of FDH with formaldehyde. The majority of the immobilized FDH molecules are responsible for the formaldehyde conversion and reduction of NAD^+.

Nanoparticles commonly act as a semiconductor material which are used as a supportive material in the development of an electrochemical biosensor. The modified AuNPs/[EMIM][OTF]/CHIT electrode displayed good biocompatibility and excellent electrochemical conductivity. As a result, the use of composite materials based on the integration of the membrane with some other materials to combine properties of the individual components has gained increasing attention [27]. Consequently, the immobilization of the FDH provided the highest signal response, which indicated that rapid increases of the peak current of MB accumulated due to the interaction of FDH and the substrate on the electrochemical cell. Due to some special characterization of ionic liquids, such as wide potential gaps (a voltage range between which the electrolyte is not oxidized or reduced) and high electrical conductivity, hydrophobicity, and insolubility in water. The reduced FDH donates the excess electron to the AuNPs/[EMIM][Otf]/CHIT together with the MB nanocomposite membrane to reduce the redox property. The MB oxidizes by transferring the electron to the external circuit due to efficient electron transfer and the good redox property of the prepared nanocomposite bio-membrane.

The direct reduction of NAD^+ at the bare electrode is not suited for analytical application due to the slow electrode kinetics and low potential material, so preparation of a modified electrode with catalytic functionality is of practical significance. Since the electro-catalytic property of the modified electrode is obviously affected by the physical and chemical characteristics of the modifiers on the electrode surface, designing a membrane preparation method is essential. The factors are evaluated by electrochemical techniques based on the affected process of modification and chitosan property. The main advantage of using NAD^+ dependent dehydrogenase-based biosensors is that oxygen (O_2) does not interfere in formaldehyde detection because it does not participate in the reaction.

Rinaudo [14] has reported that chitosan is the only pseudo-natural cationic polymer in which the NH_2 can be added with positive charge to increase solubility, while the polysaccharide has several ionizable groups that can act as a polyelectrolyte in acidic media. This unique characteristic has made the condition of chitosan be easily manipulated through pH control. FDH could be incorporated into AuNPs/CHIT via electrostatic forces. Au nanoparticles are characterized by a porous structure with hundreds of empty channels. It has reported that proteins are absorbed onto the membrane through binding of FDH's carbonyl groups interacting with AuNP's vicinal hydroxyl groups via electrostatic interaction [28]. The electrostatic interaction between oppositely-charged membranes (CHIT) and nanomaterials (ionic liquid and AuNPs) are usually strong and stable. The compatibility of AuNPs makes it excellent material for enzyme immobilization. Additionally, immobilized enzymes are more stable and easier to be reused than free enzymes.

In summary, CHIT has been used for the effective immobilization of molecules through electrostatic attraction in order to improve the stability and deposited onto the GCE. AuNPs increased the surface area of immobilization. Meanwhile, the ionic liquid [EMIM][Otf] acts as an ionic solvent which diffuses easily due to its wide solubility in the solutions, especially during electrochemical measurements. Combining all of the characteristic above, FDH/AuNPs/[EMIM][OTF]/CHIT indicated great potential in electrochemical activity for formaldehyde detection. Thus, the developed electrochemical method was detected with different concentration via the change in potential values.

3.5. *Reproducibility Assay*

A reproducibility assay is ian mportant characterization of the biosensors, showing whether the biosensor can be reproduced using the same materials and procedures. The reproducibility of the modified FDH/AuNPs/[EMIM][Otf]/CHIT/GCE in formaldehyde detection are almost similar ($p < 0.05$), implying that the reproducibility of such electrodes are high. A similar reproducibility assay was observed with different concentrations (1, 4, and 8 ppm) of formaldehyde (Figure 8). The response of the biosensors developed is reproducible, and the relative standard deviation of sensor responses below 1% ($n = 10$). Based on the result, the hypothesis is accepted where the reproducibility of the modified electrodes is high.

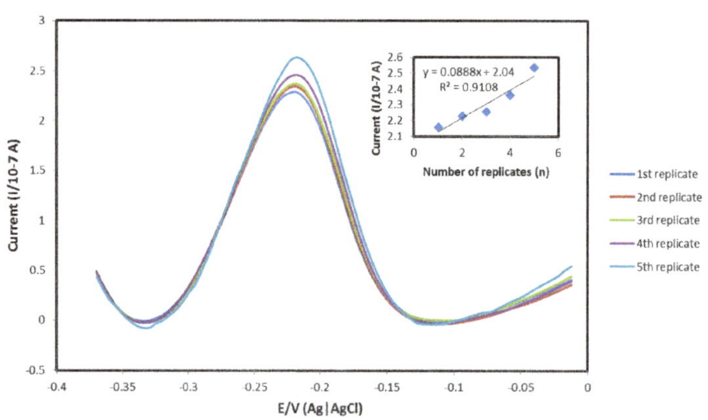

Figure 8. The reproducibility patterns of constant concentration of formaldehyde based on FDH/AuNPs/[EMIM][Otf]/CHIT/GCE was performed at pH 6.5 and temperature of 25 ± 1 °C. The concentration of formaldehyde used was 8.0 ppm.

3.6. *Real Sample Analysis*

Spike Recovery Test and Stability

In order to validate and verify the applicability of the developed biosensor, the detection of formaldehyde in some fish samples were studied. The electrochemical method was applied to two different fish samples, which are Malabar Red Snapper (*Lutjanus malabaricus*) and Longtail Tuna (*Thunnus tonggol*). The recovery rate was calculated to be 81.2% to 82.2%, showing the high accuracy rate of the developed method. It showed good standard relative deviation (RSD) which is less than 1% (Table 3). The spike recovery test was performed to validate the accuracy of sample values from invalidated fish samples. A blank *Lutjanus malabaricus* and *Thunnus tonggol* were spiked with 8.00 ppm of formaldehyde. According to Mathias et al. [23], the recovery percentage should be above 80% to represent high accuracy. The stability is one of the most important characteristics for commercial application of any biosensor system. The operational stability test demonstrated that the steady state response did not decrease for at least 7 h (corresponding to approximately 70 measurements). Furthermore, the developed biosensors showed good recovery rate stability in 50 mM of phosphate buffer, at pH 6.5; the response remaining stable for more than one month for all types of bio-recognition elements used.

Table 3. Properties of recovery rate.

Samples	Recovery (%)	RSD (%)
Lutjanus malabaricus	81.2	0.64
Thunnus tonggol	82.2	0.32

4. Conclusions

Electrochemical methods have proved to be an effective and inexpensive way for monitoring formaldehyde content due to their high sensitivity, reliability, rapidity, and economy. An novel electrochemical biosensor is developed based on FDH/AuNPs/[EMIM][Otf]/CHIT/GCE using MB as a redox indicator. AuNPs are dispersed onto chitosan and ionic liquid, which have enhanced the surface for the immobilization of FDH which increases the detection sensitivity of formaldehyde. The results indicated that the AuNPs provided a nano-sized environment for the close interaction between the enzyme (FDH) and the modified electrode, which are essential for efficient direct electron transfer. The developed formaldehyde biosensor has several advantages over conventional method such as good sensitivity and stability. The detection limit is 0.1 ppm, with linear coefficiency (r^2) of 0.9787 and recovery rate from 81.2% to 82.2%. These results suggested that the developed biosensor offers a simple, rapid, sensitive, highly selective, wide detection range, and a convenient method for formaldehyde monitoring in the fish-based research industry.

Acknowledgments: This work was supported by grants from the University Malaysia Sabah Research Grant Scheme, SBK0024-SG-2012.

Author Contributions: Aini, B.N. and Siddique, S. conceived and designed the experiments; Aini, B.N. performed the experiments; Aini, B.N. and Siddique, S. analyzed the data; Ampon, K. contributed reagents/materials/analysis tools; Aini, B.N. and Siddique, S. wrote the paper.

Conflicts of Interest: The authors declare no conflict of interest.

References

1. Marzuki, N.I.; Bakar, F.A.; Salleh, A.B.; Heng, L.Y.; Yusof, N.A.; Siddiquee, S. Electrochemical Biosensor Immobilization of Formaldehyde Dehydrogenase with Nafion for Determination of Formaldehyde from Indian Mackerel (Rastrelliger kanagurta) Fish. *Curr. Anal. Chem.* **2012**, *8*, 534–542. [CrossRef]

2. Food Safety News. Formaldehyde Detected in Supermarket Fish Imported from Asia. Retrieved from Food Safety and Quality Department Official Website. Available online: http://www.foodsafetynews.com/2013/09/formaldehyde-detected-in-supermarket-fish-imported-from-asia/#.VHq50zGUckO (accessed on 11 September 2013).
3. Ozoner, S.K.; Erhan, E.; Yilmaz, F.; Ergenekon, P.; Anil, I. Electrochemical biosensor for detection of formaldehyde in rain water. *J. Chem. Technol. Biotechnol.* **2013**, *88*, 727–732. [CrossRef]
4. Marzuki, N.I.; Bakar, F.A.; Salleh, A.B.; Heng, L.Y.; Yusof, N.A.; Siddiquee, S. Development of Electrochemical Biosensor for Formaldehyde Determination Based on Immobilized Enzyme. *Int. J. Electrochem. Sci.* **2012**, *7*, 6070–6083.
5. Occupational Health and Safety Amendment Regulations 2014. Victorian WorkCover Authority (VWA), June 2014. Available online: http://www.legislation.vic.gov.au/ (accessed on 13 September 2014).
6. Wang, Q.; Tang, H.; Xie, Q.; Tan, L.; Zhang, Y.; Li, B.; Yao, S. Room-temperature ionic liquids/multi-walled carbon nanotubes/chitosan composite electrode for electrochemical analysis of NADH. *Electrochim. Acta* **2007**, *52*, 6630–6637. [CrossRef]
7. Food Safety and Quality Department. Food Regulations 1985. Retrieved from Food Safety and Quality Department Official Website. Available online: http://fsq.moh.gov.my/v4/index.php/perundangan2/food-regulations-1985 (accessed on 12 October 2014).
8. Noordiana, N.; Fatimah, A.B.; Farhana, Y.C. Formaldehyde content and quality characteristics of selected fish and seafood from wet markets. *Int. Food Res. J.* **2011**, *18*, 125–136.
9. Bechmann, I.E. Determination of formaldehyde in frozen fish with formaldehyde dehydrogenase using a flow injection system with an incorporated gel-filtration chromatography column. *Anal. Chim. Acta* **1996**, *320*, 155–164. [CrossRef]
10. Ngamchana, S.; Surareungchai, W. Sub-millimolar determination of formalin by pulsed amperometric detection. *Anal. Chim. Acta* **2004**, *510*, 195–201. [CrossRef]
11. Yeh, T.S.; Lin, T.C.; Chen, C.C.; Wen, H.M. Analysis of free and bound formaldehyde in squid and squid products by gas chromatography-mass spectrometry. *J. Food Drug Anal.* **2013**, *21*, 190–197. [CrossRef]
12. Kumar, M.N. Review: A review of chitin and chitosan applications. *React. Funct. Polym.* **2000**, *46*, 1–27. [CrossRef]
13. Krajewska, B. Application of chitin and chitosan-based materials for enzyme immobilizations: A review. *Enzyme Microb. Technol.* **2004**, *35*, 126–139. [CrossRef]
14. Rinaudo, M. Chitin and chitosan: Properties and applications. *Prog. Polym. Sci.* **2006**, *31*, 603–632. [CrossRef]
15. Siddiquee, S.; Yusof, N.A.; Salleh, A.B.; Tan, S.G.; Bakar, F.A. Electrochemical DNA biosensor for the detection of Trichoderma harzianum based on a gold electrode modified with a composite membrane made from an ionic liquid, ZnO nanoparticles and chitosan, and by using acridine orange as a redox indicator. *Microchim. Acta* **2011**, *172*, 357–363. [CrossRef]
16. Masuda, M.; Motoyama, Y.; Kuwahara, J.; Nakamura, N.; Ohno, H. A paradoxical method for NAD^+/NADH accumulation on an electrode surface using a hydrophobic ionic liquid. *Biosens. Bioelectron.* **2013**, *39*, 334–337. [CrossRef] [PubMed]
17. Siddiquee, S.; Nor Azah, Y.; Salleh, A.B.; Tan, S.G.; Fatimah, A.B.; Lee, Y.H. DNA hybridization based on Trichoderma harzianum gene probe immobilization on self-assembled monolayers on a modified gold electrode. *Sens. Actuators B Chem.* **2010**, *147*, 198–205. [CrossRef]
18. Bareket, L.; Rephaeli, A.; Berkovitch, G.; Nudelman, A.; Rishpon, J. Carbon nanotubes based electrochemical biosensor for detection of formaldehyde released from a cancer cell line treated with formaldehyde-releasing anticancer prodrugs. *Bioelectrochemistry* **2010**, *77*, 94–99. [CrossRef] [PubMed]
19. Yao, H.; Li, N.; Xu, S.; Xu, J.Z.; Zhu, J.J.; Chen, H.Y. Electrochemical study of a new methylene blue/silicon oxide nanocomposition mediator and its application for stable biosensor of hydrogen peroxide. *Biosens. Bioelectron.* **2005**, *21*, 372–377. [CrossRef] [PubMed]
20. Bareket, L.; Rephaeli, A.; Berkovitch, G.; Nudelman, A.; Rishpon, J. Carbon nanotubes based electrochemical biosensor for detection of formaldehyde released from a cancer cell line treated with formaldehyde-releasing anticancer prodrugs. *Bioelectrochemistry* **2010**, *77*, 94–99. [CrossRef] [PubMed]
21. Lei, C.X.; Hu, S.Q.; Gao, N.; Shen, G.L.; Yu, R.Q. An amperometric hydrogen peroxide biosensor based on immobilizing horseradish peroxidase to a nano-au monolayer supported by sol-gel derived carbon ceramic electrode. *Bioelectrochemistry* **2004**, *65*, 33–39. [CrossRef] [PubMed]

22. Qian, J.; Liu, Y.; Liu, H.; Yu, T.; Deng, J. Immobilization of horseradish peroxidase with a regenerated silk fibroin membrane and its application to a tertrathiafulvalene-mediating H_2O_2 sensor. *Biosens. Bioelectron.* **1997**, *12*, 1213–1218. [CrossRef]
23. Mathias, P.C.; Haydena, J.A.; Laha, T.J.; Hoofnagle, A.N. Evaluation of matrix effects using a spike recovery approach in a dilute-and-inject liquid chromatography–tandem mass spectrometry opioid monitoring assay. *Clin. Chim. Acta* **2014**, *437*, 38–42. [CrossRef] [PubMed]
24. Dennison, M.J.; Hall, J.M.; Turner, A.P.F. Direct monitoring of formaldehyde vapour and detection of ethanol vapour using dehydrogenase-based biosensors. *Analyst* **1996**, *12*, 1769–1774. [CrossRef]
25. Herschkovitz, Y.; Eshkenazi, I.; Campbell, C.E.; Rishpon, J. An electrochemical biosensor for formaldehyde. *J. Electroanalyt. Chem.* **2000**, *491*, 182–187. [CrossRef]
26. Khlupova, M.; Kuznetsov, B.; Demkiv, O.; Gonchar, M.; Csoregi, E.; Shleev, S. Intact and permeabilized cells of the yeast Hansenula polymorpha as bioselective elements for amperometric assay of formaldehyde. *Talanta* **2007**, *71*, 934–940. [CrossRef] [PubMed]
27. Ling, Y.P.; Heng, L.Y. A Potentiometric Formaldehyde Biosensor Based on Immobilization of Alcohol Oxidase on Acryloxysuccinimide-modified Acrylic Microspheres. *Sensors* **2010**, *10*, 9963–9981. [CrossRef] [PubMed]
28. Dias, S.L.P.; Fujiwara, S.T.; Gushikem, Y.; Bruns, R.E. Methylene blue immobilized on cellulose surfaces modified with titanium dioxide and titanium phosphate: Factorial design optimization of redox properties. *J. Electroanal. Chem.* **2002**, *531*, 141–146. [CrossRef]

14

Amperometric Biosensor Based on Zirconium Oxide/Polyethylene Glycol/Tyrosinase Composite Film for the Detection of Phenolic Compounds

Nor Monica Ahmad [1,2,*], Jaafar Abdullah [2], Nor Azah Yusof [2], Ahmad Hazri Ab Rashid [3], Samsulida Abd Rahman [3] and Md. Rakibul Hasan [4]

1 School of Chemistry and Environment, Faculty of Applied Science, UiTM Kuala Pilah, 72 000 Negeri Sembilan, Malaysia
2 Department of Chemistry, Faculty of Science, Universiti Putra Malaysia, 43400 Serdang, Selangor, Malaysia; jaafar@science.upm.edu.my (J.A.); azahy@science.upm.edu.my (N.A.Y.)
3 Industrial Biotechnology Research Centre, SIRIM Berhad, 1, Persiaran Dato' Menteri, P.O. Box 7035, Section 2, 40700 Shah Alam, Selangor, Malaysia; ahazri@sirim.my (A.H.A.R.); sulida@sirim.my (S.A.R.)
4 Nanotechnology & Catalysis Research Centre, Institute of Postgraduate Studies, University of Malaya, 50603 Kuala Lumpur, Malaysia; rakibacctdu@gmail.com
* Correspondence: normonica@gmail.com

Academic Editors: Donatella Albanese and Roberto Pilloton

Abstract: A phenolic biosensor based on a zirconium oxide/polyethylene glycol/tyrosinase composite film for the detection of phenolic compounds has been explored. The formation of the composite film was expected via electrostatic interaction between hexacetyltrimethylammonium bromide (CTAB), polyethylene glycol (PEG), and zirconium oxide nanoparticles casted on screen printed carbon electrode (SPCE). Herein, the electrode was treated by casting hexacetyltrimethylammonium bromide on SPCE to promote a positively charged surface. Later, zirconium oxide was mixed with polyethylene glycol and the mixture was dropped cast onto the positively charged SPCE/CTAB. Tyrosinase was further immobilized onto the modified SPCE. Characterization of the prepared nanocomposite film and the modified SPCE surface was investigated by scanning electron microscopy (SEM), Electrochemical Impedance Spectroscopy (EIS), and Cyclic voltamogram (CV). The developed biosensor exhibits rapid response for less than 10 s. Two linear calibration curves towards phenol in the concentrations ranges of 0.075–10 μM and 10–55 μM with the detection limit of 0.034 μM were obtained. The biosensor shows high sensitivity and good storage stability for at least 30 days.

Keywords: tyrosinase; zirconium oxide; phenol detection

---

1. Introduction

Phenol formation in the aquatic environment not only comes from natural processes but also from anthropogenic processes resulting from the direct discharge from industries [1]. The main natural processes of phenol formation are the decomposition of organic matter or synthesis by fungi and plants [2]. In terms of anthropogenic processes, phenols have widely been used in industries such as the production of plastic, textile, pharmaceutical, petroleum, pesticides, herbicides, insecticides, and fungicides [3].

The undesirability of the existence of phenols in river water is due to their strong action, high degree of poisonousness to aquatic life, in addition to their unpleasant tastes and odors. Phenolic compounds are a group of polluting chemicals that are easily absorbed by animals and humans through the skin and mucous membranes. These substances are toxic to most organs and tissues, especially in the lungs, liver, kidneys, and genitourinary system [4].

Even with a lower concentration, phenols are considered to be dangerous substances and have life-threatening toxicities. Phenols have been listed as major toxic pollutants by the United States Environmental Protection Agency (EPA) and many other countries around the world [4]. The European Union has established maximum permission level of phenols in water for human consumption which is within the concentration range of 0.1 and 0.5 $mg \cdot L^{-1}$.

Phenolic compounds are one of the major contaminants in waters. Thus, the ability to detect its presence represents a benefit to the protection of public health and the environment. Currently, there are many methods for the detection of phenol in the environment, such as reversed phase liquid chromatography [5], spectrophotometric [2,6], and high performances liquid chromatography [7,8]. However, these methods involve expensive instrumentation, require skill personnel to handle the instrumentation, and necessitate complicated pre-processing of sample, all of which make these methods unsuitable for field monitoring [9].

In contrast, electrochemical sensors offer numerous advantages over conventional methods because of the simplicity, sensitivity, rapidity and less, if any, tedious pre-treatment for samples. The key challenges in the development of biosensors are to improve and diversify techniques for protein entrapment in order to achieve better performance and stability. In view of this challenge, there is a genuine need for new technologies, such as the utilization of nanomaterials for the improvement of the analytical performances of developed sensors. This is because most of the samples are taken from natural resources which normally contain very little amounts of phenol content; as such, a very low detection limit of the environmental biosensor will enhance the capability of the biosensor for in situ applications.

Zirconium oxide has been reported for the past few years for the detection of many analytes, such as the detection of *Escherichia coli* [10], choline [11], hydrogen peroxide [12–14], urea [15], and glucose [16].

The metal oxide offers good compatibility and a high isoelectric point. Thus, it provides a template for the electrostatic interaction between enzyme, polymer, and surfactant. As a result, the cross-linker, such as glutaraldehyde, could be avoided in the enzyme immobilization step. The use of glutaraldehyde at excess amounts usually will cause the conformation change of an enzyme and therefore result in the enzyme becoming denatured [16,17].

The development of phenolic biosensors based on metal oxides have been explored by many researchers; for example, a zinc oxide derived tyrosinase biosensor which has been shown to exhibit good sensitivity and a lower detection limit of 0.05 μM [18]. In considering another example, iron oxide has been applied in the development of a biosensor by incorporating a multi-walled carbon nanotube and polyaniline electrodeposited onto a gold electrode; in doing so, it was found that the biosensor showed better performance with high sensitivity and had a low detection limit of 0.03 μM [19].

Figure 1 illustrates the possible assembling process of a CTAB (hexacetyltrimethylammonium bromide)/PEG (polyethylene glycol)-ZrO_2/tyrosinase composite on screen printed carbon electrode. Firstly, CTAB provides a positive charge on the surface of the electrode, and then it is electrostatically bound to oxygen in polyethylene glycol. At pH 6, zirconium oxide (ZrO_2) tends to form a negative surface charge [13], which later binds to a tyrosinase enzyme. Furthermore, ZrO_2 has an affinity towards proteins since amine and carboxyl groups in the enzyme act as a ligand to ZrO_2 [17]. Therefore, the idea of this study is to explore the advantage of ZrO_2 nanoparticles in combination with polyethylene glycol for the development of a phenolic biosensor which has high sensitivity, selectivity, simple technique, and fast detection.

In this research, polyethylene glycol, zirconium oxide nanoparticles, and hexacetyltrimethylammonium bromide had been used as a matrix since the synergistic effect of them in combination ensures the stability of the matrix and also will produce a phenolic biosensor with a comparable performance against the current studies. Polyethylene glycol (PEG) is a neutral non-ionic polymer with no charge on its backbone [20]; it contains an oxygen atom along its backbone, and therefore an electron pair is moving around the atom. As the electrons are moving along the atom, an electric current occurs and may improve the conductivity of the nanocomposite [21]. Herein, hexacetyltrimethylammonium bromide (CTAB) acts as a surfactant making a nonpolar chain of CTAB that interacts with the neutral polyethylene glycol.

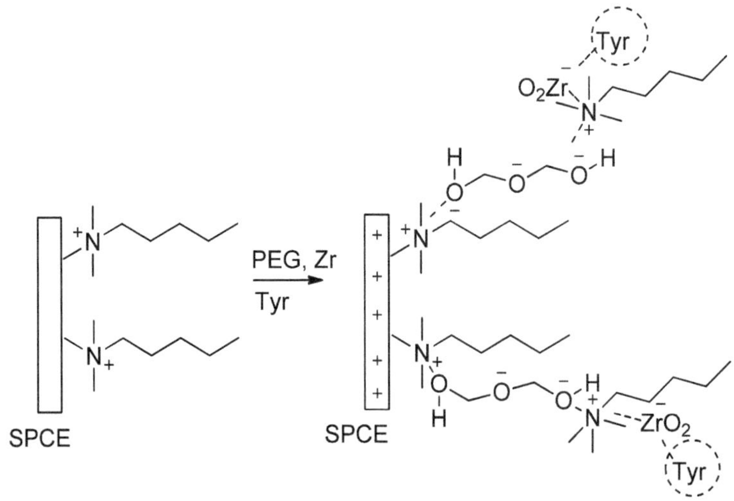

Figure 1. Possible assembling process of CTAB (hexacetyltrimethylammonium bromide)/PEG polyethylene glycol)-ZrO_2/tyrosinase on screen printed carbon electrode. SPCE, screen printed carbon electrode.

2. Materials and Methods

2.1. Reagents

Tyrosinase from mushrooms (T3824-25KU), phenol, hexacetyltrimethylammonium bromide (CTAB), Polyethylene glycol (PEG), and zirconium oxide nanoparticles (ZrO_2) (size less than 100 nm) were purchased from Sigma. Ascorbic acid (Unilab, Mumbai, India), uric acid (Sigma, St. Louis, MO, USA), hydrogen peroxide (Merck, Kenilworth, NJ, USA), glucose (Univar, Downers Grove, IL, USA), magnesium sulfateheptahydrate (Fluka, St. Louis, MO, USA), calcium chloride hydrate (Univar), iron (III) chloride hexahydrate (sigma-Aldrich), *p*-cresol (Sigma), 4-chlorophenol (Sigma), and *o*-kresol (Aldrich, St. Louis, MO, USA) were analytical grade and dissolved in phosphate buffer upon being used. All chemicals were freshly prepared prior to use. All aqueous solutions were prepared using deionized water.

2.2. Apparatus

Cyclic voltammetric, electrochemical impedance spectroscopy, and amperometric measurements were performed using potentiostat (Autolab) using a two electrode system. Working electrodes were modified using CTAB/PEG-ZrO_2 with Ag/AgCl acting as a reference electrode and a Pt wire acting as the counter electrode. All electrochemical experiments were carried out in 5 mL of 0.050 mM phosphate buffer (pH 6.0). Scanning electron microscope- Energy-dispersive X-ray spectroscopy (SEM-EDX) was carried out using Carlzeiss Supra 40 VP FESEM. Fourier transform infrared spectroscopy (FTIR)analysis was conducted using Perkin Elmer Spectrum 100.

2.3. Preparation of Enzyme Electrode

A solution of hexacetyltrimethyl ammonium bromide (54 mg/mL) was prepared in 0.5 M NaCl pH 8.0. CTAB solution (2.5 μL) was drop casted onto the surface of a working electrode and allowed to dry at room temperature for 1 h. Zirconium oxide powder (18 mg) was dispersed in the phosphate buffer solution (pH 8). On the other hand, 18 μL of polyethylene glycol was dissolved in 0.1 M NaCl (pH 5.4). Next, the latter two solutions were mixed at a certain ratio and pipetted on top of the modified electrode with CTAB. Then, 2.0 uL of ZrO_2/PEG was dropped onto the electrode surface. Finally, 2.0 μL of tyrosinase (10 mg/mL) was pipetted onto the electrode and allowed to dry at 4 °C overnight.

2.4. Optimization and Performance Studies of the Biosensor

A series of optimization studies were carried out, including tests to determine the effect of applied potential, pH buffer, concentration of nanoparticles, and influence of the PEG-ZrO_2 layer. The study was conducted using cyclic voltamogram and amperometric techniques. Phenol substrate was diluted from 10 μM to the final concentration using a phosphate buffer solution (pH 6). Electrochemical studies, including cyclic voltammetric, amperometric, and impedance measurements, were done using SPCE, SPCE/CTAB, SPCE/CTAB/PEG, and SPCE/CTAB/PEG-ZrO_2.

3. Results and Discussion

3.1. Characterization of the Modified SPCE

The interaction between nanosized ZrO_2 and polyethylene glycol to the tyrosinase could be studied by comparing the FTIR spectra of the ZrO_2, pure tyrosinase, polyethylene glycol, and PEG-ZrO_2/tyrosinase, as shown in Figure 2. As can be noted in pure tyrosinase (spectrum b), peaks from 1750 to 1600 cm^{-1}, 1600 to 1500 cm^{-1}, and 1350 to 1200 cm^{-1} are assigned as amide I, amide II, amide III, respectively [22]. When tyrosinase interacted with ZrO_2 (spectrum c), the spectrum did not change dramatically, which indicates the metal oxide does not alter the native structure of the enzyme.

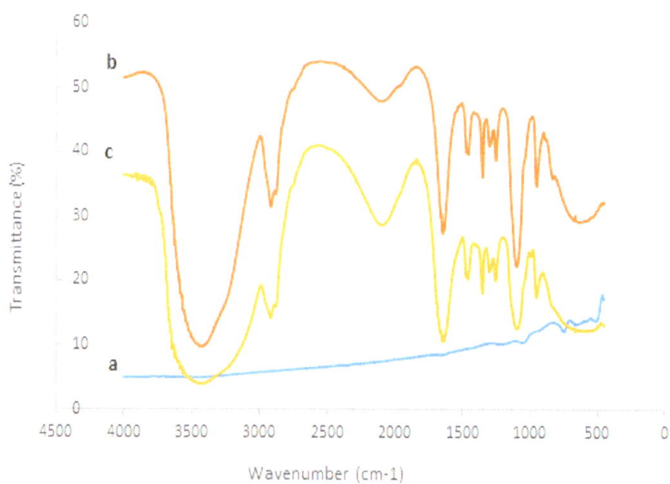

Figure 2. Fourier transform infrared spectroscopy spectra of (**a**) ZrO_2; (**b**) pure tyrosinase; (**c**) PEG-ZrO_2/tyrosinase.

A scanning election microscopy (SEM) image of a CTAB/PEG/ZrO_2 nanocomposite film is shown in Figure 3. It was found that the CTAB/PEG/ZrO_2 modified electrode exhibits uniform and tiny holes over the whole surface. Energy-dispersive X-ray spectroscopy (EDX) was used to analyze the elemental composition of the modifiers on the SPCE. The spectrum (Figure 3C) shows the presence of carbon (C), oxygen (O), sodium (Na), phosphorus (P), chlorine (Cl), bromine (Br), and zirconium (Zr) on the modified electrode, which indicates the successful deposition of CTAB/PEG/ZrO_2 on the electrode. However, when the enzyme was immobilized on the composite (Figure 4), a larger coagulant appeared, thereby showing that the pores on the surface had been totally covered by the enzyme. Data analyzed by EDX proved that the zirconium was successfully added into the nanocomposite (Figure 4B,C)

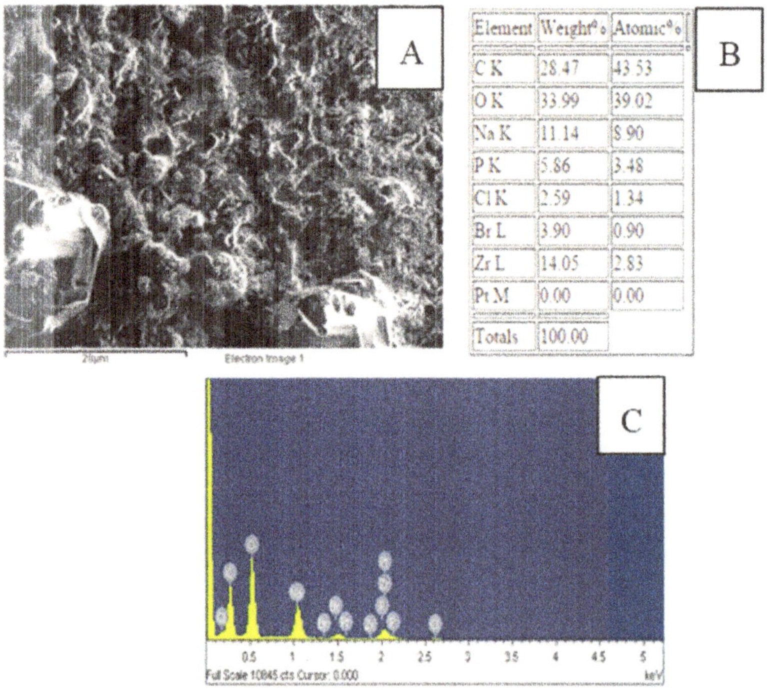

Element	Weight%	Atomic%
C K	28.47	43.53
O K	33.99	39.02
Na K	11.14	8.90
P K	5.86	3.48
Cl K	2.59	1.34
Br L	3.90	0.90
Zr L	14.05	2.83
Pt M	0.00	0.00
Totals	100.00	

Figure 3. Scanning electron microscopy (SEM) photographs (**A**); table of EDX analysis; (**B**) and spectrum of SPCE/PEG-ZrO_2 (**C**).

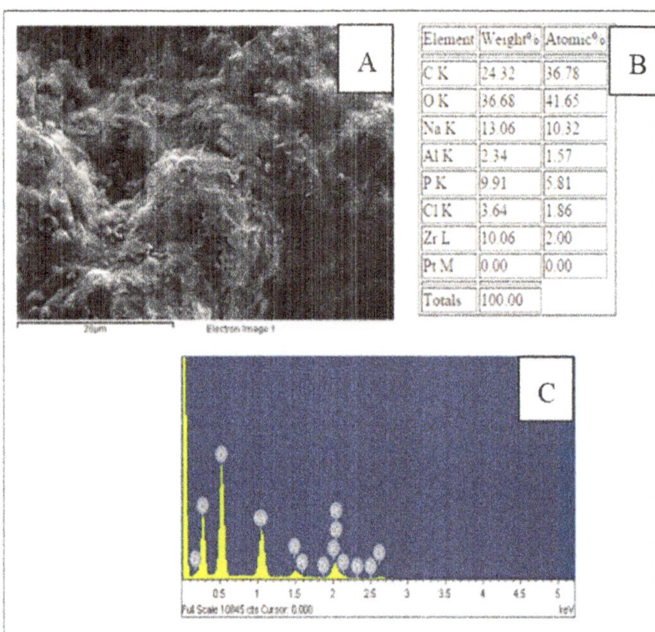

Element	Weight%	Atomic%
C K	24.32	36.78
O K	36.68	41.65
Na K	13.06	10.32
Al K	2.34	1.57
P K	9.91	5.81
Cl K	3.64	1.86
Zr L	10.06	2.00
Pt M	0.00	0.00
Totals	100.00	

Figure 4. SEM photographs (**A**); EDX data; (**B**); and spectrum of SPCE/PEG-ZrO_2/tyrosinase (**C**).

3.2. *Electrochemical Studies*

Electrochemical impedance spectroscopy (EIS) is a common method to investigate the interfacial properties of a modified electrode surface during the stepwise-assembly processes. Figure 5 displays the Nyquist plots of the EIS of the bare electrode (electrode A), SPCE modified CTAB (electrode B), SPCE modified CTAB/PEG (electrode C), and SPCE modified CTAB/PEG-ZrO_2 (electrode D), respectively.

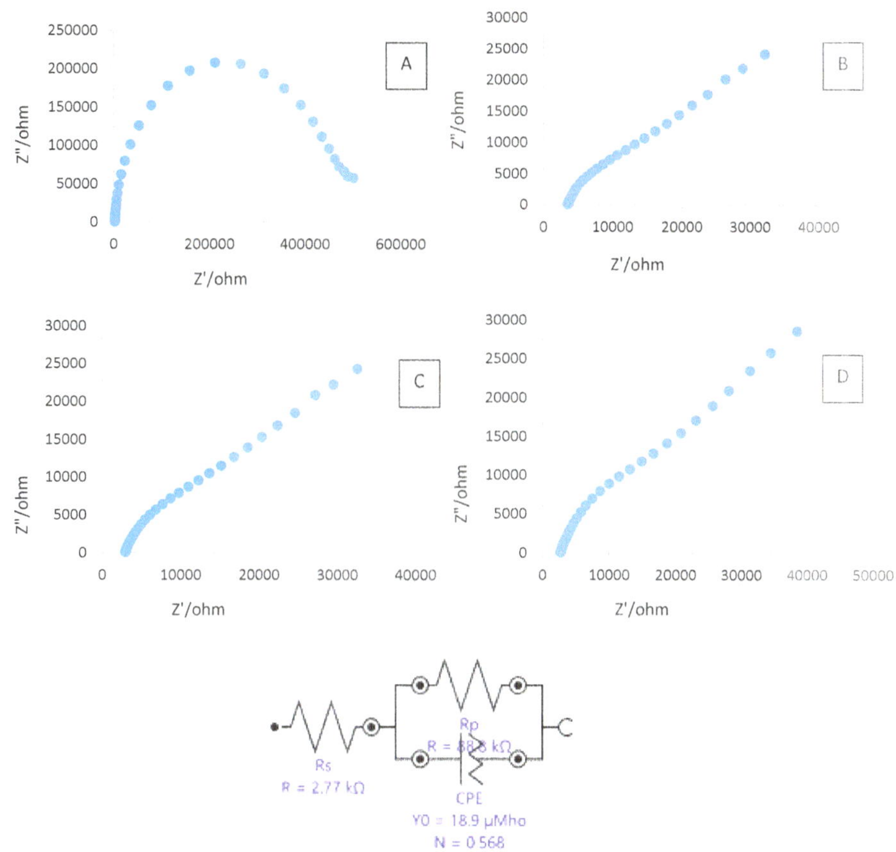

Figure 5. Electrochemical impedance spectroscopy (EIS) of: (**A**) bare SPCE; (**B**) SPCE/CTAB; SPCE/CTAB/PEG; (**C**) and SPCE/CTAB/PEG-ZrO_2 (**D**) in 5.0 mM $K_4Fe(CN)_6$ containing 0.1 M KCl as a supporting electrolyte.

The simulated values of charge transfer resistance (R_{CT}) at the bare unmodified electrode, SPCE with CTAB, SPCE casting with CTAB/PEG, and SPCE casting with CTAB/PEG-ZrO_2 were 473,180 Ω, 99,645 Ω, 88,762 Ω, and 88,077 Ω, respectively. After modification of the SPCE with CTAB, charge transfer resistance was found to decrease, thereby showing that the conductivity has been improved, and was further decreased when PEG was added to the electrode. Upon addition of the zirconium oxide to the composite, charge transfer resistance was found to change by a slight decrease, thus showing that the material enhanced the conductivity of the modified electrode. Theoretically, ZrO_2 nanoparticles behave as a nanoscale electrode, boosting electron conveyance between the surface of electrode and ferrocyanide ions. Q similar finding was also reported by other researchers [10] where the presence of nano-ZrO_2 was found to increase the effective electroactive surface area, resulting in enhancement of the diffusion of redox species on the electrode surface. The value of R_{CT} shows a decreased resistance when zirconium oxide was added to the bare Indium Tin Oxide (ITO) electrode. In another study [11], the value of R_{CT} shows a decreased resistance when a zirconium oxide/multi-walled carbon nanotube was added to the glassy carbon electrode. Furthermore, Zhao et al. [13] stated that the addition of ZrO_2 into the nonconductive chitosan decreased the resistance value, as indicated in the Nyquist plot. This behavior is due to ZrO_2 being a semiconductor material, as such, the electron transfer from $[(FeCN)_6{}^{3-/4-}]$ to the electrode surface becomes easier.

3.3. *Cyclic Voltamogram*

The electrochemical behavior of the different modified electrodes was investigated using 0.05 M phosphate buffer solution PBS (pH 6), consisting of 0.1 M KCl at the scan rate of 0.01 V/s. Figure 6 shows the cyclic voltamogram (CV) of tyrosinase immobilized on SPCE (curve a), tyrosinase immobilized on SPCE/CTAB/PEG (curve b), and tyrosinase immobilized on SPCE/CTAB/ZrO_2-PEG (curve c). A poor reduction peak current was observed when tyrosinase was immobilized on an unmodified electrode. A similar finding was also reported by Apetrei et al. (2015) [23]. Instead, a clear and better reduction peak current occurred at a lower potential when zirconium and polyethylene glycol were used as supporting matrix, which provided a higher surface area and good conductivity. The effect of the scan rate (Figure 7) from 10 mVs^{-1} to 80 mVs^{-1} on the biosensor response in the presence of 10 μM phenol in 0.05 M phosphate buffer solution (pH 6.0) was also investigated. The peak currents were linearly proportional to the scan rates, thereby indicating a redox property of the modified electrodes [12] and surface-controlled electrode process [14].

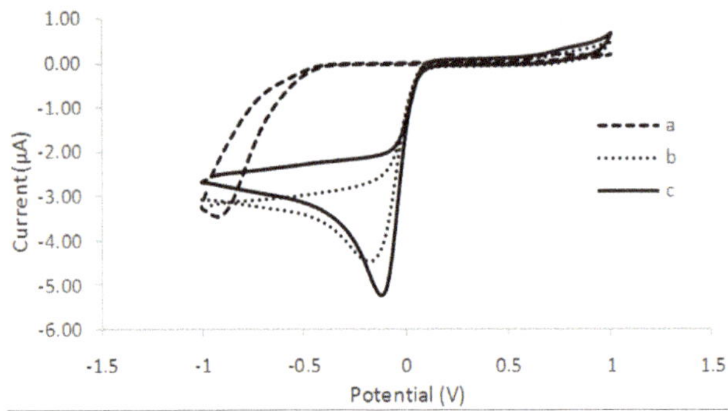

Figure 6. Cyclic voltamogram of (**a**) SPCE/tyrosinase; (**b**) SPCE/CTAB/PEG/tyrosinase; and (**c**) SPCE/CTAB/ZrO_2-PEG/tyrosinase in the presence of 10 μM phenol in 50 mM phosphate buffer solution (PBS) pH 6.0.

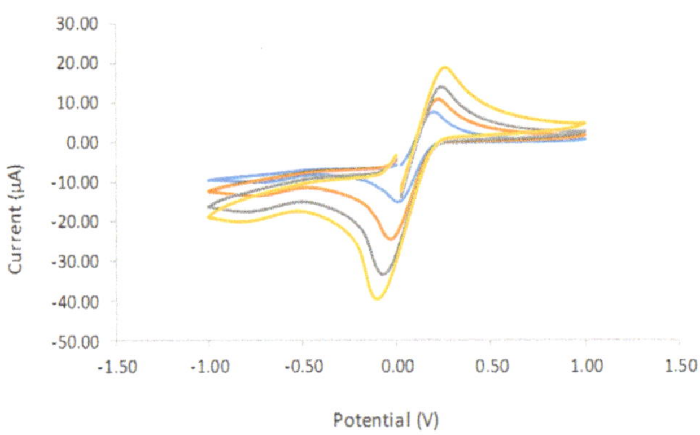

Figure 7. Cyclic voltamogram study on the effect of the scan rate from 0.01 V/s until 0.09 V/s in 5.0 mM $K_4Fe(CN)_6$ containing 0.1 M KCl as a supporting electrolyte. 3.5. Optimization of Experimental Parameters

In this work, the electrochemical measurements have been performed using a chronoamperometric technique to observe the performance of the immobilized tyrosinase on PEG-ZrO_2 composite film. Tyrosinase is a copper containing enzyme that catalyzes the oxidation of phenol group to *o*-quinone, which is commonly used in the detection of phenolic compounds. The oxidation of phenols by tyrosinase can be presented according to the following reactions:

$$\text{Phenol} + \text{tyrosinase} \rightarrow \text{catechol} \quad (1)$$

$$\text{Catechol} + \text{tyrosinase} \rightarrow o\text{-quinone} + H_2O \quad (2)$$

$$o\text{-quinone} + H^+ + 2e^- \rightarrow \text{catechol} \quad (3)$$

The oxidation of phenol by tyrosinase has two steps: phenol is oxidized to catechol (*o*-benzenediol), and then further oxidized by tyrosinase to *o*-quinone. The liberated quinone species can also be electrochemically reduced, and the reaction can be measured at a lower potential [24,25]. Thus, this provides the additional advantage of the enzymatic electrochemical recycling of the substrate, giving rise to signal amplification.

In this work, the effect of applied potential was investigated (Figure 8A) in the potential range of −0.05 V to −0.4 V vs. AgCl, and the optimum response of the immobilized tyrosinase on PEG-ZrO_2 composite film was observed at the applied potential of −0.2 V vs. AgCl. Thus, the applied potential of −0.2 V was chosen for further study. The influence of pH on the biosensor response is shown in Figure 8B. The maximum current response was observed at pH 6.0. This is in accordance with the work reported by Xue et al. [26], Cheng [27], and Liu et al. [28] which indicate that the immobilization of enzymes does not drastically alter their pH response characteristics. Thus this pH was chosen for subsequent studies.

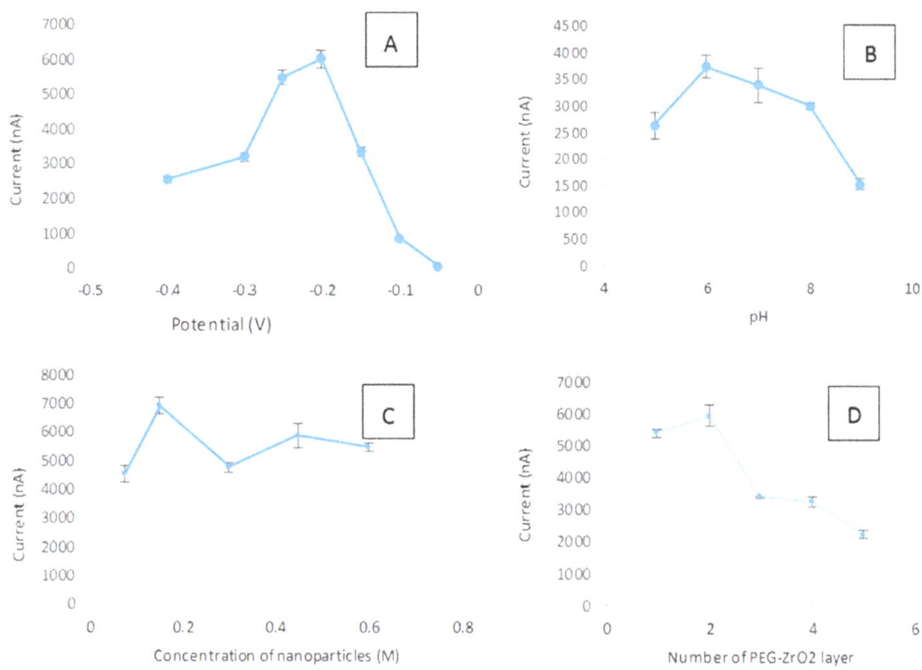

Figure 8. The effect of applied potential (**A**); pH buffer (**B**); concentration of nanoparticles (**C**); and number of PEG-ZrO_2 layers on modified SPCE (**D**). Phenol concentration and applied potential were fixed, respectively, at 10 μM and −0.2 V vs. AgCl.

The effect of the concentration of the metal oxide incorporated into the nanocomposite film was also optimized, as shown in Figure 8C. It can be noted that the concentration of 0.075 M ZrO_2 nanoparticles was sufficient to facilitate the electron transfer since the higher concentrations of metal oxide show reduced current signals. The effect of the film thickness of the composite film on the biosensor response was also studied in this work. Figure 8D shows the different current responses produced when a different number of layers was applied on the electrode surface. The biosensor response decreased with the increase in film thickness [29–32]. This phenomenon suggests that the thicker film that formed on the surface of the electrode caused the interfacial charge transfer between the SPCE and substrate to become difficult [9]. The enzyme has the capability to transfer electrons during oxidation and reduction when there is only a thin film on the electrode surface. With thicker PEG-ZrO_2 films, the distance between the biomolecules and the electrodes are fully occupied with the thick matrix, and it becomes more difficult for the electron transfers to occur [20]. Therefore, by considering the activity and sensitivity of CTAB/ZrO_2-PEG/tyrosinase towards phenol, the optimum thickness of one layer was selected for the subsequent experiment.

3.4. *Interference Studies*

The selectivity of the prepared sensor based on SPCE/CTAB/PEG-ZrO_2/tyrosinase was also investigated by measuring the amperometric response towards 4 μM phenol in the presence of some possible interference ions. Table 1 shows the change in current response in the presence of interfering substances. It can be noted that uric acid, glucose, Mg^{2+}, Ca^{2+}, and Fe^{3+} did not show any significant interfering effect on the determination of phenol. However, ascorbic acid and H_2O_2 were shown to cause interference. This might be related to ascorbic acid being one of the enzyme inhibitors, which might reduce the tyrosinase activity.

Table 1. Effect of some interference species on the sensor response.

Interferent	Coexisting Level	Change of Current Response (%)
Ascorbic acid	3 μM	−5.78
Uric acid	300 μM	−0.69
H_2O_2	50 μM	5.18
Glucose	1000 μM	4.65
Mg^{2+}	40 μM	2.88
Ca^{2+}	40 μM	3.20
Fe^{3+}	40 μM	1.14

3.5. *Analytical Performance of the Developed Biosensor*

In this study, the performance of the developed sensor for the detection of phenol was investigated under optimum conditions in the concentration range of 0.075 μM to 120 μM. Table 2 presents the analytical characteristic of biosensors reported in literature for phenolic detection. The calibration curve was performed separately for the lower range (0.075–10 μM) and higher range (10–55 μM), respectively. It was observed that above the concentration of 55 μM, the sensor response reached the maximum value, thus indicating the saturation point. The reduction currents are linear to the concentration of phenol ranging from 0.075 to 10 μM and 10 to 55 μM with correlation coefficients 0.999 (Figure 9) and 0.992 (Figure 10), respectively, with the detection limit of 0.034 μM ($S/N = 3$). The sensitivity of SPCE/CTAB/PEG-ZrO_2/tyrosinase obtained was 219.5 (mA/M), which is slightly higher than previous work using zinc oxide nanoparticles [18]. The response time of the biosensor was found to be less than 10 s. This fast response time is comparable with others studies [9,18] and might be contributed by the zirconium oxide, which promotes better conductivity of the modified electrode [10,12].

The reproducibility of the biosensor fabrication was investigated by measuring the response of the sensor towards a fixed concentration of phenol (10 μM) using different electrodes. Three different enzyme electrodes were tested and the relative standard deviation (RSD) value was calculated to be 6.88%. The repeatability of the sensor was also evaluated (Figure 11A), and the RSD of 8.8% was observed for twenty successive assays of phenol (10 μM). The storage stability of the enzyme electrodes when stored at 4 °C was investigated, and it was found to be stable for at least 30 days (Figure 11B).

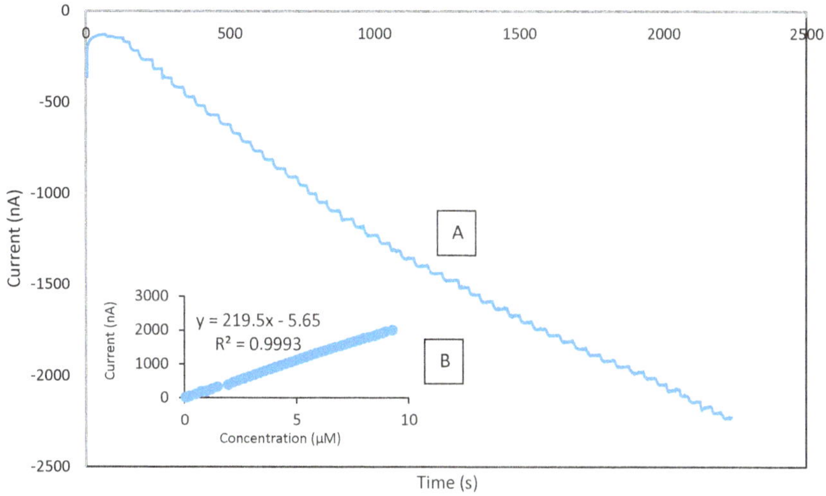

Figure 9. Typical current-time response curve (**A**); and calibration curves of phenol (**B**) obtained with SPCE/CTAB/PEG-ZrO_2/Tyr on screen printed carbon electrode with the phenol concentration range of 0.075–10 µM.

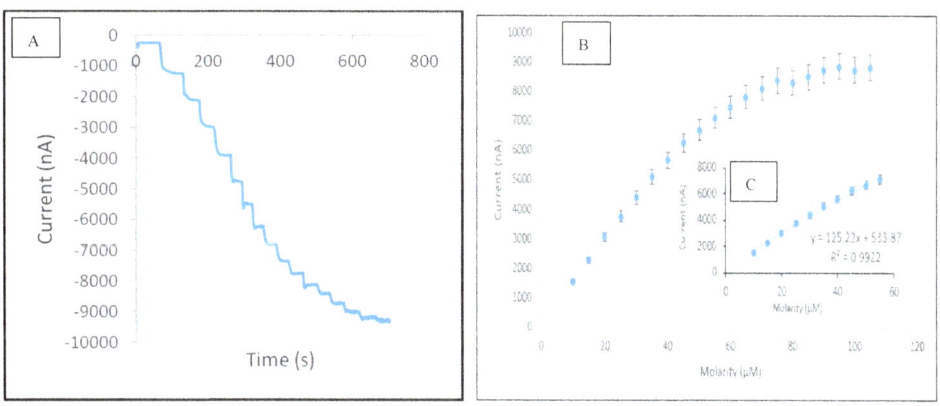

Figure 10. Typical current-time response curve (**A**); calibration curves for the concentration of phenol range 10–120 µM (**B**); and concentration of phenol range 10–55 µM (**C**) obtained with SPCE/CTAB/PEG-ZrO_2/Tyr.

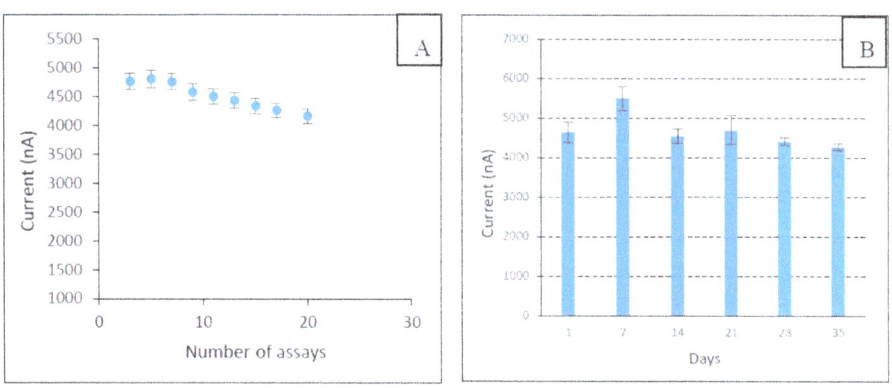

Figure 11. The repeatability of the developed biosensor (**A**) and storage stability of the fabricated biosensor (**B**).

Table 2. Analytical characteristic of biosensors reported in literature for phenolic detection.

Composite System	Linear Range (μM)	Applied Potential (V)	Detection Limit (μM)	Response Time (s)	Reference
Zinc oxide/catechol	0.15–65	−0.2	0.05	10	[18]
Iron oxide/coliform	0.01–39	−0.2	0.005	5	[27]
Bismuth oxide/catechol	0.01–8	−0.2	0.05	8	[9]
Graphene oxide-gold nanoparticle/catechol	0.083–23	−0.25	0.024	6	[33]
Iron oxide/MWCNT/PANI Au/guaicol/polyphenol	0.1-10 10–500	−0.2	0.03	3	[19]
Zirconium oxide	0.075–10 10–55	−0.2	0.034	10	This work

3.6. Selectivity Study

Several phenolic compounds (phenol, 4-chlorophenol, and *p*-kresol) were tested by the proposed biosensor. Table 3 presents the response characteristics of the enzyme electrode towards different phenolic compounds. The value of the apparent Michaelis-Menten constant provides the information on the affinity of an enzyme for its substrate, where a smaller value indicates a stronger substrate binding and higher catalytic activity. In this study, the apparent Michaelis-Menten constant values (K_M^{app}) for the CTAB/PEG-ZrO_2/tyrosinase towards phenol, catechol, and 4-chlorophenol were studied and tabulated in Table 3.

The lowest K_M^{app} value was found for *p*-cresol. This observation is slightly better than the observation from the biosensor based on polycrystalline bismuth oxide films for *p*-cresol (36 μM) [9]. The biosensor with a lower K_M^{app} indicates that it has the capability to detect a substrate at both a very low and high concentration and has higher affinity towards the substrate, which allows it to perform a wider linear range [25]. On the other hand, the K_M^{app} for phenol was found to be 61.42 μM, which is fairly similar to the results from the biosensor based on iron oxide-coated carbon nanotubes (58.6 μM) [27] and better than the results reported using polycrystalline bismuth oxide films (319 μM) [9].

Table 3. The response characteristics of the SPCE/CTAB/PEG/tyrosinase composite film to phenolic compound.

Phenol Compound	Linear Range (μM)	Correlation Coefficient (R^2)	Detection Limit (μM)	K_M^{app} (μM)
Phenol	0.5–9.5 10.0–55.0	0.9900 0.9993	0.0379 0.1003	61.42 193.33
4-chlorophenol	1.5–7.0	0.9942	0.2372	3650.00
p-kresol	0.025–1.0 1.0–12.0	0.9999 0.9997	0.0175 0.5232	1.50 5.25

3.7. Analysis of Spiked Real Water Samples

The performances of the biosensors have been tested with the analysis of spiked real samples. Water samples were taken from three different rivers in Kuala Lumpur and were brought to the laboratory without any pre-treatment. Water samples were spiked with a known concentration of phenol (0.6 μM) and measured using the developed biosensor and the standard spectrophotometric method, respectively. Table 4 presents the result of the water samples recovered. The results demonstrate both the biosensor and the spectrophotometric method. As shown in Table 4, the calculated values of $|t|$ are less than the tabulated t for two degrees of freedom ($N1 + N2 - 2$) at the 95% confidence level (which is 2.920), so there is no statistical difference in the results by the two methods. This result shows that the two methods used for the determination of phenol in the spiked water samples were in good agreement and comparable.

Table 4. Determination of spiked phenol in the matrix of river water ($n = 3$).

River Water	Total Phenolic Content by Present Method (μM) Mean ± SD ($n = 3$)	Total Phenolic Content by Standard Spectrophotometric Method (μM) Mean ± SD ($n = 3$)	*T*-Test Value
River 1	0.5839 ± 0.0127	0.6675 ± 0.0092	1.5500
River 2	0.5891 ± 0.0003	0.6242 ± 0.0139	1.2448
River 3	0.5897 ± 0.0002	0.5833 ± 0.0416	0.0771

Note: The critical value, $t_4 = 2.92$ ($p = 0.05$).

4. Conclusions

This study presents a very simple and inexpensive method for phenolic determination in water samples. Despite the simplicity and common materials used, a considerably low detection limit was obtained. This method is considered to be a good platform for future modifications using other materials. In the future, the method should be modified by introducing novel materials, such as ionic liquid or quantum dots, for exploring the effects of new and different materials.

Acknowledgments: This work was supported by "Geran Dana Pembudayaan Penyelidikan (RAGS) 2013" (600-RMI/RAGS 5/3 (31/2013)). Special thanks to Bioprocess Department Sirim Berhad, Shah Alam for giving permission to use Autolab potentiostat throughout this study. The funds for covering the costs to publish in open access have been granted by the Ministry of Higher Education, Malaysia (Mybrain15).

Author Contributions: N.M.A. performed the experiments, collected and analyzed the data, and wrote the manuscript. J.A. analyzed the data and primarily provided the ideas in the introduction and discussion sections. N.A.Y. helped to analyze the data for the interferences and characterization section of the results. A.H. and S.A.R. contributed to enzyme and phenol preparation. R.H. contributed to the data interpretations for electrochemical impedance spectroscopy.

Conflicts of Interest: The authors declare no conflict of interest.

Abbreviations

The following abbreviations are used in this manuscript:

MDPI	Multidisciplinary Digital Publishing Institute
DOAJ	Directory of open access journals
TLA	Three letter acronym
LD	linear dichroism

References

1. Michalowicz, J.; Duda, W. Phenols-sources and toxicity. *Pol. J. Environ. Stud.* **2007**, *16*, 347–362.
2. Lavilla, I.; Gil, S.; Costas, M.; Bendicho, C. Dispersive liquid-liquid microextraction combined with microvolume spectrophotometry to turn green the 5530 APHA standard method for determining phenols in water and wastewater. *Talanta* **2012**, *98*, 197–202. [CrossRef] [PubMed]
3. Santana, C.M.; Ferrera, Z.S.; Padron, M.E.T.; Rodrigiez, J.J.S. Methodologies for the extraction of phenolic compounds from environmental samples: New Approaches. *Molecules* **2009**, *14*, 298–320. [CrossRef] [PubMed]
4. Zheng, Z.; Tian, L.; Li, Z.; Jia, L.; Zhang, X.; Xia, M.; Hu, Y. Whole-cell method for phenol detection based on the color reaction of phenol with 4-aminoantipyrine catalyzed by CotA laccase on endospore surfaces. *Biosens. Bioelectron.* **2015**, *69*, 162–166. [CrossRef] [PubMed]
5. Asan, A.; Isildak, I. Determination of major phenolic compounds in water by reversed-phase liquid chromatography after pre-column derivatization with benzoyl chloride. *J. Chromatogr. A* **2003**, *988*, 145–149. [CrossRef]
6. Nassiri, M.; Zahedi, M.M.; Pourmortazavi, S.M.; Yousefzade, M. Optimization of dispersive liquid-liquid microextraction for preconcentration and spectrophotometric determination of phenols in Chabahar Bay seawater after derivatization with 4-aminoantipyridine. *Mar. Pollut. Bull.* **2014**, *86*, 512–517. [CrossRef] [PubMed]

7. Ou, J.; Hu, L.; Hu, L.; Li, X.; Zou, H. Determining of phenolic compounds in river waterwith on-line coupling bisphenol A imprinted monolithic pre-column with high performance liquid chromatography. *Talanta* **2006**, *69*, 1001–1006. [CrossRef] [PubMed]
8. Feng, Q.; Zhao, L.; Lin, J.M. Molecularly imprinted polymer as micro-solid phase extraction combined with high performance liquid chromatography to determine phenolic compounds in environmental water samples. *Anal. Chim. Acta* **2009**, *650*, 70–76. [CrossRef] [PubMed]
9. Shan, D.; Zhang, J.; Xue, H.G.; Zhang, Y.C.; Cosnier, S.; Ding, S.N. Polycrystalline bismuth oxide films for development of amperometric biosensor for phenolic compound. *Biosens. Bioelectron.* **2009**, *24*, 3671–3676. [CrossRef] [PubMed]
10. Solanki, P.R.; Kaushik, A.; Chavdan, P.M.; Maheshwari, S.N.; Malhotra, B.D. Nanostructured zirconium oxide based genosensor for Escherichia coli detection. *Electrochem. Commun.* **2009**, *11*, 2272–2277. [CrossRef]
11. Pundir, S.; Chauhan, N.; Narang, J.; Pundir, C.S. Amperometric choline biosensor based on multiwalled carbon nanotubes/zirconium oxide nanoparticles electrodeposited on glassy carbon electrode. *Anal. Biochem.* **2012**, *427*, 26–32. [CrossRef] [PubMed]
12. Liu, B.; Cao, Y.; Chen, D.; Kong, J.; Deng, J. Amperometric biosensor based on nanoporous ZrO_2 matrix. *Anal. Chim. Acta* **2003**, *478*, 59–66. [CrossRef]
13. Zhao, G.; Feng, J.J.; Xu, J.J.; Chen, H.Y. Direct electrochemistry and electrocatalysis of heme proteins immobilized on self-assembled ZrO_2 film. *Electrochem. Commun.* **2005**, *7*, 724–729. [CrossRef]
14. Liu, S.; Dai, Z.; Chen, H.; Ju, H. Imobilization of hemoglobin on zirconium dioxide nanoparticles for preparation of a novel hydrogen peroxide biosensor. *Biosens. Bioelectron.* **2004**, *19*, 963–969. [CrossRef] [PubMed]
15. Sumana, G.; Das, M.; Srivasta, S.; Malhotra, B.D. A novel urea biosensor based on zirconia. *Thin Solid Films* **2010**, *519*, 1187–1191. [CrossRef]
16. Yang, Y.; Yang, H.; Yang, M.; Liu, Y.; Shen, G.; Yu, R. Amperometric glucose biosensor based on a surface treated nanoporous ZrO_2/Chitosan composite film as immobilization matrix. *Anal. Chim. Acta* **2004**, *525*, 213–220. [CrossRef]
17. Chang, M.Y.; Juang, R.S. Stability and reactivity of acid phosphatase immobilized on composite beads of chitosan and ZrO_2 powders. *Int. J. Biol. Macromol.* **2007**, *40*, 224–231. [CrossRef] [PubMed]
18. Li, Y.F.; Liu, Z.M.; Liu, Y.L.; Yang, Y.H.; Shen, G.L.; Yu, R.Q. A mediator-free phenol biosensor based on immobilizing tyrosinase on ZnO nanoparticles. *Anal. Biochem.* **2006**, *349*, 33–40. [CrossRef] [PubMed]
19. Rawal, R.; Chawla, S.; Devender, S.; Pundi, C.S. An amperometric biosensor based on laccase immobilized onto Fe_3O_4NPs/cMWCNT/PANI/Au electrode for determination of phenolic content in tea leaves extract. *Enzym. Microb. Technol.* **2012**, *51*, 179–185. [CrossRef] [PubMed]
20. Qiao, K.; Hu, N. Direct electron transfer and electrocatalysis of myoglobin loaded in layer-by-layer fils assembled with nonionic poly(ethylene glycol) and ZrO_2 nanoparticles. *Bioelectrochemistry* **2009**, *75*, 71–76. [CrossRef] [PubMed]
21. Arshak, K.; Velusamy, V.; Korostynska, O.; Stasiak, K.O.; Adley, C. Conducting polymers and their applications to biosensors: Emphasizing on foodborne pathogen detection. *IEEE Sens. J.* **2009**, *9*, 1942–1951. [CrossRef]
22. Shi, C.; Dai, Y.; Liu, Q.; Xie, Y.; Xu, X. The FT-IR spectrometric analysis of the changes of polyphenol oxidase II secondary structure. *J. Mol. Struct.* **2003**, *644*, 139–144. [CrossRef]
23. Apetrei, I.M.; Apetrei, C. The biocomposite screen-printed biosensor based on immobilization of tyrosinase onto the carboxyl functionalised carbon nanotube for assaying tyramine in fish products. *J. Food Eng.* **2015**, *149*, 1–8. [CrossRef]
24. Lu, L.; Zhang, L.; Zhang, X.; Huan, S.; Shen, G.; Yu, R. A novel tyrosinase biosensor based on hydroxyapatite-chitosan nanocomposite for the detection of phenolic compounds. *Anal. Chim. Acta* **2010**, *665*, 146–151. [CrossRef] [PubMed]
25. Apetrei, C.; Rodriguez-Mendez, M.L.; De Saja, J.A. Amperometrictyrosinase based biosensor using an electropolymerized phosphate-doped polypyrrole film as an immobilization support.Application for detection of phenolic compounds. *Electrochim. Acta* **2011**, *56*, 8919–8925. [CrossRef]
26. Xue, H.; Shen, Z. A highly stable biosensor for phenols prepared by immobilizing polyphenol oxidase into polyaniline-polyacrylonitrile composite matrix. *Talanta* **2000**, *57*, 289. [CrossRef]

27. Cheng, Y.; Liu, Y.; Huang, J.; Li, K.; Xian, Y.; Zhang, W.; Jin, L. Amperometrictyrosinase biosensor based on Fe_3O_4 nanoparticles-coated carbon nanotubes nanocomposite for rapid detection of coliforms. *Electrochim. Acta* **2009**, *54*, 2588–2594. [CrossRef]
28. Liu, Z.; Wang, J.; Xie, D.; Chen, G. Polyaniline-coated Fe_3O_4 nanoparticles-carbon-nanotube composite and its application in electrochemical biosensing. *Small Nano Micro* **2008**, *4*, 462–466. [CrossRef] [PubMed]
29. Vedrine, C.; Fabiano, S.; Tran-Minh, C. Amperometric tyrosinase based biosensor using an electrogeneratedpolythiophene film as an entrapment support. *Talanta* **2003**, *59*, 535–544. [CrossRef]
30. Shan, D.; Cosnier, S.; Mousty, C. Layered double hydroxides: An attractives material for electrochemical biosensor design. *Anal. Chem.* **2003**, *75*, 3872–3879. [CrossRef] [PubMed]
31. Han, E.; Shan, D.; Xue, H.G.; Cosnier, S. Hybrid Material based on chitosan and layered double hydroxides: Characterization and application to the design of amperometric phenol biosensor. *Biomacromolecules* **2007**, *8*, 971–975. [CrossRef] [PubMed]
32. Fan, Q.; Shan, D.; Xue, H.G.; He, Y.Y.; Cosnier, S. Amperometric phenol biosensor based on laponite clay–chitosan nanocomposite matrix. *Biosens. Bioelectron.* **2007**, *22*, 816–821. [CrossRef] [PubMed]
33. Song, W.; Li, D.W.; Li, Y.T.; Li, Y.; Long, Y.T. Disposable biosensor based on graphene oxide conjugated with tyrosinase assembled gold nanoparticles. *Biosens. Bioelectron.* **2011**, *26*, 3181–3186. [CrossRef] [PubMed]

15

Impedimetric Label-Free Immunosensor on Disposable Modified Screen-Printed Electrodes for Ochratoxin A

Francesca Malvano [1], Donatella Albanese [1,*], Alessio Crescitelli [2], Roberto Pilloton [3] and Emanuela Esposito [2]

1 Department of Industrial Engineering, University of Salerno, 84084 Fisciano SA, Italy; fmalvano@unisa.it
2 Institute for Microelectronics and Microsystems of the National Council of Research (CNR), 80131 Napoli, Italy; alessio.crescitelli@cnr.it (A.C.); emanuela.esposito@cnr.it (E.E.)
3 Institute of Atmospheric Pollution Research of the National Council of Research (CNR), 00015 Roma, Italy; roberto.pilloton@cnr.it
* Correspondence: dalbanese@unisa.it

Academic Editor: Jeff D. Newman

Abstract: An impedimetric label-free immunosensor on disposable screen-printed carbon electrodes (SPCE) for quantitative determination of Ochratoxin A (OTA) has been developed. After modification of the SPCE surface with gold nanoparticles (AuNPs), the anti-OTA was immobilized on the working electrode through a cysteamine layer. After each coating step, the modified surfaces were characterized by cyclic voltammetry (CV) and electrochemical impedance spectroscopy (EIS). The capacitance was chosen as the best parameter that describes the reproducible change in electrical properties of the electrode surface at different OTA concentrations and it was used to investigate the analytical parameters of the developed immunosensor. Under optimized conditions, the immunosensor showed a linear relationship between 0.3 and 20 ng/mL with a low detection limit of 0.25 ng/mL, making it suitable to control OTA content in many common food products. Lastly, the immunosensor was used to measure OTA in red wine samples and the results were compared with those registered with a competitive ELISA kit. The immunosensor was sensitive to OTA lower than 2 μg/kg, which represents the lower acceptable limit of OTA established by European legislation for common food products.

Keywords: immunosensor; screen printed electrodes; Ochratoxin A; electrochemical impedance spectroscopy

---

1. Introduction

Mycotoxins are a large and varied group of mold-secondary metabolites with common features because they are all produced by fungi and have toxic effects against vertebrates and other organisms. Mycotoxins affect a broad range of agricultural products, including cereals, cereal-based foods, dried fruits, wine, milk, coffee beans, cocoa, or meat products, which are the basis of the economies of many developing countries [1]. Moreover, mycotoxins are presently considered as the most important chronic dietary risk factor, higher than food additives or pesticide residues [2].

Ochratoxin A (OTA) is one of the most abundant mycotoxins that contaminates food products; it is found in tissue and organs of animals, including human blood and breast milk, and is known to produce nephrotoxic, teratogenic, carcinogenic, and immune toxic activity in several animal species [3]. OTA affects humans mainly through consumption of improperly stored food products, causing cancer.

The International Agency of Research on Cancer (IARC) has classified OTA as a possible carcinogenic compound for humans since it causes immune suppression and immune toxicity [4].

From the mid-2000s, approximately 100 countries (covering 85% of the world's inhabitants) had specific regulations or detailed guidelines for the occurrence of mycotoxins in food [2]. The European Union has established with the Regulation (EC) No 1881/2006, stating the acceptable limits for OTA in many products at high risk of contamination: OTA is allowed in very small concentrations (about 0.5–10 μg/Kg) depending on the kind of food [5]. These regulatory limits force all Member States to monitor and control mycotoxin levels in foodstuffs in order to reduce the intake of this toxic compound.

The methods most frequently used for OTA determination are thin-layer chromatography (TLC), high-performance liquid chromatography (HPLC), coupled to fluorescence or mass spectrometry detectors [6]. The chromatographic techniques are highly sensitive and specific, but require well-equipped laboratory facilities, time-consuming pretreatment steps, and highly-trained personnel that strongly limit the routine implementation of chromatography-based approaches [7]. Immune assays can be used as cheaper and quicker alternatives to chromatographic methods for mycotoxin detection. Competitive enzyme-linked immune sorbent assay (ELISA) is the most common commercial immune assay used for OTA detection in the food sector based on spectrophotometric reading, however, it suffers the drawbacks of time-consuming (for example, 50 min for I'screen Ochra Elisa kit (Tecna-Trieste, Italy); 90 min for OTA ELISA, (Abraxis LLC, Warminster, PA, USA), and the narrow dynamic range up to 16 ng/mL.

In recent years there has been a strong interest in the development of immunosensors based on the antigen-antibody interaction, but novel specific ligands (e.g., aptamers) are emerging.

Among all of the possible immunosensors (electrochemical, optical, microgravimetric) the electrochemical ones rank highly owing to their sensitivity, low cost, simplicity and, in some cases, miniaturization, portability, and integration in automated devices [8].

In the literature are reported two different types of electrochemical OTA immunosensors: label- and label-free-based. For the labelled immunosensors, the interaction between OTA and anti-OTA, based on direct and/or indirect competitive immunoassay, is detected by the use of enzymes exploiting the classical electrochemical techniques, such as amperometric, potentiometric, and conductimetric methods [9–13].

This immunosensor exhibits a detection limit ranging from 0.008 [12] to 0.12 [10] ng/mL with a dynamic range up to 250 ng· mL [13].

The application of electrochemical impedance spectroscopy (EIS), as a transduction technology, enables the label-free detection and quantification of the immune complex and, thus, for the development of biosensors for food hazards [14,15]. EIS is a powerful informative and non-destructive technique due to the small voltage excitation used during detection, which can be used to study the electrical properties of the sensing device interface and tracing the reactions occurring on it [16,17].

Different impedimetric label-free OTA affinity biosensors have been described previously by immobilization of monoclonal antibody and aptamers on the surface of gold or platinum electrodes [18–21]. This impedimetric immunosensor exhibits detection limit ranging from 0.01 [19] to 2 [20] ng/mL, with and a dynamic range up to 25 ng/mL [21].

In recent years the applications of disposable screen-printed carbon electrodes (SPCEs), characterized by low-cost fabrication and mass production, have attracted an increasing interest for the development of labelled immunosensors (especially enzyme immunosensors) but it is noteworthy that few studies [22,23] on electrochemical label-free immunosensors integrated onto SPCEs have been developed.

Exploiting the advantages of gold nanoparticles (AuNPs), which have been extensively used as matrices for the immobilization of macromolecules, such as proteins, enzymes, and antibodies, in addition to providing a microenvironment similar to what obtained under physiological conditions [24], it is possible to design a new electrochemical sensor by the modification of a working electrode surface. Moreover, AuNPs have attracted considerable attention in electroanalysis because of their excellent physical and chemical properties, such as high surface to volume ratio, good electrical properties, strong adsorption ability, and good surface properties. Electrodeposition of metallic nanoparticles on an electrode surface is a better process than deposition from solution, as the former is comparatively easier, faster, and generates a more stable surface. In addition, electrochemical deposition allows Au(III) to be addressed only on a polarised working electrode as Au(0) not on auxiliary or reference electrodes. Compared to gold electrodes, the electrodeposition of metallic nanoparticles or aggregated clusters (simply abbreviated as nanoparticles in this paper) on SPEs is more advantageous because of the unique properties offered by the metallic nanoparticles as described earlier [25]. Moreover the gold deposition on the electrode avoids poisoning and cross-contamination, which interferes with the analysis. These problems are absent in disposable SPCEs. Consequently, the combination of screen-printing and electrodeposition of metallic nanoparticles is a very promising technique for the mass production of electrochemical sensors with enhanced sensitivity [25].

For this reason, the aim of this work is the development of a label-free impedimetric immunosensor for OTA detection, realized on an AuNP-modified SPCE. EIS and CV were used to characterize each step of electrode modification and the analytical performances of the immunosensors developed. Finally the possibility to use a fast and cheap disposable biosensor like that proposed in this study could represent a key factor for the monitoring of mycotoxins in food products.

2. Materials and Methods

2.1. *Chemicals*

Glutaraldehyde solution ($C_5H_8O_2$, 50 wt % in H20), cysteamine (C_2H_7NS, ⩽98%), gold (III) chloride hydrate ($HAuCl_4$, 99.9%), sulfuric Acid (H_2SO_4, 99.9%), ethanolamine ($NH_2CH_2CH_2OH$, >99.5%), potassium hexacyanoferrate (III) ($[Fe(CN)_6]^{3-}$, >99%), and Ochratoxin A were purchased from Sigma-Aldrich (Milano, Italy). Potassium ferrocyanide ($[Fe(CN)_6]^{4-}$) was obtained from Carlo Erba reagent (Milano, Italy). Anti-Ochratoxin A antibody (Anti OTA, 1 mg/mL) was purchased from Abcam (Cambridge, UK), NaH_2PO_4, Na_2HPO_4, NaCl, and KCl used in the preparation of phosphate-buffered saline (PBS: 0.1 M KCl, pH 7.4) were also obtained from Sigma Aldrich (Milano, Italy). I'screen Ochra ELISA kit for the detection of Ochratoxin A was purchased from Tecna (Italy).

2.2. *Apparatus*

The electrochemical measurements were carried out with a computer-controlled Autolab PGSTAT 204 Potentiostat (Metrohm), equipped with an impedance module (FRA32M) and the experimental data were analysed with Nova software (Metrohm). Screen-printed carbon electrodes (SPCEs), based on a three-electrode layout (working/auxiliary/reference; Figure 1A), were produced in three screen-printing steps as described in Albanese et al. [26]. Specifically, a first layer of a carbon/graphite ink (G-Went, Pontypool, UK) was deposed to define the conducting tracks, the working and auxiliary electrodes. The second was a silver/silver chloride ink (Acheson Colloiden B.V., Scheemda, The Netherlands), used as a pseudo-reference electrode. The third layer consisted in an insulating ink (G-Went, Pontypool, UK). Between the first and the second screen-printing steps, the strips were cured at 80 °C for 25 min to dry off residual solvents and cure the patterned pastes after every step of screen-printing. The diameter of the working electrode was 2.8 mm. Scanning electron microscopy (SEM) images were obtained on a Raith Turnkey 150 SEM.

2.3. *Immunosensor Manufactoring*

2.3.1. Preparation of Gold-Modified SPCEs

The gold deposition on the homemade SPCEs was conducted after an electrochemical treatment at 1.7 V vs. Ag/AgCl as a reference electrode for 360 s in PBS.

The electrochemical AuNP deposition was carried out using a solution of 1 M $HAuCl_4$ in 0.5 M H_2SO_4 under a constant potential of −0.4 V vs. Ag/AgCl in a range of 50–400 s.

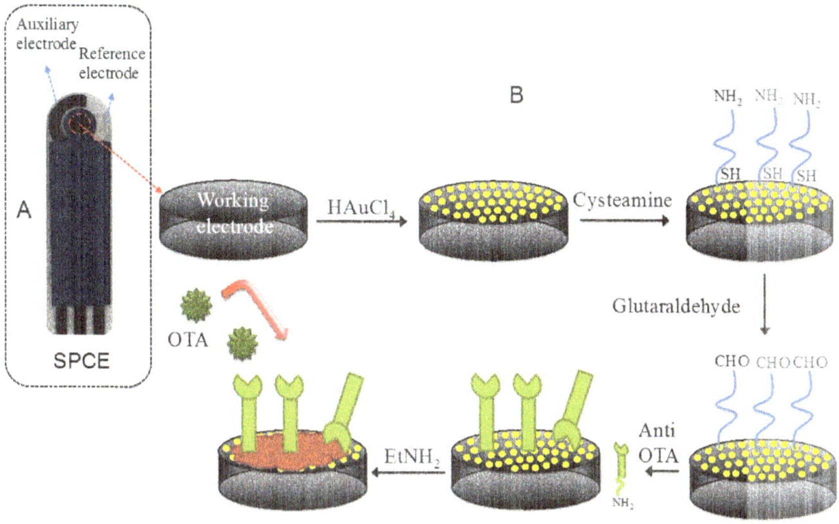

Figure 1. (**A**) Screen-printed carbon electrode layout; and (**B**) steps used for the fabrication of the immunosensor.

2.3.2. Electrochemical Deposed Multilayer (EDM)

EDM was employed to create thiol layers attached onto AuNPs. Cysteamine 20 mM was dropped onto the AuNPs modified working electrode and a constant potential of 1.2 V vs. Ag/AgCl for 20 min was applied. After the electrode was thoroughly rinsed with water, to remove physically-adsorbed cysteamine, 100 µL of glutaraldehyde solution 12% (v/v) were dropped onto the modified working electrode for 1 h and then, again, rinsed with water.

2.3.3. Antibody Immobilization

Different concentrations of anti-OTA solution (1 µg/mL, 5 µg/mL, 10 µg/mL) were dropped onto the modified electrode for 30 min at room temperature, then the electrode was rinsed in PBS to remove unbound antibodies. After the immobilization step, ethanolamine 1 M (pH 8.5) for 15 min was used to block unreacted active sites. The schematic diagram of immunosensor fabrication is shown in Figure 1B.

2.4. Experimental Measurement

EIS and CV measurements were used to characterize each step of the electrode modification.

For the impedance measurements, a sinusoidal AC potential (10 mV) in the frequency range from 0.1 to 10^4 Hz was superimposed to 0.00 mV (vs. reference electrode) DC potential. The impedance spectra were plotted in the form of Nyquist plots, where the complex impedance is displayed as the sum of the real and imaginary components (Z′ and Z″ respectively), and in the form of Bode diagram where the total impedance of the system (Z) is plotted versus frequency. All measurements were performed in a solution of 1 mM ferri/ferrocyanide redox couple ($[Fe(CN)_6]^{4-/3-}$, 1:1) in PBS, pH 7.5, as background electrolyte at room temperature.

The voltammetric measurements were performed from −0.6 to 0.6 V vs. Ag/AgCl with a scan rate of 0.05 V/s; the redox couple used for the CV was the same as that used for impedance measurements.

For the OTA analysis, 20 µL of OTA at different concentrations in PBS were dropped onto the working area of the immunosensor and incubated for 20 min. Before the impedance measurements, the immunosensor was rinsed thoroughly with copious amounts of PBS.

2.5. *Preparation of Wine Samples for OTA Measurement*

The preparation of red wine samples was conducted according to the procedure described in the I'screen Ochra ELISA kit. 5 mL of wine was added to 5 mL of 1 M HCl and 10 mL of dichloromethane; the solution was shaken in a low-speed shaker (400 rpm) for 15 min and centrifuged at 2200 rpm for 15 min. Five millilitres of solvent phase was added to 2.5 mL of the 0.13 M sodium bicarbonate solution; the solution was shaken for 30 s. The upper aqueous phase was recovered and centrifuged to remove solvent traces and finally diluted two times with sodium bicarbonate solution.

This procedure was replicated for the three different OTA (1.5 ng/mL, 5 ng/mL, and 10 ng/mL) spiked wine samples. The OTA results obtained by the immunosensors were compared with those measured with the competitive ELISA kit for OTA.

3. Results

3.1. *Characterization of the Electrode Modifying Process*

The electrodeposition of AuNPs on the electrode surface was strongly affected by the electrodeposition time, which have been optimized to obtain the best analytical performances in our device. As Figure 2 shows, an increase of the electrodeposition time from 50 to 300 s leads to significant current increase, while an effect that plateaued at a longer deposition time is observed (inset Figure 2). Therefore, an electrodeposition time of 300 s was selected as optimum.

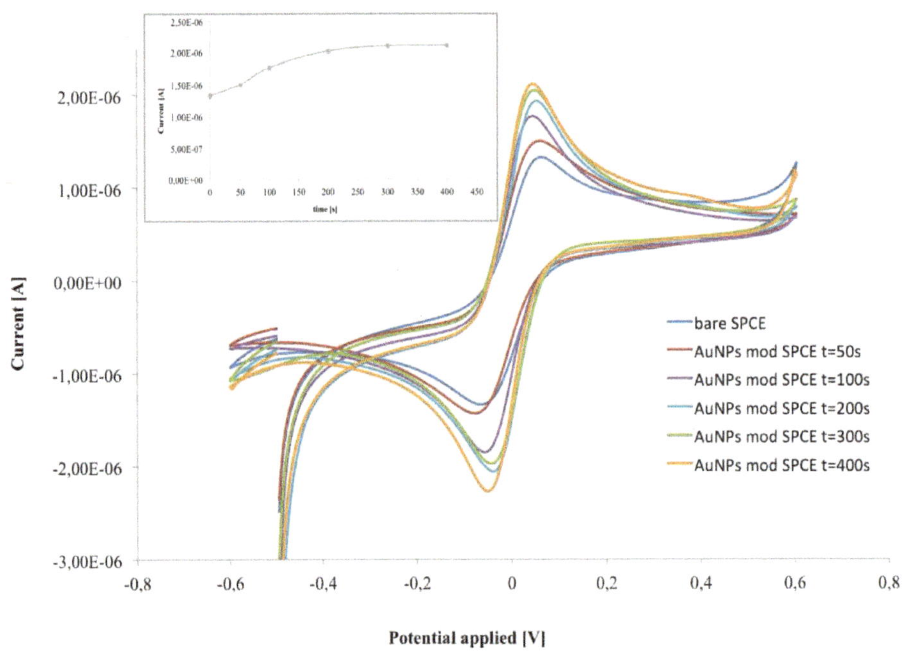

Figure 2. CV of bare and AuNP-modified SPCE at different deposition times. Inset: current intensity of the anodic peak at different deposition times, in 1 mM ferri/ferrocyanide redox couple ($[Fe(CN)_6]^{4-/3-}$, 1:1) in PB, pH 6.8.

As expected, the working electrode modified with AuNPs exhibited the characteristic increase of the anodic and cathodic peaks, thus confirming the successful modification process. Moreover increasing the electrodeposition time from 50 to 300 s, larger peak currents and a smaller peak-to-peak potential separations (ΔE) were observed. In particular, the optimized AuNP deposition time increased the electrochemical performance of the electrode with anodic current of 2.1 μA and ΔE = 91 mV for AuNPs/SPCE, in contrast to 1.3 μA and ΔE = 135 mV for SPCE (Figure 2). This behaviour was attributed to the enhanced electrochemical activity of the AuNPs, which allowed the increase of the electrode active area and shifted the peak potential near to 0 V giving rise to a smaller peak-to-peak separation.

This fact suggests a slight improvement in the electrocatalytic properties of the electrode produced by the addition of the AuNPs, which facilitated the electron-transfer process [27].

SEM images (Figure 3) of the carbon working electrode before and after the gold electrodeposition had been carried out, in order to verify the presence of the AuNPs. As expected, the surface of the bare carbon electrode shows the typical flake-shaped graphite particles along with large cavities. When the electrode is biased to deposit (reduce) the gold, the tips, the reliefs, and depressions of the SPCE surface suffer from a heterogeneous distribution of electric charge that promotes the formation of a heterogeneous dimension of Au particles, besides considering that a high time of deposition favours the interfusion of NPs in larger gold ones so the nano-structure was destroyed. Cluster agglomeration of AuNPs and single NPs are evident in Figure 3b,c. Moreover the quantity of deposed gold on carbon printed surface (122 pg per electrode) has been calculated from the deposition current (0.6 μA) and time (300 s), considering the Faraday constant = 96,485.34 C/mol, the number of electrons (3) involved in the reduction of Au(III) to Au(0), and the atomic weight of Au (196.96 D). AuNPs deposed on SPCE resulted in a cheap gold surface since it was obtained with a smaller quantity of gold than the expensive commercial solid gold electrodes.

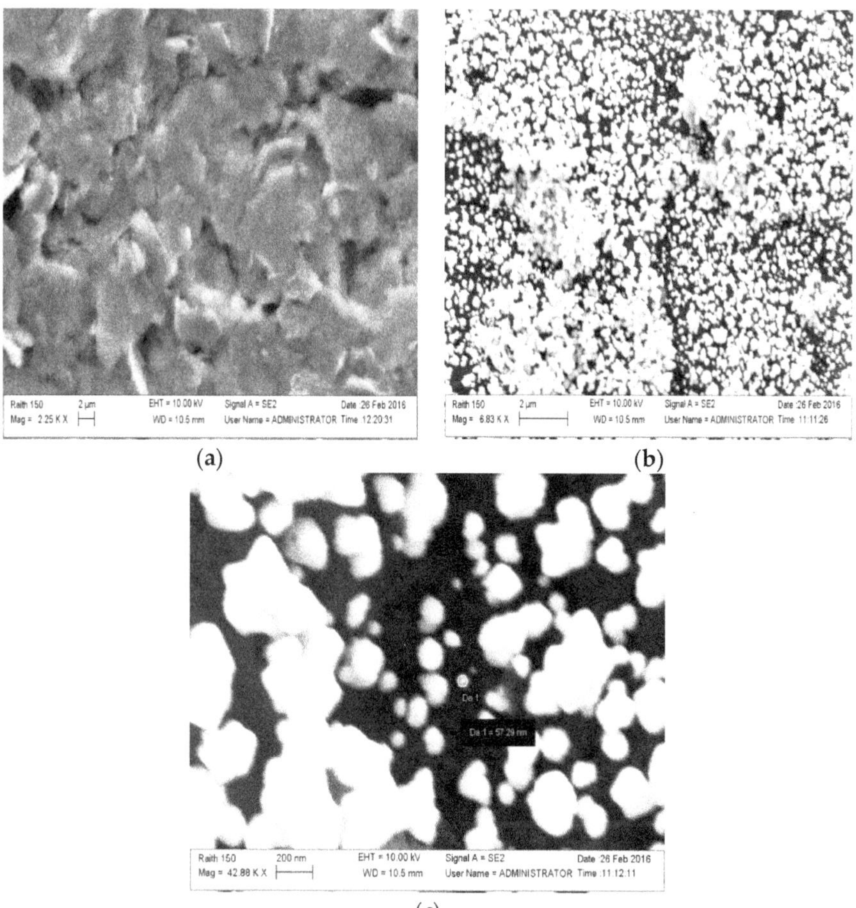

Figure 3. SEM surface images of (**a**) a bare carbon electrode; and (**b**,**c**) a carbon electrode after gold electrodeposition.

Experimental complex plane impedance spectra for the bare SPCE and SPCE-AuNPs are shown in Figure 4. The almost linear and close-to-vertical spectra, observed for both electrodes, is caused by a faster mass-transfer limited process due to electron flow from the electrode surface in the bulk solution. This behaviour indicates a purely capacitive response of the electrode properties [28]. When the AuNPs are deposed, a decrease of curve slope was observed.

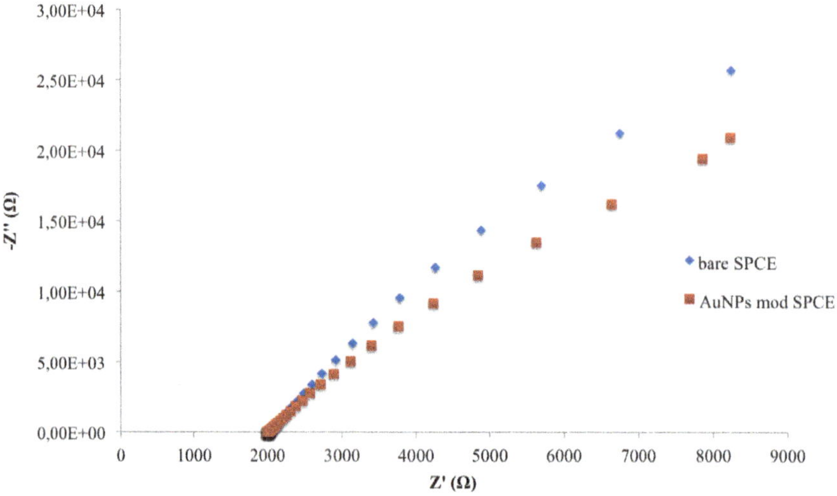

Figure 4. Nyquist plots in impedance measurements of bare and AuNP-modified SPCEs.

In order to characterize the behaviour of the sensing layers, EIS and CV measurements have been carried out during each step of the immunosensor construction (Figures 5 and 6).

The cysteamine layers, as well as the consecutive immobilization of anti-OTA and ethanolamine, caused a significant decrease of the electron transfer rate, measured by CV, with a lowering of both anodic and cathodic peaks due to hindering effects of the layers [29,30] (Figure 5).

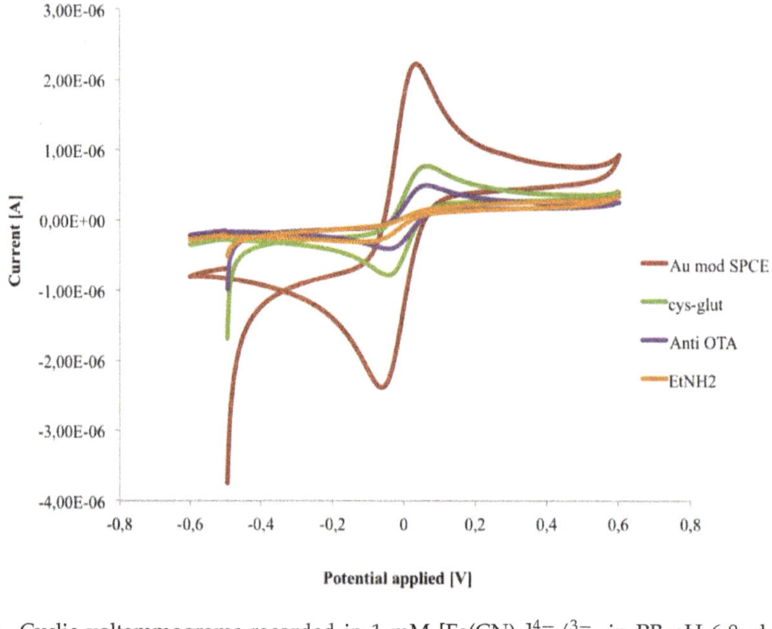

Figure 5. Cyclic voltammograms recorded in 1 mM $[Fe(CN)_6]^{4-/3-}$, in PB pH 6.8, during the fabrication of the immunosensor.

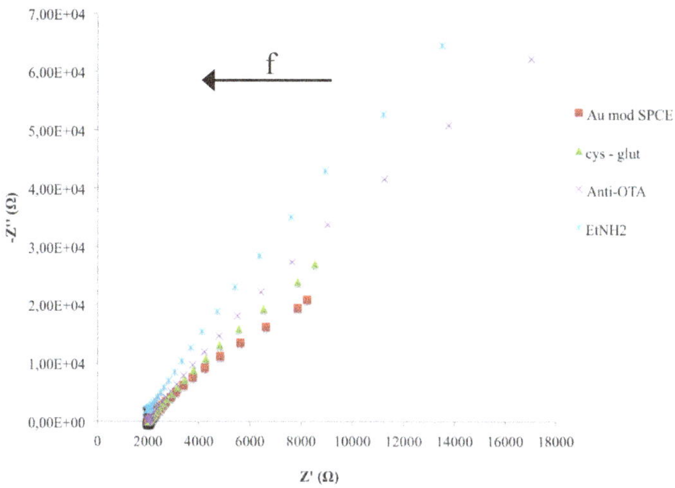

Figure 6. Nyquist plots in impedance measurements during the fabrication of the immunosensor.

Impedance spectra, during the immunosensor fabrication, represented as the change of the two impedance components (Z′ resistive component, Z″ capacitive component), as a function of frequency, were shown in Figure 6. The increase of both Z components is due to a change in the electron-transfer resistance caused by the biocomposite layer on the surface of the electrode that also induces a capacitance decrease because of the increased distance in the plate separation between the surface of the electrode and electrolyte solution. Moreover it is evident that a significant change of impedance components occurs only at low frequencies.

For a better description of the change caused by the immobilization steps on the impedance properties of the immunosensor, the Bode plot (total impedance in function of frequency) have been reported (Figure 7). While no differences were shown at the higher frequency region (inset of Figure 7) significant total impedance changes were shown from 0.1 to 1 Hz.

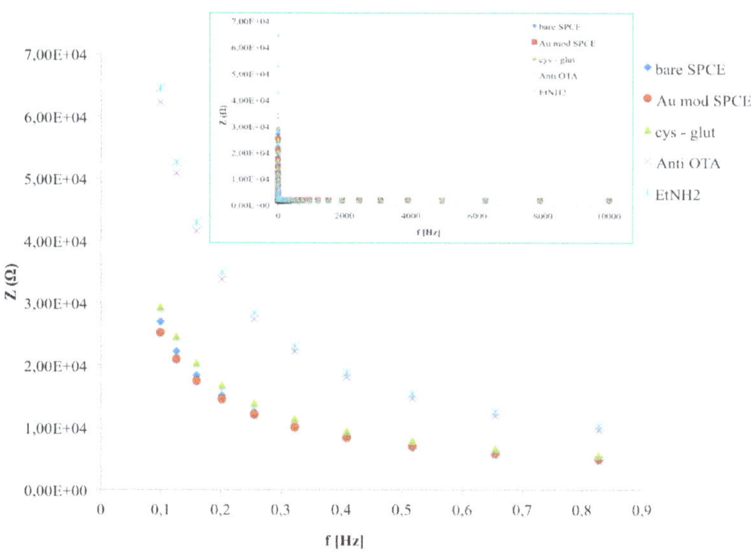

Figure 7. Bode plots in impedance measurements after all immunosensor fabrication steps in the frequency range 0.1–1 Hz. The inset shows Bode plots in the frequency range 0.1–10,000 Hz.

In this range no significant differences were observed when the cysteamine layer was attached to AuNPs, in contrast to the immobilization of anti-OTA molecules, which gives rise to a substantial total impedance increase. No changes in impedance value were observed after the blocking of active sites with $EtNH_2$.

The Nyquist plots of the developed immunosensor after the incubation with three different OTA concentrations are reported in Figure 8. In the given frequency range, the binding of OTA with anti-OTA affects the sensor impedance signal; in particular, we observe a decrease in the capacitive component (–Z″) of total impedance at low frequencies. According to other studies [31–34], on impedimetric immunosensors, the making of the immunocomplex induces a capacitance decrease, which can be directly related to the amount of analyte to be quantified.

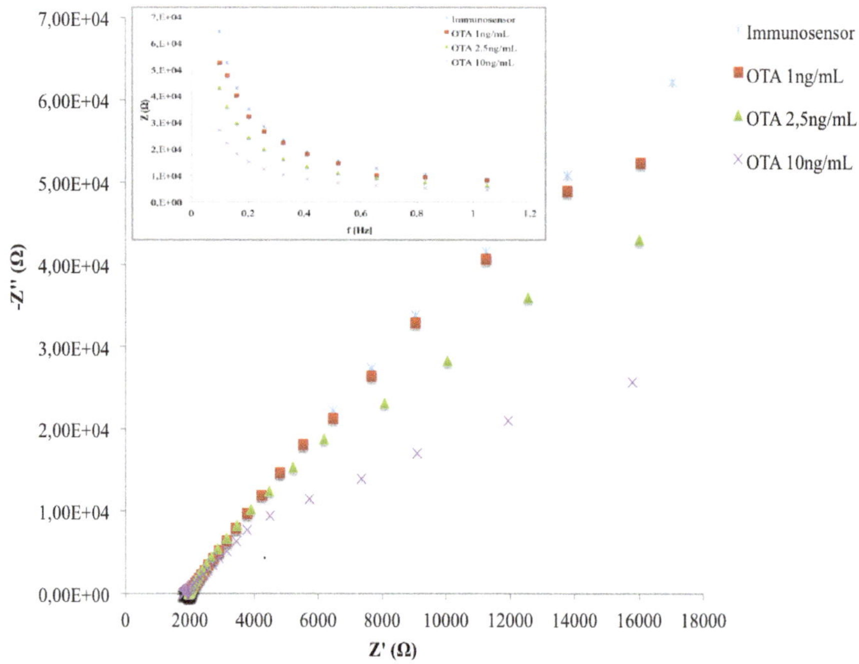

Figure 8. Nyquist plot in impedance measurements of the immunosensor before and after the interaction with different OTA concentrations.

As shown in the inset of Figure 8, the maximum differences among the Bode plots corresponding to different OTA amounts were observed at 0.1 Hz. The latter was chosen as the operating frequency for all impedance measurements during the analytical performances of the immunosensor.

3.2. Optimization of Anti-OTA Concentration.

The influence of the antibody concentration on the immunosensor analytical performance was investigated. For this reason, immunosensors were developed by the immobilization of three different amounts of anti-OTA (1 μg/mL, 5 μg/mL, 10 μg/mL) and the capacitance (C) was measured for OTA from 0.3 ng/mL to 40 ng/mL, after an incubation time of 20 min. The capacitance of the system was calculated according to Yang et al. [33], using the following equation:

$$C = -\frac{1}{2\pi f Z''} \quad (1)$$

where f is the operating frequency (Hz), and Z″ is the capacitive component of the total impedance.

Throughout the whole study, the change in capacitance (denoted as ΔC), taken as a measure before and after immunoreaction, is calculated by the following equation:

$$\Delta C = C_{anti\ OTA-OTA} - C_{anti\ OTA} \tag{2}$$

where $C_{anti\ OTA-OTA}$ is the value of the capacitance after OTA coupling to the anti-OTA and $C_{anti\ OTA}$ represents the value of the capacitance of the native immunosensor.

For the immunosensor with 1 μg/mL anti-OTA no significant changes in capacitance was measured before and after the immunocomplex in the range of OTA investigated. The calibration curves of the OTA immunosensors with 5 μg/mL and 10 μg/mL anti-OTA, obtained by plotting the logarithmic value of OTA concentrations versus ΔC, are shown in Figure 9, As reported in our previous study [29], lower antibody amounts allow detecting lower OTA concentrations; in particular, for 5 μg/mL anti-OTA, the immunosensor shows a significant ΔC in the range from −0.52 to 1.30 log OTA (0.3 to 20 ng/mL), while ΔC changes only for values higher than 0.69 log OTA (5 ng/mL) with 10 μg/mL anti-OTA. Moreover, higher antibody amounts allow obtaining higher sensitivity and a higher capacitance signal (see inset Figure 9) due to the higher antigen-binding capacity.

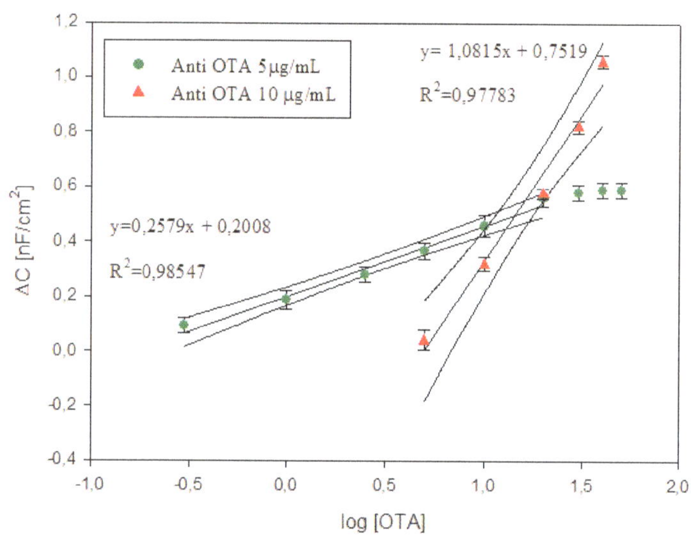

Figure 9. Calibration curves of OTA immunosensors at 5 μg/mL and 10 μg/mL anti-OTA. Data represent the average values of five immunosensors with error bars and 95% confidence curves. The inset shows the measured capacitance in the range of OTA investigated for the immunosensors with 5 μg/mL and 10 μg/mL anti-OTA.

The detection limit (LOD), calculated using the sum of average blank solution and three times the standard deviation, was 0.37 ng/mL and 5.42 ng/mL for immunosensor with 5 μg/mL and 10 μg/mL, respectively. The comparison of the analytical performance of the label-free immunosensors on screen-printed AuNP-modified carbon electrodes developed in this study with the other impedimetric immunosensor reported in the literature is reported in Table 1. Since no previous studies have been published on the label-free immunosensor on screen-printed carbon electrodes which shows capacitive behaviour, we have compared the results with resistive immunosensors developed on Au and Pt electrodes. In the Table 1 the sensitivity of our immunosensors has been calculated using the change in total impedance as a function of different OTA amounts (data not reported). The analytical parameters obtained by our label-free impedimetric immunosensors are suitable for the analytical determination of OTA in the range of interest for food matrices. In addition, considering that the electrodes used for the current fabrication of impedimetric immunosensors are pure gold electrodes (e.g., thin-film gold electrodes require 2270 pg of gold) our impedimetric immunosensors are cheaper, because of the use of disposable SPCE modified with a very small quantity of gold (calculated to be 122 pg of gold per electrode).

Table 1. Comparison among impedimetric OTA label-free biosensors.

Schematic Immunosensor Assembly	Sensitivity (kΩ mL/ng)	Linear Range (ng/mL)	LOD (ng/mL)	Sensitivity x LOD	References
Pt/PANI-PV-SO^{3-}/Ab	0.56	2–10	2.00	1.12	[20]
Au/TA/GA/BSA/Ab–MNP	6.50	0.05–1	0.01	0.06	[19]
Au/4-CP/Ab	20.25	1–20	0.50	10.12	[18]
Au/MBA/ProtA-G/Ab	14.03	0.010-5	0.010	0.14	[29]
Au/MBA/Ab	377.78	0.005–0.050	0.005	1.89	[29]
SPCE/AuNPs/Cys-Glut/Ab(5 μg/mL)	2.56	0.3–20	0.37	0.64	This work
SPCE/AuNPs/Cys-Glut/Ab(10 μg/mL)	3.09	5–40	5.42	7.72	This work

PANI-PV-SO^{3-}: Polyaniline–polyvinylsulfonate; TA: Thiolamine SAM; GA: Glutaraldehyde; MNP: Magnetic Nanoparticles. *4-CP: 4-Carboxyphenyl; MPA: 4 Mercaptobenzoic acid; Ab: OTA Monoclonal Antibody.*

The reproducibility calculated on five different immunsensors showed a good relative standard deviation (RSD) for both immunosensors: 5.18% for 5 μg/mL anti-OTA and 2.5 ng/mL OTA, 5.69% for 10 μg/mL anti-OTA and 20 ng/mL OTA. The feasibility of applying the proposed immunosensor for the detection of OTA in wine was studied. Since the maximum OTA concentration permitted by European Commission (EC) No 1881/2006 is 2 μg/kg we have tested the immunosensor at 5 μg/mL anti-OTA. Finally, the storage stability was also determined. For this purpose different immunosensors were stored for three weeks at 4 °C without chemical preservatives and characterized at regular interval times. After the investigated storage period, the immunosensors showed a negligible loss of activity.

Red wine samples were spiked with three different concentrations of OTA, and analysed by the developed immunosensors and a competitive ELISA kit for OTA detection. The sample preparation used was the same for both the analytical methods. The results, reported in Table 2, show a comparable performance for both methods and, thus, the capability of the immunosensor is a fast analytical technique for the control of OTA in food samples.

Table 2. OTA results in red wine samples obtained by ELISA and the developed impedimetric immunosensor.

	Spiked Concentration (μg/L)	Found Concentration (μg/L)	Recovery (%)
ELISA	1.50	1.49	99.77
	5.00	6.12	122.45
	10.00	9.90	98.96
Impedimetric immunosensor	1.50	1.36	94.56
	5.00	4.99	99.79
	10.00	10.29	102.91

4. Conclusions

The first immunosensor for OTA detection based on EIS with a modified SPCE is reported. The surface of ca arbon electrode was modified with electrochemical gold deposition, which has demonstred a very cheap way to obtain gold-like behaving electrodes using a very small quantity of the metal (122 pg per electrode). Thus, a label-free impedimetric immunosensor for Ochratoxin A detection was developed on Au modified SPCE and EIS was used to analyze the analytical immunosensor performance. Capacitance was chosen as the best parameter that describes the electrical changes of the electrode surface due to the immunoreaction between anti-OTA and OTA at different concentrations. The developed immunosensor, with its very low detection limit and high sensitivity, exploits the advantages of cheapness, simplicity, and versatility of the SPCE and its results are suitable for fast OTA measurement in food matrices.

Author Contributions: F.M. performed the experiments, collected and analysed the data. D.A. defined the research line and analysed the data. F.M. and D.A. wrote the manuscript. R.P. contributed to the manuscript writing and data evaluation. A.C. and E.E. performed the SEM images and interpreted the data.

Conflicts of Interest: The authors declare no conflict of interest.

References

1. Shepard, G.S.; Berthiller, F.; Burdaspal, C.; Crews, M.A.; Jonker, M.A.; Krska, R.; MacDonald, S.; Malone, R.J.; Maragos, C.; Sabino, M.; et al. Developments in mycotoxin analysis: An update for 2010–2011. *World Mycotoxin J.* **2012**, *5*, 3–30. [CrossRef]
2. Van Egmond, H.P.; Schothorst, R.C.; Jonker, M.A. Regulations relating to mycotoxins in food: Perspectives in a global and European context. *Anal. Bioanal. Chem.* **2007**, *389*, 147–157. [CrossRef] [PubMed]
3. Kaushik, A.; Solanki, P.R.; Ansari, A.A.; Ahmad, S.; Malhotra, B.D. A nanostructured cerium oxide film-based immunosensor for mycotoxin detection. *Nanotechnology* **2009**, *20*, 055105. [CrossRef] [PubMed]
4. Ansari, A.A.; Kaushik, A.; Solanki, P.R.; Malhotre, D.B. Nanostructured zinc oxide platform for mycotoxin detection. *Bioelectrochemistry* **2010**, *77*, 75–81. [CrossRef] [PubMed]
5. Vidal, C.; Bonel, L.; Ezquerra, A.; Hernandez, S.; Bertolin, J.R.; Cubel, C.; Castillo, J.R. Electrochemical affinity biosensors for detection of mycotoxins: A review. *Biosens. Bioelectron.* **2013**, *49*, 146–158. [CrossRef] [PubMed]
6. Maragos, C.M.; Busman, M. Rapid and advanced tool for mycotoxin analysis: A review. *Food Addit. Contam. Part A Chem. Anal. Control Expo. Risk Assess.* **2010**, *27*, 688–700. [CrossRef] [PubMed]
7. Krska, R.; Ullrich, P.S.; Molinelli, A.; Sulyok, M.; MacDonald, S.; Crews, C. Mycotoxin analysis: An update. *Food Addit. Contam. Part A Chem. Anal. Control Expo. Risk Assess.* **2008**, *25*, 152–163. [CrossRef] [PubMed]
8. Farrè, M.; Kantiani, L.; Perez, S.; Barcelò, D. Sensors and biosensors in support of EU Directives. *Trends Anal. Chem.* **2009**, *28*, 170–185. [CrossRef]
9. Prieto-Simòn, B.; Campàs, M.; Marty, J.L.; Noguer, T. Novel highly-performing immunosensor-based strategy for ochratoxin A detection in wine samples. *Biosens. Bioelectron.* **2008**, *23*, 995–1002. [CrossRef] [PubMed]
10. Vidal, J.C.; Bonel, L.; Ezquerra, A.; Duato, P.; Castillo, J.R. An electrochemical immunosensor for ochratoxin A determination in wines based on a monoclonal antibody and paramagnetic microbeads. *Anal. Bioanal. Chem.* **2012**, *403*, 1585–1593. [CrossRef] [PubMed]
11. Heurich, M.; Kadir, M.K.A.; Tothill, I.E. An Electrochemical Sensor Based on Carboxymethylated Dextran Modified Gold Surface for Ochratoxin A Analysis. *Sens. Actuators B. Chem.* **2011**, *156*, 162–168. [CrossRef]
12. Perrotta, P.R.; Arèval, F.J.; Vettorazzi, N.R.; Zòn, M.A.; Fernàndez, H. Development of a very sensitive electrochemical magneto immunosensor for the direct determination of ochratoxin A in red wine. *Sens. Actuators B Chem.* **2012**, *162*, 327–333. [CrossRef]
13. Alarcòn, S.H.; Micheli, L.; Palleschi, G.; Compagnone, D. Development of an electrochemical Immunosensor for Ochratoxin A. *Anal. Lett.* **2004**, *37*, 1545–1558. [CrossRef]
14. Primiceri, E.; Chiriacò, M.S.; de Feo, F.; Santovito, E.; Fusco, V.; Maruccio, G. A multipurpose biochip for food pathogen detection. *Anal. Methods* **2016**, *8*, 3055–3060. [CrossRef]
15. Wang, Y.; Ye, Z.; Ying, Y. New Trends in Impedimetric Biosensors for the Detection of Foodborne Pathogenic Bacteria. *Sensors* **2012**, *12*, 3449–3471. [CrossRef] [PubMed]
16. Barsoukov, E. *Impedance Spectroscopy: Theory, Experiment and Applications*, 2nd ed.; John Wiley and Sons: Hoboken, NJ, USA, 2005.
17. Katz, E.; Willner, I. Probing Biomolecular Interactions at Conductive and Semiconductive Surfaces by Impedance Spectroscopy: Routes to Impedimetric Immunosensors, DNA-Sensors, and Enzyme Biosensors. *Electroanal* **2003**, *15*, 913–947. [CrossRef]
18. Radi, A.E.; Munoz-Berbel, X.; Latesc, V.; Martyc, J.L. Label-free impedimetric immunosensor for sensitive detection of ochratoxin A. *Biosens. Bioelectron.* **2009**, *24*, 1888–1892. [CrossRef] [PubMed]
19. Zamfir, L.G.; Geana, I.; Bourigua, S.; Rotariu, L.; Bala, C.; Errachid, A.; Jaffrezic-Renault, N. Highly sensitive label-free immunosensor for ochratoxin A based on functionalized magnetic nanoparticles and EIS/SPR detection. *Sens. Actuators B Chem.* **2011**, *159*, 178–184. [CrossRef]

20. Muchindu, M.; Iwuoha, E.; Pool, E.; West, N.; Jahed, N.; Baker, P.; Waryo, T.; Williams, A. Electrochemical ochratoxin A Immunosensor System Develop on Sulfonated Polyaniline. *Electroanal* **2010**, *23*, 122–128. [CrossRef]
21. Chrouda, A.; Sbartai, A.; Bessueille, F.; Renaud, L.; Maaref, A.; Jaffrezic-Renault, N. Electrically addressable deposition of diazonium-functionalized antibodies on boron-doped diamond microcells for the detection of ochratoxin A. *Anal. Methods* **2015**, *7*, 2444–2451. [CrossRef]
22. Lin, C.H.; Wu, C.C.; Kuo, Y.F. A high sensitive impedimetric salbutamol immunosensor based on the gold nanostructure-deposited screen-printed carbon electrode. *J. Electroanal. Chem.* **2016**, *768*, 27–33. [CrossRef]
23. Lien, T.T.N.; Takamura, Y.; Tamiya, E.; Vestergaard, M.C. Modified screen printed electrode for development of a highly sensitive label-free impedimetric immunosensor to detect amyloid beta peptides. *Anal. Chim. Acta* **2015**, *892*, 69–76. [CrossRef] [PubMed]
24. Liu, S.; Leech, D.; Ju, H. Application of Colloidal Gold in Protein Immobilization, Electron Transfer, and Biosensing. *Anal. Lett.* **2003**, *36*, 1–19. [CrossRef]
25. Mistry, K.K.; Layek, K.; Mahapatra, A.; RoyChaudhuri, C.; Saha, H. A review on amperometric—Type immunosensors based on screen-printed electrodes. *Analyst* **2014**, *139*, 2289–2311. [CrossRef] [PubMed]
26. Albanese, D.; Liguori, C.; Paciello, V.; Pietrosanto, A. Winemaking Process Monitoring Based on a Biosensor Automatic System. *IEEE Trans. Instrum. Meas.* **2011**, *60*, 1909–1915. [CrossRef]
27. Regiart, M.; Pereira, S.V.; Bertolino, F.A.; Garcia, C.D.; Raba, J.; Aranda, P.R. An electrochemical immunosensor for anti-T. cruzi IgM antibodies, a biomarker for congenital Chagas disease, using a screen-printed electrode modified with gold nanoparticles and functionalized with shed acute phase. *Microchim. Acta* **2016**. [CrossRef]
28. Bernalte, E.; Marín-Sánchez, C.; Pinilla-Gil, E.; Brett, C.M.A. Characterisation of Screen-Printed Gold and Gold Nanoparticle-Modified Carbon Sensors by Electrochemical Impedance Spectroscopy. *J. Electroanal Chem.* **2013**, *709*, 70–76. [CrossRef]
29. Malvano, F.; Albanese, D.; Pilloton, R.; Di Matteo, M. A high sensitive impedimetric label free immunosensor for Ochratoxin A measurement in cocoa beans. *Food Chem.* **2016**, *212*, 688–694. [CrossRef]
30. Geng, P.; Zhang, X.; Meng, W.; Wang, Q.; Zhang, W.; Jin, L.; Feng, Z.; Wu, Z. Self-assembled monolayers-based immunosensor for detection of Escherichia Coli using electrochemical impedance spectroscopy. *Electrochim. Acta* **2008**, *53*, 4663–4668. [CrossRef]
31. Yin, T.; Wei, W.; Yang, L.; Gao, X.; Gao, Y. A novel capacitive immunosensor for transferrin detection based on ultrathin alumina sol–gel-derived films and gold nanoparticles. *Sens. Actuators B Chem.* **2006**, *117*, 286–294. [CrossRef]
32. Rahman, A.; Shiddiky, M.J.A.; Park, J.S.; Shim, Y.B. An impedimetric immunosensor for the label-free detection of bisphenol A. *Biosens. Bioelectron.* **2007**, *22*, 2464–2470. [CrossRef] [PubMed]
33. Yang, G.J.; Huang, J.L.; Meng, W.J.; Shen, M.; Jiao, X.A. A reusable capacitive immunosensor for detection of Salmonella spp. Based on grafted ethylene diamine and self-assembled gold nanoparticles manolayer. *Anal. Chim. Acta* **2009**, *647*, 159–166. [CrossRef] [PubMed]
34. Li, J.; Wu, Z.; Wang, H.; Shen, G.; Yu, R. A reusable capacitive immunosensor with a novel immobilization procedure based on 1,6-hexanedithiol and nano-Au self-assembled layers. *Sens. Actuators B Chem.* **2005**, *110*, 327–334. [CrossRef]

16

Multi-Wire Tri-Gate Silicon Nanowires Reaching Milli-pH Unit Resolution in One Micron Square Footprint

Enrico Accastelli [1], Paolo Scarbolo [2], Thomas Ernst [3], Pierpaolo Palestri [2], Luca Selmi [2] and Carlotta Guiducci [1,*]

1 Institute of Bioengineering, École Polytechnique Fédérale de Lausanne (EPFL), 1015 Lausanne, Switzerland; enrico.accastelli@epfl.ch
2 DIEGM, Università degli Studi di Udine, 33100 Udine, Italy; scarbolo.paolo@spes.uniud.it (P.S.); palestri@uniud.it (P.P.); luca.selmi@uniud.it (L.S.)
3 Laboratoire d'Électronique et de Technologie de l'Information (LETI), Commissariat à l'Énergie Atomique et aux Énergies Alternatives (CEA), 38054 Grenoble Cedex 9, France; thomas.ernst@cea.fr
* Correspondence: carlotta.guiducci@epfl.ch

Academic Editors: Mark A. Reed and Mathias Wipf

Abstract: The signal-to-noise ratio of planar ISFET pH sensors deteriorates when reducing the area occupied by the device, thus hampering the scalability of on-chip analytical systems which detect the DNA polymerase through pH measurements. Top-down nano-sized tri-gate transistors, such as silicon nanowires, are designed for high performance solid-state circuits thanks to their superior properties of voltage-to-current transduction, which can be advantageously exploited for pH sensing. A systematic study is carried out on rectangular-shaped nanowires developed in a complementary metal-oxide-semiconductor (CMOS)-compatible technology, showing that reducing the width of the devices below a few hundreds of nanometers leads to higher charge sensitivity. Moreover, devices composed of several wires in parallel further increase the exposed surface per unit footprint area, thus maximizing the signal-to-noise ratio. This technology allows a sub milli-pH unit resolution with a sensor footprint of about 1 μm^2, exceeding the performance of previously reported studies on silicon nanowires by two orders of magnitude.

Keywords: silicon nanowires; tri-gate transistors; ISFET; pH sensors; 1/f noise

1. Introduction

Reducing the size of electronic devices affects the signal-to-noise ratio (SNR). Structures with improved gate-to-channel coupling, indicated as multi-gate devices, were conceived for traditional solid-state systems to overcome this issue [1]. In particular, the feature of these devices, enhanced subthreshold swing, reduced short-channel effects such as drain-induced barrier lowering (DIBL) and, consequently, resulted in an improved scalability [2–4]. As a matter of fact, the introduction of multi-gate device architectures has so far effectively sustained Moore's law and kept up the pace of technological advancement in the electronics industry.

In the field of bioanalytics, the large-scale integration of CMOS chips exposing arrays of liquid-gate FET pH-sensors has shown its potential in applications such as DNA sequencing [5], and holds the promise to innovate DNA quantification based on quantitative PCR [6–8]. If the paradigm of nanoscale multi-gate devices improved as well the SNR of liquid-gate sensors, it would be possible to reduce the sensor size and consequently increase the throughput of analytical systems.

Silicon-based multi-gate structures, commonly indicated as nanoribbons (SiNRs) and nanowires (SiNWs), have been proposed as bio and chemical sensors [9–29] . Although a few works indicate that improved macromolecular sensing can be achieved with smaller devices [30], no consensus has been reached on the effect of size reduction on pH sensitivity as well as the role of device technology, device layout, bias and signal readout [31,32]. In what follows, we show that tri-gate silicon nanoribbons with rectangular cross-section exhibit an enhanced sensitivity *vs.* pH when decreasing their width below a few hundreds of nanometers. We perform noise characterization for devices of different size and biasing, proposing a multi-wire configuration to achieve higher SNR. The resolution that can be achieved with a sensor footprint of one micrometer square corresponds to a 0.8‰ shift in pH, which is equivalent to approximately 100 electrons in the case of silicon dioxide interfaces. This performance is two orders of magnitude better than the one obtained with planar devices [33,34].

We developed tri-gate devices on Silicon-On-Insulator (SOI) substrates based on self-aligned CMOS-compatible top-down processes, with accuracy down to 5 nm. The use of a semi-industrial process ensures a high level of control over process variations and enables the fabrication of high-density individually connected SiNRs with a well-defined orientation and a wide range of widths and lengths. Such features still represent a challenge for bottom-up technologies [35].

2. Experimental Section

2.1. *Technology and Fabrication Process*

The n+/p/n+ SiNRs are fabricated on SOI wafers and patterned by means of a top-down hybrid deep ultraviolet (DUV) and e-beam lithography followed by a reactive ion etching (RIE). The fabrication process was entirely developed at CEA-LETI. The wafers are composed of a 200 nm silicon layer on top of a 400 nm thick SiO_2 insulating bulk oxide layer (BOX). The silicon top layer is first thinned by chemical mechanical polishing (CMP) and then by several steps of silicon thermal oxidation/desoxidation to obtain a 50 nm silicon top layer, which defines the thickness (tNR) of the SiNRs. Devices with feature sizes above 300 nm are patterned using deep ultraviolet (DUV), while e-beam lithography is employed for smaller dimensions. Once patterned, the undesired material is etched away by reactive ion etching (RIE). A high quality 3 nm SiO_2 gate oxide is grown using thermal dry oxidation. In order to obtain n-type devices, the SiNRs are doped by boron implantation (1×10^{18} cm^{-3}). A sacrificial polysilicon gate is used as a hard mask to dope the source and drain terminals with phosphorous (1×10^{19} cm^{-3}), thus effectively defining the SiNR length. The entire chip surface, with the exception of the contact pads and the SiNR, is passivated by a multi-layer insulator composed of 50 nm of Si_3N_4, 300 nm of tetraethyl orthosilicate (TEOS) and 200 nm of phosphosilicate glass (PSG) (Figure 1b). This multilayer insulator is designed to withstand the liquid environment and to avoid the propagation of pin-holes in the passivation that could short-circuit the electrolyte with the contact lines [36].

2.2. *Ag/AgCl Reference Electrode Fabrication*

The Ag/AgCl electrodes are obtained by a galvanostatic oxidation on silver tubes. The silver tubes are dipped in 0.1 M HNO_3 for about 1 min, in order to clean and activate the surface, and then rinsed with deionized water. After the surface activation, the silver wire is connected to a working electrode (anode); a platinum wire is connected to a counter electrode (cathode) and both of them are dipped into a solution of 0.1 M KCl. A current density of 2.5 mA/cm^2 is applied at the anode for a time that depends on the desired thickness of the AgCl layer (5 μm in this work). At the end of the oxidation, the Ag/AgCl tubes are dipped into a solution of 0.1 M KCl for at least 4 hours prior to use. The performances in terms of voltage drift have been compared with respect to commercial Ag/AgCl (see Supplementary Figure S10).

2.3. *Microfluidics*

The microchannels are obtained with a chemical-resistant double-coated tape (3M 9086), patterned by laser micromachining. The height of the channels is thereby defined by the thickness of the tape

(190 μm). A poly(methyl methacrylate) (PMMA) cap with holes drilled in the locations of inlets and outlets is placed on top of the tape to seal the channels, and the inlet and outlet tubes are inserted.

A syringe pump (Harvard Apparatus) is used to flux the solution of interest into the microfluidics. Due to the double-coated tape system, the microfluidics can easily be removed by incubating the chip in 2-Propanol alcohol overnight. The chip can, therefore, be cleaned more thoroughly and re-used. Figure 1b shows an SEM image of a used device after the cleaning procedure.

2.4. Electrical Characterization

The electrical characterization of the devices was performed by means of a semiconductor parameter analyzer (SPA, Agilent 4156C) used both in sweep and sampling modes, controlled by LabVIEW VIs and MATLAB scripts via a GPIB interface.

2.5. pH Sensing Experiments

The SiNR chips are cleaned by successive washing steps of ethanol/acetone/ethanol (10 min each), separated by rinsing with deionized water and drying with N_2. After the cleaning procedure of the chip surface, the microfluidic module is mounted and the chip is ready for the experiment. The solutions at different pH are interspersed by 10 μM KCl (pH_{KCl} ~6.8) injections. Each injection is 15 min long, at fixed flow rate of 5 μL/min. At the end of each injection, the syringe pump is stopped and the solution is changed.

The different pH solutions are prepared starting with 10 mM phosphate buffered saline (PBS) containing 100 mM KCl, which is added to stabilize the Ag/AgCl RE. The solutions are adjusted to the desired pH by adding either a strong acid (H_2SO_4) or a strong base (NaOH), so that the difference in the ionic strength of the solutions results to be negligible.

3. Results and Discussion

3.1. pH Sensitivity of Single SiNR Devices as a Function of Their Width

The fabricated chip features 75 SiNRs with thickness (t_{NR}) of 50 nm and different widths (W_{NR}) and lengths (L_{NR}) (Figure 1a,b). Devices with identical L_{NR} and different W_{NR} (and vice versa) were fabricated with the specific aim of studying the effect of size on the device noise and sensitivity, both in terms of $\Delta V_{TH}/\Delta pH$ and $\Delta I_{D\text{-}S}/\Delta pH$.

The SiNR chip is coupled with a microfluidic module that employs Ag/AgCl reference electrodes (REs) and allows subsequent injections of different solutions into sub-5 μL microchannels (Figure 1c) [37].

The SiNRs can be operated either by the solid-state back-gate or by the liquid front-gate (Figure 1d). The back-gating approach consists in applying a gate voltage ($V_{BG\text{-}S}$) between the silicon substrate and the source terminal. Instead, in the case of front-gating, a voltage $V_{FG\text{-}S}$ is applied between the electrolyte solution, biased by Ag/AgCl REs, and the source terminal, while the back-gate is short-circuited with the source contact. As shown in our previous work [37], the front-gating configuration with grounded back-gate prevents from any parasitic coupling between the electrolyte solution and the environment.

Figure 2 shows the $I_{D\text{-}S}$-$V_{FG\text{-}S}$ and $I_{D\text{-}S}$-$V_{D\text{-}S}$ characteristics of a SiNR in front-gating bias. The SiNR shows a MOSFET behavior, with threshold voltage (V_{TH}) of approximately 1.5 V and a sub-threshold swing (SS) of about 100 mV/dec. The V_{TH} does not show any systematic trend *vs.* W. Typical $I_{D\text{-}S,ON}/I_{D\text{-}S,OFF}$ ratio in virgin devices is of about 10^4, and can be as good as 10^6, while the leakage in Figure 2a (red curve) is more representative of a device that has been extensively used in liquid environment. Note that the leakage may have different sources, both inside and outside the active device area, but in any case does not affect our sensitivity data that is taken well above V_{TH}. A slightly negative differential output resistance is sometimes observed at large V_{GS} (Figure 2b) probably due to a small drift *vs.* time (also visible in Figure 3b and discussed later on), that lowers $I_{D\text{-}S}$

while sweeping the $V_{D\text{-}S}$ with an integration time of 20 ms and 151 bias points per $I_{D\text{-}S}$-$V_{D\text{-}S}$ curve. A V_{DS} of 1.5V was selected to maximize the absolute change of the drain current with the pH without incurring in reliability issues (see also Supplementary Figure S1) and because it is favorable in terms of SNR with respect to lower V_{DS} values [38].

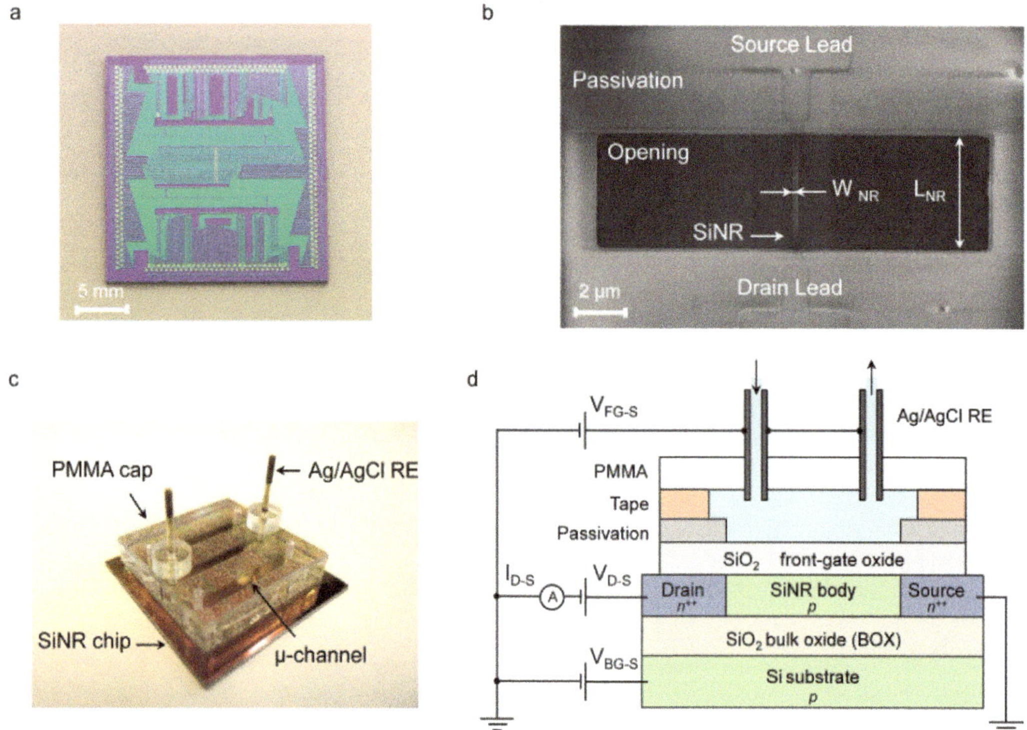

Figure 1. (**a**) Optical image of the chip; (**b**) SEM image of a Silicon NanoRibbon (SiNR). Top view of a device with W_{NR} = 87 nm and L_{NR} = 4250 nm. The source and drain leads are passivated, while the body of the device is exposed. The length of each SiNR corresponds to the opening in the passivation; (**c**) Optical image of the microfluidics setup; (**d**) Cross section of the fabricated device and a sketch of the measurement setup (not to scale).

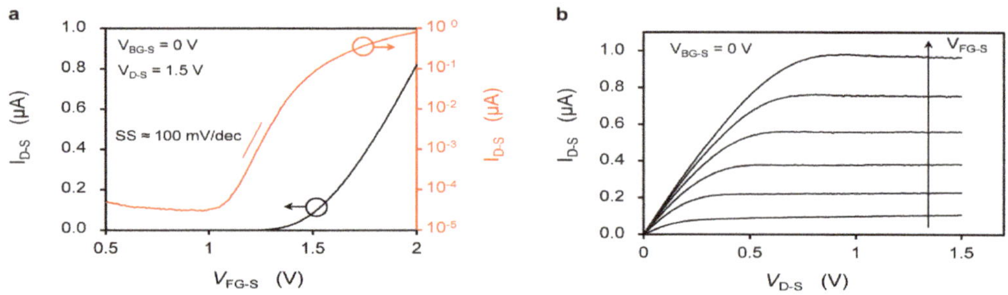

Figure 2. (**a**,**b**) Characterization of a SiNR with length (L_{NR}) of 2375 nm and a width (W_{NR}) of 290 nm. The electrolyte is 100 µM KCl. (**a**) Drain current ($I_{D\text{-}S}$) *vs.* gate voltage ($V_{FG\text{-}S}$) plotted in linear (left *y* axis) and logarithmic (right *y* axis) scale; (**b**) Drain current ($I_{D\text{-}S}$) *vs.* drain voltage ($V_{D\text{-}S}$) plotted for different constant gate voltages ($V_{FG\text{-}S}$), ranging from 1.5 V to 2.0 V, with a step of 0.1 V.

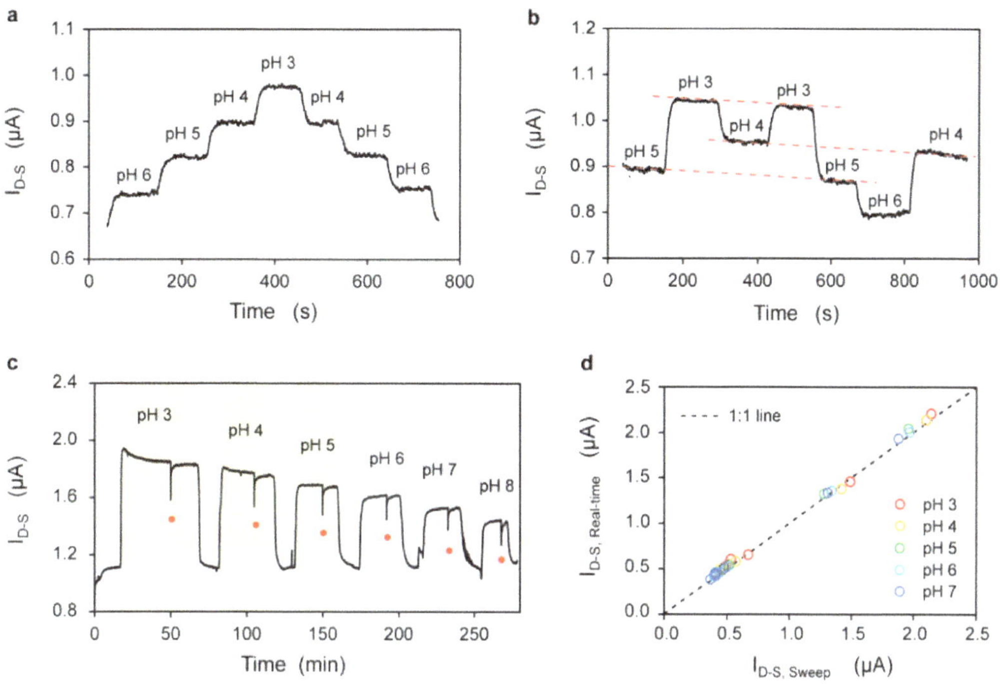

Figure 3. (**a**) Drain current ($I_{D\text{-}S}$) observed at fixed voltage bias upon injection of decreasing/increasing series of pH values; (**b**) Drain current ($I_{D\text{-}S}$) observed at fixed voltage bias upon injection of randomize series of pH values. The three parallel red dotted lines highlight the drift affecting the $I_{D\text{-}S}$; (**c**) Drain current ($I_{D\text{-}S}$) measurement upon injection of solutions with different pH values and identical ionic strength. The red dots indicate when the $I_{D\text{-}S}$-$V_{FG\text{-}S}$ characterization is performed; (**d**) Average $I_{D\text{-}S}$ observed at fixed polarization ($I_{D\text{-}S,Real\text{-}time}$) *vs.* the $I_{D\text{-}S}$ extracted from the $I_{D\text{-}S}$-$V_{FG\text{-}S}$ sweeps ($I_{D\text{-}S,Sweep}$) from a set of SiNRs. A 1:1 line is plotted as reference. All measurements of the figure refer to the same device which has a W_{NR} of 50 nm and a L_{NR} of 2375 nm.

In our setup the liquid-gate terminal is common to all the devices while the source and drain contacts can be individually addressed for each SiNR device, allowing the current of the single devices to be measured independently.

Figure 3a shows the drain current of a SiNR measured in real-time upon the injection of solutions with decreasing and then increasing values of pH. According to the site binding theory [39–41], solutions with different pH values in contact with the gate oxide induce changes in the surface charge of the front-gate oxide as an effect of the deprotonation (protonation) of the silanol groups in the presence of OH^- (H^+) ions in the electrolyte. In particular, the surface of the front-gate oxide becomes negatively charged when it is in contact with electrolyte solutions with pH values higher than its isoelectric point (pI $\approx$ 2 in the case of SiO_2). The change in surface charge affects the surface potential, which in turn modifies the conductance of the device when subjected to a constant voltage bias. The device is biased above threshold ($V_{FG\text{-}S} - V_{TH} \approx 0.5$ V) and in saturation regime ($V_{D\text{-}S} = 1.5$ V), thus increasing the absolute value and the linearity of the current response in terms of $\Delta I_{D\text{-}S}/\Delta$pH with respect to the subthreshold regime (see Supplementary Figure S1). Moreover, the devices are biased to work in the saturation regime to maximize the dynamic range. As expected in the case of an *n*-type device, the drain current decreases with increasing pH, as more and more negative charges accumulate at the oxide surface, thus depleting the electrons in the channel. The device shows little hysteresis between the forward and backward pH sweeps (see Supplementary Figure S2). Non-monotonically increasing/decreasing pH series (Figure 3b) show that the conductance of the device depends on pH and experiences a linear drift, which does not show any relevant correlation with the pH values.

Figure 3c,d compares the device current evaluated either by keeping the device at a fixed voltage bias, or by performing a sequence of $I_{D\text{-}S}$-$V_{FG\text{-}S}$ characteristics. Two conditioning injections at acidic and basic pH (pH 3 and pH 8, respectively) are performed at the beginning of the experiment in order to prime the front-gate oxide surface, and with the effect of improving the subthreshold slope (typically from between 150 and 200 mV/dec down to 100 mV/dec) and setting it to a stable value. For the rest of the entire experiment, the subthreshold slope remains constant, leading to a rigid shift of the $I_{D\text{-}S}$-$V_{FG\text{-}S}$ characteristics upon pH injections (see Supplementary Figure S3). In order to cope with the dependence of the device current with the ionic force of the electrolyte (see Supplementary Figure S4), the pH solutions were prepared to have the same ionic strength (100 mM). The monitoring of the drift was performed by exposing the device to subsequent injections of a saline solution (10 μM KCl) alternated with the solutions at different pH.

In this experiment, the device has been kept at the above mentioned bias ($V_{FG\text{-}S} - V_{TH} \approx 0.5$ V, $V_{D\text{-}S} = 1.5$ V) (current *vs.* time plotted in Figure 3c), with the exception of the time points indicated by the red dots on the plot, when the device has been subjected to a series of three $V_{FG\text{-}S}$ sweeps (from 0 V to 2 V). The plot on Figure 3d shows a 1:1 correlation between the current measured at a fixed bias $I_{D\text{-}S,Real\text{-}time}$ (averaged over 5 min) and the current extracted from the $I_{D\text{-}S}$-$V_{FG\text{-}S}$ corresponding to the same bias ($I_{D\text{-}S,Sweep}$).

In our measurements the current drift is not affected by the size of the devices; rather, it can be ascribed to the wear out of the Ag/AgCl reference electrode, and possibly to the relatively thin nanowire top-oxide (3 nm).

The experiment described in Figure 3c has been performed on several nanowires to assess their pH sensitivity, both in terms of the change of the threshold voltage $\Delta V_{TH}/\Delta pH$ (Figure 4a,b) and in terms of the normalized current signal $\Delta I'_{D\text{-}S}/\Delta pH$ (Figure 4c,d), where $I'_{D\text{-}S} = I_{D\text{-}S}/[(W_{NR} + 2 \cdot t_{NR})/L_{NR}]$ is the current normalized by the form factor. Figure 4a shows the shift of $I_{D\text{-}S}$-$V_{FG\text{-}S}$ characteristics for one of the devices ($W_{NR} = 170$ nm and $L_{NR} = 2375$ nm). The threshold voltage of the *n*-type device increases due to the accumulated negative charges at the interface between the gate oxide and the electrolyte. The threshold voltage sensitivity $\Delta V_{TH}/\Delta pH$ for a set of SiNRs with different widths and identical length ($L_{NR} = 2375$ nm) located close to each other on the chip area is shown in Figure 4b. The average voltage shift is about 30 mV/pH, in agreement with other previous works using SiO_2 as gate oxide [42–44]. The voltage shift does not depend on the device width (Figure 4b), as shown previously [31], while it has a well-proven dependence on the buffer capacity of the gate insulator [39].

The sensitivity in terms of current signal as a function of the device width is shown in Figure 4c,d. In this analysis the effect of the source (R_S) and drain (R_D) parasitic series resistances on the performance of SiNRs devices has been taken into account by extracting their value and compensating for the corresponding voltage losses (see Supplementary Figure S5). The sensitivity of $\Delta I'_{D\text{-}S}/\Delta pH$ is not constant, but instead increases for decreasing width (W_{NR}), due to the larger device transconductance g'_m (Figure 4c). The sensitivity for devices with different widths and different lengths is plotted in Figure 4d as a function of the width, indicating that the length does not affect the sensitivity for the considered range (350–4250 nm). SiNRs with width below few hundreds of nanometers exhibit a higher transconductance.

Interestingly, this result is in contrast with other works [32], in which a linear dependence of the transconductancewith the factor $(W_{NR} + 2 \cdot t_{NR})/L_{NR}$ is found. The enhancement of the transconductance with smaller W_{NR} could be a signature of marked corner effects, typical of devices with high body doping and rectangular cross-section [45], as opposed to low-doped trapezoidal wires [32].

The next section analyzes the noise characteristics of the SiNRs, which is essential to evaluate the dependence of the sensor performance on their size and, ultimately, to determine the smallest pH change detectable per unit footprint surface.

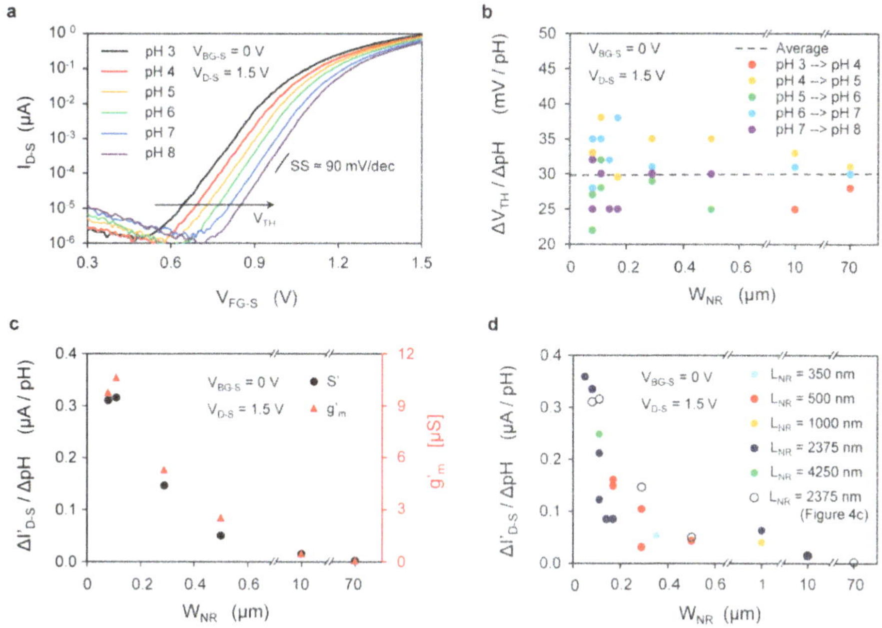

Figure 4. (**a**) Drain current ($I_{D\text{-}S}$) *vs.* front-gate voltage ($V_{FG\text{-}S}$) characteristics for a device with W_{NR} = 170 nm and L_{NR} = 2375 nm exposed to different pH; (**b**) Threshold voltage shifts over different pH, calculated at $I_{D\text{-}S}$ = 1 nA and plotted against W_{NR}; (**c**) pH sensitivity ($\Delta I'_{D\text{-}S}/\Delta$pH) and normalized transconductance (g'_m), plotted against the SiNR width (W_{NR}). The length L_{NR} of the devices is constant (L_{NR} = 2375 nm); (**d**) Normalized-current sensitivity (S′ = $\Delta I'_{D\text{-}S}/\Delta$pH) plotted against the SiNR width (W_{NR}), for devices with different length (L_{NR}), located on the same chip, all extracted at the same $V_{FG\text{-}S} - V_{TH}$ = 0.5 V.

3.2. Noise Characterization of the SiNRs

At low frequencies, the noise of SiNWs and SiNRs is dominated by flicker noise [22,25,46,47], which is characterized by a power spectral density that is proportional to $f^{-\gamma}$ where f is the frequency and $0.7 < \gamma < 1.3$ [48]. The flicker noise leads to a degradation of the SNR that is more important for devices having smaller gate areas [49].

In what follows, we characterize the noise at different bias points for three SiNRs, ranging from 110 nm to 10 μm in width, by performing the fast Fourier transform (FFT) [50] of $I_{D\text{-}S}$ sampled at f_S = 10 Hz. A spectral filtering technique [51] has been employed to compensate for the distortions caused by aliasing, which can impact the scaling exponents of $f^{-\gamma}$ noises (see Supplementary Figure S6) [51–54].

Figure 5a shows the current noise power spectral density (S_{ID}) for a SiNR (L_{NR} = 2375 nm, W_{NR} = 110 nm) biased in subthreshold ($V_{FG\text{-}S}$ = 0.9 V), weak inversion ($V_{FG\text{-}S}$ = 1.0 V and 1.1 V) and above threshold ($V_{FG\text{-}S}$ = 1.7 V), respectively. The S_{ID} of the silicon nanoribbon follows the expected $1/f$ behavior at low frequency, with larger noise at high $V_{FG\text{-}S}$.

On the other hand, Figure 5b shows that when considering the ratio between noise power and squared signal, working above threshold leads to higher SNR. In support of this observation, Figure 5c reports $S_{ID}/I_{D\text{-}S}{}^2$ *vs.* $I_{D\text{-}S}$ for different sampling frequencies, showing that working at larger currents lead to smaller noise-to-signal ratio. These results are consistent with previously reported works [55], in which the SNR is maximized at the peak transconductance. Moreover, the plot shows that the quantity $S_{ID}/I_{D\text{-}S}{}^2$ and $(g_m/I_{D\text{-}S})^2$ follow the same trend *vs.* $I_{D\text{-}S}$ (see also Supplementary Figure S7), thus supporting the validity of the carrier-number fluctuation (ΔN) arising from the dynamic trapping and de-trapping of free carriers within the gate oxide as the dominating factor of the flicker noise [48,49].

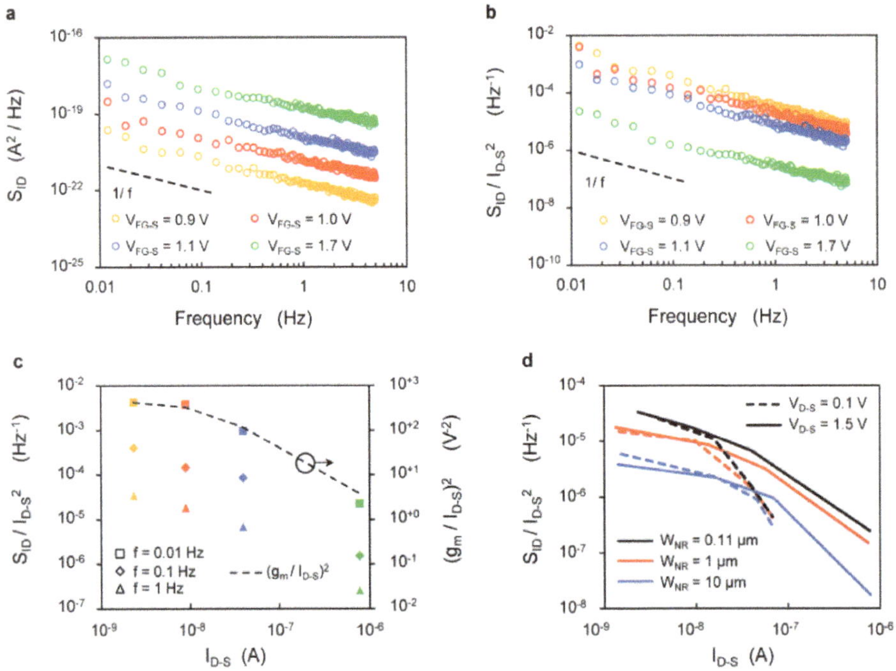

Figure 5. (**a**–**c**) Noise characteristics of a SiNR with length L_{NR} = 2375 nm, width W_{NR} = 110 nm and drain voltage $V_{D\text{-}S}$ = 1.5 V. (**a**) Low-frequency drain current noise spectral density (S_{ID}) characteristics; (**b**) $S_{ID}/I_{D\text{-}S}^2$ plotted against frequency; (**c**) $S_{ID}/I_{D\text{-}S}^2$ plotted for different frequencies (f = 0.01 Hz, f = 0.1 Hz and f = 1 Hz) as a function of $I_{D\text{-}S}$, compared with the $(g_m/I_{D\text{-}S})^2$ ratio (dotted line, right axis); (**d**) $S_{ID}/I_{D\text{-}S}^2$ plotted as a function of $I_{D\text{-}S}$ for SiNRs with same length (L_{NR} = 2375 nm) and different widths (W_{NR} = 110 nm, W_{NR} = 1 μm and W_{NR} = 10 μm) biased to work in saturation ($V_{D\text{-}S}$ = 1.5 V, solid lines) and linear regime ($V_{D\text{-}S}$ = 0.1 V, dotted lines), at a frequency f = 1 Hz.

Finally, Figure 5d compares the three SiNRs with different widths in terms of the $S_{ID}/I_{D\text{-}S}^2$ factor. In the low current region, the SNR depends only weakly on the drain voltage. Instead, in strong inversion, the saturation regime ensures a lower noise-to-signal ratio.

In conclusion, since nano-sized transistors occupying smaller areas suffer more from intrinsic noise, those approaches aimed at increasing the array density of a chip by employing tinier pH sensors must take into account the degradation of the SNR, which would ultimately negatively affect the resolution in pH. In what follows, we show that multi-wire transistors can reduce this limit and thus allow smaller area per sensing pixel with improved resolution.

3.3. Multiple-Wire Devices

In this section, we show that devices consisting of multiple nanowires connected in parallel exceed the performance of single devices occupying the same footprint area, and we compare their performances with existing planar and tri-gate devices. In fact, multi-wires devices benefit, on one hand, from the enhanced sensitivity of narrower silicon structures and, on the other hand, from the lower noise provided by their larger interface area [56]. Moreover, previous works have shown the superior inter-device uniformity of multi-wire devices when compared to single SiNR [57]. As a consequence, multi-wire devices alleviate the variability of electrical parameters such as V_{TH}, SS and g_m.

The four common-source devices characterized in this work exhibit independent drain contacts for each finger, which allows us to compare the performance of the single-wire with that of two-, three- and four-wire devices (Figure 6, cartoon A, B, C and D respectively). The devices were biased above threshold ($V_{FG\text{-}S} - V_{TH} \approx 1$ V) and in saturation regime ($V_{D\text{-}S}$ = 1.5 V). The results show an increase of the maximum transconductance with the number of SiNR fingers (Figure 6a). However, these values are smaller than the sum of the transconductance of individual wires, mainly due to the slightly different threshold voltage of the considered four wires, which results in a degradation of the average g_m. As shown in Figure 4c, the current sensitivity is directly linked to the transconductance of the device and, therefore, it also increases with the number of fingers.

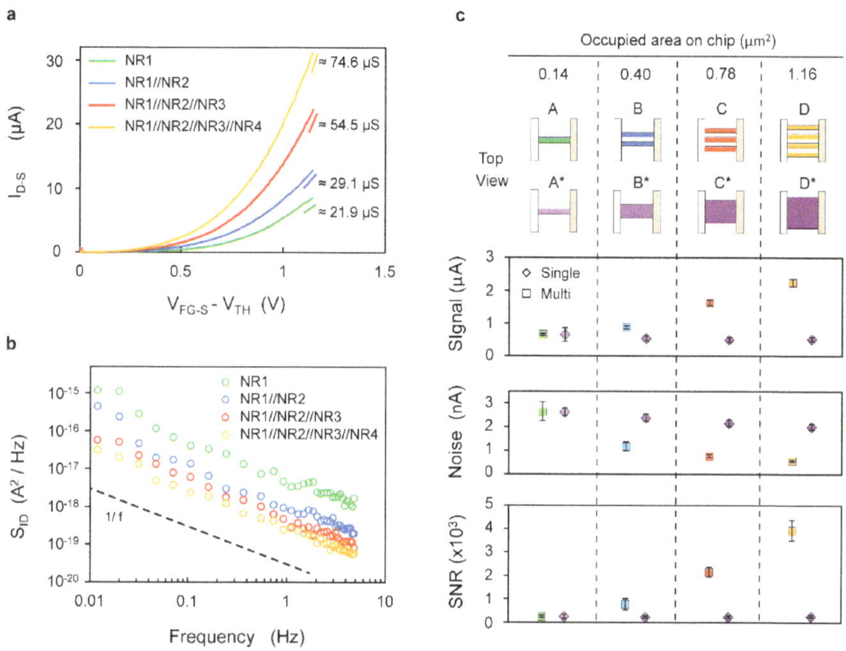

Figure 6. (**a–c**) The SiNRs have dimensions as follows: $W_{NR1,2}$ = 60 nm, $W_{NR3,4}$ = 110 nm with $L_{NR1,2,3,4}$ = 2375 nm. (**a**) Drain current ($I_{D\text{-}S}$) *vs.* overdrive voltage ($V_{FG\text{-}S} - V_{TH}$) characteristics; the value of the transconductance extracted at $V_{FG\text{-}S} - V_{TH}$ = 1.1 V is indicated on the right; (**b**) Low-frequency current noise spectral density (S_{ID}) characteristics (**c**) Signal, rms noise (as obtained by integrating S_{ID} over 1Hz bandwidth centered around 1Hz) and SNR values for multi-finger devices (□) and for single SiNR occupying the same area on chip (◊) with color-coded cartoon representation of the devices with the indication of the occupied area, considering a distance of 50 nm between fingers.

Figure 6b reports the current noise as a function of the frequency for devices with increasing number of fingers showing an improvement for devices featuring larger area, as expected from S_{ID} scaling rules. As for Figure 5, the spectra have been compensated for aliasing distortions (Figure S6, Supplementary). Figure 6c reports the Signal, Noise and SNR for devices of increasing occupied area featuring multiple nanowires (□). The Signal value corresponds to the measured g_m of the device multiplied by $\Delta V_{TH}/\Delta pH$ (assumed to be 30 mV/pH, according to Figure 4b) and the related error bars are defined based on the variability over the timescale of an experiment (a few hours). The Noise value of multi-wire devices is obtained by calculating the square root of the integral of the noise spectrum S_{ID} in 1 Hz bandwidth centered at 1 Hz. The corresponding error bars are calculated from the prediction bounds of the interpolated spectrum (Figure S8, Supplementary).

The analysis of sensitivity and noise characteristics allows us to evaluate the resolution of the devices, *i.e.*, the smallest detectable pH change. The resolution (δpH) is calculated as pH change giving a signal-to-noise ratio SNR = 3:

$$SNR = \frac{\Delta I_{D-S}/\,\Delta pH}{\sqrt{\int S_{ID} df}} = 3 \tag{1}$$

Since in Figure 4c we see that $\Delta I_{DS}/\Delta pH = g_m\, \Delta V_{TH}/\Delta pH$, we can also compute

$$SNR = g_m \frac{\Delta V_{TH}/\Delta pH}{\sqrt{\int S_{ID} df}} = \frac{\Delta V_{TH}/\Delta pH}{\sqrt{\int S_V df}} \tag{2}$$

where $S_V = S_{ID}/g_m^2$ is the voltage noise power spectral density. The noise-equivalent pH value is obtained by dividing the noise level (square root of the integral of the current noise spectra over the measurement frequency bandwidth) by the current sensitivity ($\Delta I_{D\text{-}S}/\Delta pH$). A resolution of ~0.8‰ of pH change is achieved in a 1 Hz bandwidth, centered at 1 Hz, by a four-fingers device occupying approximately 1.16 μm^2. In terms of the lowest detectable change of electron surface density at the gate interface, the achieved pH resolution corresponds to 1.78×10^{-17} C/μm^2.

This result is close to the lowest reported value obtained with tri-gate nanowires (0.5‰ of a pH shift in a 1 Hz bandwidth centered at 10 Hz) employing a device with a 7 μm^2 footprint [25]. Nevertheless, in the context of ever increasing array density of integrated pH sensors, the most indicative parameter is the resolution that can be achieved in a unit of occupied footprint area on the chip. In this regard, our results outperform the previous works (0.0008 pH *vs.* 0.0005$\cdot\sqrt{(7)}$ = 0.0013 pH change with 1 μm^2 footprint device) [25], despite our more conservative choice of the SNR level to define the resolution (SNR = 3) and of a lower central frequency (f_C) for the bandwidth (1 Hz *vs.* 10 Hz). When evaluated under the same conditions (SNR = 1, f_C = 10 Hz), our system outperforms the state-of-the-art by two orders of magnitude.

In order to compare the performance of multi-wire design with single nanoribbon devices, the trend of single SiNRs of equivalent area (A*, B*, C* and D*) has been reported in Figure 6c (◊). In this case, the Signal values have been derived from Figure 4d, with the error bars taking into account the interpolation error of the fitted trend. The Noise values (◊ Noise plot Figure 6c) are evaluated on the basis of the noise characterization of single ribbon devices (Figure 5d, $V_{D\text{-}S}$ = 1.5 V) and the corresponding error bars take into account the interpolation error (Figure S9, Supplementary). This suggests that the SNR of multi-wire devices increases with the area with a steeper trend than single nanoribbons and, in particular, a device occupying 1.16 μm^2 is characterized by a SNR that is 15 times higher than the one of a single nanoribbon of identical footprint area.

Clearly, the resolution could be further improved by increasing the density of interconnected nanowires per device, and by sampling at higher frequencies [58]. Moreover, the employment of high-*k* gate dielectrics such as Al_2O_3 and HfO_2 [16,31] would induce a larger change of surface potential upon a pH change, leading to a higher signal transduced by the sensor.

4. Conclusions

The performances including an improved sensitivity of nano-sized tri-dimensional silicon devices as detectors of surface charge in electrolyte environment have been investigated. The tri-gate configuration gives silicon nanoribbons undeniable advantages with respect to planar devices and, in particular, in this work we show that ribbons with width below a few hundreds of nanometers show enhanced conductivity properties, ultimately leading to higher sensitivity.

The enhanced performance characteristic of narrower wires can be combined with the lower noise granted by the larger gate area of multiple nanowires connected in parallel. Moreover, multi-wire devices assure improved inter-device uniformity in terms of the conductance characteristics.

In conclusion, we have shown that tri-dimensional, multi-wire devices constitute a successful approach to scale down the size of the single pH sensor, achieving unprecedented pH resolution per unit occupied footprint area. This feature is of particular interest in integrated pH-based bioanalytics on CMOS technology such as DNA sequencing and quantitative PCR, which lean toward sensor arrays of ever-increasing density. Our technology relies on highly-controlled top-down CMOS-compatible fabrication processes, which are required in large-scale integration.

Acknowledgments: This work has been funded by the Swiss Nano-Tera project ISyPeM (128852) and by the SNSF (Swiss National Science Foundation) project Bio3D (200021 140554). The authors wish to thank Federico Pittino for helpful discussions and Julien Buckley for his contribution to the design of the silicon nanoribbons.

Author Contributions: Enrico Accastelli and Carlotta Guiducci conceived and designed the experiments. Enrico Accastelli performed the experiments. Thomas Ernst was responsible for the fabrication of the devices. Enrico Accastelli, Paolo Scarbolo, Pierpaolo Palestri, Carlotta Guiducci, Luca Selmi equally contributed to analyze the data, devise extraction, compensation and normalization procedures for signal and noise. Enrico Accastelli and Carlotta Guiducci wrote the main part of the manuscript and all authors contributed to writing and revision of the manuscript. Carlotta Guiducci planned the project, directed the research and contributed for materials/analysis tools. All authors contributed to the discussion of the results and revised the manuscript.

Conflicts of Interest: The authors declare no conflict of interest.

References

1. James, D. Intel Ivy Bridge unveiled—The first commercial tri-gate, high-k, metal-gate CPU. In Proceedings of the IEEE Custom Integrated Circuits Conference, San Jose, CA, USA, 9–12 September 2012; pp. 1–4.
2. Agrawal, N.; Kimura, Y.; Arghavani, R.; Datta, S. Impact of Transistor Architecture (Bulk Planar, Trigate on Bulk, Ultrathin-Body Planar SOI) and Material (Silicon or III-V Semiconductor) on Variation for Logic and SRAM Applications. *IEEE Trans. Electron. Devices* **2013**, *60*, 3298–3304. [CrossRef]
3. Colinge, J.P. *FinFETs and Other Multi-Gate Transistors*; Springer: New York, NY, USA, 2008.
4. Sun, X.; Moroz, V.; Damrongplasit, N.; Shin, C.; Liu, T.-J.K. Variation Study of the Planar Ground-Plane Bulk MOSFET, SOI FinFET, and Trigate Bulk MOSFET Designs. *IEEE Trans. Electron Devices* **2011**, *58*, 3294–3299. [CrossRef]
5. Rothberg, J.M.; Hinz, W.; Rearick, T.M.; Schultz, J.; Mileski, W.; Davey, M.; Leamon, J.H.; Johnson, K.; Milgrew, M.J.; Edwards, M.; *et al.* An integrated semiconductor device enabling non-optical genome sequencing. *Nature* **2011**, *475*, 348–352. [CrossRef] [PubMed]
6. Duarte-Guevara, C.; Lai, F.-L.; Cheng, C.-W.; Reddy, B., Jr.; Salm, E.; Swaminathan, V.; Tsui, Y.-K.; Tuan, H.C.; Kalnitsky, A.; Liu, Y.-S.; *et al.* Enhanced Biosensing Resolution with Foundry Fabricated Individually Addressable Dual-Gated ISFETs. *Anal. Chem.* **2014**, *86*, 8359–8367. [CrossRef] [PubMed]
7. Guiducci, C.; Spiga, F.M. Another transistor-based revolution: On-chip qPCR. *Nat. Methods* **2013**, *10*, 617–618. [CrossRef] [PubMed]
8. Toumazou, C.; Shepherd, L.M.; Reed, S.C.; Chen, G.I.; Patel, A.; Garner, D.M.; Wang, C.-J.A.; Ou, C.-P.; Amin-Desai, K.; Athanasiou, P.; *et al.* Simultaneous DNA amplification and detection using a pH-sensing semiconductor system. *Nat. Methods* **2013**, *10*, 641–646. [CrossRef] [PubMed]
9. Bunimovich, Y.L.; Shin, Y.S.; Yeo, W.-S.; Amori, M.; Kwong, G.; Heath, J.R. Quantitative real-time measurements of DNA hybridization with alkylated nonoxidized silicon nanowires in electrolyte solution. *J. Anal. Chem. Soc.* **2006**, *128*, 16323–16331. [CrossRef] [PubMed]
10. Cui, Y.; Wei, Q.Q.; Park, H.K.; Lieber, C.M. Nanowire nanosensors for highly sensitive and selective detection of biological and chemical species. *Science* **2001**, *293*, 1289–1292. [CrossRef] [PubMed]
11. Elfstroem, N.; Karlstroem, A.E.; Linnros, J. Silicon nanoribbons for electrical detection of biomolecules. *Nano Lett.* **2008**, *8*, 945–949. [CrossRef] [PubMed]
12. Gao, X.P.A.; Zheng, G.; Lieber, C.M. Subthreshold Regime has the Optimal Sensitivity for Nanowire FET Biosensors. *Nano Lett.* **2010**, *10*, 547–552. [CrossRef] [PubMed]
13. Gao, Z.; Agarwal, A.; Trigg, A.D.; Singh, N.; Fang, C.; Tung, C.-H.; Fan, Y.; Buddharaju, K.D.; Kong, J. Silicon nanowire arrays for label-free detection of DNA. *Anal. Chem.* **2007**, *79*, 3291–3297. [CrossRef] [PubMed]
14. Hahm, J.; Lieber, C.M. Direct ultrasensitive electrical detection of DNA and DNA sequence variations using nanowire nanosensors. *Nano Lett.* **2004**, *4*, 51–54. [CrossRef]
15. Ishikawa, F.N.; Chang, H.-K.; Curreli, M.; Liao, H.-I.; Olson, C.A.; Chen, P.-C.; Zhang, R.; Roberts, R.W.; Sun, R.; Cote, R.J.; *et al.* Label-Free, Electrical Detection of the SARS Virus N-Protein with Nanowire Biosensors Utilizing Antibody Mimics as Capture Probes. *ACS Nano* **2009**, *3*, 1219–1224. [CrossRef] [PubMed]
16. Knopfmacher, O.; Tarasov, A.; Fu, W.; Wipf, M.; Niesen, B.; Calame, M.; Schoenenberger, C. Nernst Limit in Dual-Gated Si-Nanowire FET Sensors. *Nano Lett.* **2010**, *10*, 2268–2274. [CrossRef] [PubMed]
17. Li, J.; Zhang, Y.; To, S.; You, L.; Sun, Y. Effect of Nanowire Number, Diameter, and Doping Density on Nano-FET Biosensor Sensitivity. *ACS Nano* **2011**, *5*, 6661–6668. [CrossRef] [PubMed]

18. Li, Z.; Chen, Y.; Li, X.; Kamins, T.I.; Nauka, K.; Williams, R.S. Sequence-specific label-free DNA sensors based on silicon nanowires. *Nano Lett.* **2004**, *4*, 245–247. [CrossRef]
19. Masood, M.N.; Chen, S.; Carlen, E.T.; van den Berg, A. All-(111) Surface Silicon Nanowires: Selective Functionalization for Biosensing Applications. *ACS Appl. Mater. Interfaces* **2010**, *2*, 3422–3428. [CrossRef] [PubMed]
20. Nair, P.R.; Alam, M.A. Design considerations of silicon nanowire biosensors. *IEEE Trans. Electron Devices* **2007**, *54*, 3400 3408. [CrossRef]
21. Patolsky, F.; Zheng, G.F.; Hayden, O.; Lakadamyali, M.; Zhuang, X.W.; Lieber, C.M. Electrical detection of single viruses. *Proc. Natl. Acad. Sci. USA* **2004**, *101*, 14017–14022. [CrossRef] [PubMed]
22. Rajan, N.K.; Duan, X.; Reed, M.A. Performance limitations for nanowire/nanoribbon biosensors. *Wiley Interdiscip. Rev. Nanomed. Nanobiotechnol.* **2013**, *5*, 629–645. [CrossRef] [PubMed]
23. Stern, E.; Klemic, J.F.; Routenberg, D.A.; Wyrembak, P.N.; Turner-Evans, D.B.; Hamilton, A.D.; LaVan, D.A.; Fahmy, T.M.; Reed, M.A. Label-free immunodetection with CMOS-compatible semiconducting nanowires. *Nature* **2007**, *445*, 519–522. [CrossRef] [PubMed]
24. Stern, E.; Vacic, A.; Reed, M.A. Semiconducting Nanowire Field-Effect Transistor Biomolecular Sensors. *IEEE Trans. Electron Devices* **2008**, *55*, 3119–3130. [CrossRef]
25. Tarasov, A.; Fu, W.; Knopfmacher, O.; Brunner, J.; Calame, M.; Schoenenberger, C. Signal-to-noise ratio in dual-gated silicon nanoribbon field-effect sensors. *Appl. Phys. Lett.* **2011**, *98*. [CrossRef]
26. Wang, W.U.; Chen, C.; Lin, K.H.; Fang, Y.; Lieber, C.M. Label-free detection of small-molecule-protein interactions by using nanowire nanosensors. *Proc. Natl. Acad. Sci. USA* **2005**, *102*, 3208–3212. [CrossRef] [PubMed]
27. Zhang, G.-J.; Zhang, L.; Huang, M.J.; Luo, Z.H.H.; Tay, G.K.I.; Lim, E.-J.A.; Kang, T.G.; Chen, Y. Silicon nanowire biosensor for highly sensitive and rapid detection of Dengue virus. *Sens. Actuators B Chem.* **2010**, *146*, 138–144. [CrossRef]
28. Rigante, S.; Scarbolo, P.; Wipf, M.; Stoop, R.L.; Bedner, K.; Buitrago, E.; Bazigos, A.; Bouvet, D.; Calame, M.; Schönenberger, C.; *et al.* Sensing with Advanced Computing Technology: Fin Field-Effect Transistors with High-k Gate Stack on Bulk Silicon. *ACS Nano* **2015**, *9*, 4872–4881. [CrossRef] [PubMed]
29. Buitrago, E.; Fernández-Bolaños, M.; Rigante, S.; Zilch, C.F.; Schröter, N.S.; Nightingale, A.M.; Ionescu, A.M. The top-down fabrication of a 3D-integrated, fully CMOS-compatible FET biosensor based on vertically stacked SiNWs and FinFETs. *Sens. Actuators B Chem.* **2014**, *193*, 400–412. [CrossRef]
30. Elfstrom, N.; Juhasz, R.; Sychugov, I.; Engfeldt, T.; Karlstrom, A.E.; Linnros, J. Surface charge sensitivity of silicon nanowires: Size dependence. *Nano Lett.* **2007**, *7*, 2608–2612. [CrossRef] [PubMed]
31. Bedner, K.; Guzenko, V.A.; Tarasov, A.; Wipf, M.; Stoop, R.L.; Just, D.; Rigante, S.; Fu, W.; Minamisawa, R.A.; David, C.; *et al.* pH Response of Silicon Nanowire Sensors: Impact of Nanowire Width and Gate Oxide. *Sens. Mater.* **2013**, *25*, 567–576.
32. Rajan, N.K.; Brower, K.; Duan, X.; Reed, M.A. Limit of detection of field effect transistor biosensors: Effects of surface modification and size dependence. *Appl. Phys. Lett.* **2014**, *104*. [CrossRef]
33. Fritz, J.; Cooper, E.B.; Gaudet, S.; Sorger, P.K.; Manalis, S.R. Electronic detection of DNA by its intrinsic molecular charge. *Proc. Natl. Acad. Sci. USA* **2002**, *99*, 14142–14146. [CrossRef] [PubMed]
34. Gentil, C.; Philippin, G.; Bockelmann, U. Signal enhancement in electronic detection of DNA hybridization. *Phys. Rev. E* **2007**, *75*. [CrossRef] [PubMed]
35. Yao, J.; Yan, H.; Lieber, C.M. A nanoscale combing technique for the large-scale assembly of highly aligned nanowires. *Nat. Nanotechnol.* **2013**, *8*, 329–335. [CrossRef] [PubMed]
36. Halté, C.; Delapierre, G.; Fournier, T.; Buckley, J.; Gely, M.; De Salvo, B.; Baron, T.; Vinet, F. Rapid Top-down Fabrication of Si Nanowire and Fully Automated Test Platform: Application to pH. In Proceedings of the International Conference on Wearable Micro and Nano Technologies for Personalized Health, Valencia, Spain, 21–23 May 2008.
37. Accastelli, E.; Cappi, G.; Buckley, J.; Ernst, T.; Guiducci, C. Comparison between front- and back-gating of Silicon Nanoribbons in real-time sensing experiments. In Proceedings of the IEEE Conference on Nanotechnology, Beijing, China, 5–8 August 2013; pp. 517–520.
38. Pud, S.; Li, J.; Sibiliev, V.; Petrychuk, M.; Kovalenko, V.; Offenhäusser, A.; Vitusevich, S. Liquid and Back Gate Coupling Effect: Toward Biosensing with Lowest Detection Limit. *Nano Lett.* **2014**, *14*, 578–584. [CrossRef] [PubMed]

39. Bergveld, P.; VanHal, R.; Eijkel, J. The Remarkable Similarity between the Acid-Base Properties of ISFETs and Proteins and the Consequences for the Design of ISFET Biosensors. *Biosens. Bioelectron.* **1995**, *10*, 405–414. [CrossRef]
40. Bousse, L.; Bergveld, P. The role of buried OH sites in the response mechanism of inorganic-gate pH-sensitive ISFETs. *Sens. Actuators* **1984**, *6*, 65–78. (no A and B in Sensors and Actuators at that time). [CrossRef]
41. Yates, D.E.; Levine, S.; Healy, T.W. Site-binding model of the electrical double layer at the oxide/water interface. *J. Chem. Soc. Faraday Trans. 1: Phys. Chem. Condens. Phases* **1974**, *70*, 1807–1818. [CrossRef]
42. Bergveld, P. Thirty years of ISFETOLOGY—What happened in the past 30 years and what may happen in the next 30 years. *Sens. Actuators B Chem.* **2003**, *88*, 1–20. [CrossRef]
43. Siu, W.M.; Cobbold, R. Basic Properties of the Electrolyte-SiO_2-Si System—Physical and Theoretical Aspects. *IEEE Trans. Electron Devices* **1979**, *26*, 1805–1815. [CrossRef]
44. Vu, X.T.; GhoshMoulick, R.; Eschermann, J.F.; Stockmann, R.; Offenhaeusser, A.; Ingebrandt, S. Fabrication and application of silicon nanowire transistor arrays for biomolecular detection. *Sens. Actuators B Chem.* **2010**, *144*, 354–360. [CrossRef]
45. Fossum, J.G.; Yang, J.W.; Trivedi, V.P. Suppression of corner effects in triple-gate MOSFETs. *IEEE Electron Device Lett.* **2003**, *24*, 745–747. [CrossRef]
46. Kim, S.; Rim, T.; Kim, K.; Lee, U.; Baek, E.; Lee, H.; Baek, C.-K.; Meyyappan, M.; Deen, M.J.; Lee, J.-S. Silicon nanowire ion sensitive field effect transistor with integrated Ag/AgCl electrode: pH sensing and noise characteristics. *Analyst* **2011**, *136*, 5012–5016. [CrossRef] [PubMed]
47. Zhuge, J.; Wang, R.; Huang, R.; Tian, Y.; Zhang, L.; Kim, D.-W.; Park, D.; Wang, Y. Investigation of Low-Frequency Noise in Silicon Nanowire MOSFETs. *IEEE Electron Device Lett.* **2009**, *30*, 57–60. [CrossRef]
48. Simoen, E.; Claeys, C. On the flicker noise in submicron silicon MOSFETs. *Solid State Electron.* **1999**, *43*, 865–882. [CrossRef]
49. Ghibaudo, G.; Roux, O.; Nguyen-Duc, C.; Balestra, F.; Brini, J. Improved Analysis of Low-Frequency Noise in Field-Effect Mos-Transistors. *Phys. Status Solidi A Appl. Res.* **1991**, *124*, 571–581. [CrossRef]
50. Harris, F.J. On the use of windows for harmonic analysis with the discrete Fourier transform. *Proc. IEEE* **1978**, *66*, 51–83. [CrossRef]
51. Kirchner, J.W. Publisher's note: Aliasing in 1/f(alpha) noise spectra: Origins, consequences, and remedies. *Phys. Rev. E* **2005**, *71*. [CrossRef]
52. Caloyannides, M.A. Microcycle Spectral Estimates of 1-F Noise in Semiconductors. *J. Appl. Phys.* **1974**, *45*, 307–316. [CrossRef]
53. Foster, S.; Cranch, G.A.; Tikhomirov, A. Experimental evidence for the thermal origin of 1/f frequency noise in erbium-doped fiber lasers. *Phys. Rev. A* **2009**, *79-5*, 053802-1–053802-7. [CrossRef]
54. Kasdin, N.J. Discrete Simulation of Colored Noise and Stochastic-Processes and 1/F(Alpha) Power-Law Noise Generation. *Proc. IEEE* **1995**, *83*, 802–827. [CrossRef]
55. Rajan, N.K.; Routenberg, D.A.; Reed, M.A. Optimal signal-to-noise ratio for silicon nanowire biochemical sensors. *Appl. Phys. Lett.* **2011**, *98*, 264107-1–264107-3. [CrossRef] [PubMed]
56. Clément, N.; Han, X.L.; Larrieu, G. Electronic transport mechanisms in scaled gate-all-around silicon nanowire transistor arrays. *Appl. Phys. Lett.* **2013**, *103*, 263504. [CrossRef]
57. Regonda, S.; Tian, R.; Gao, J.; Greene, S.; Ding, J.; Hu, W. Silicon multi-nanochannel FETs to improve device uniformity/stability and femtomolar detection of insulin in serum. *Biosens. Bioelectron.* **2013**, *45*, 245–251. [CrossRef] [PubMed]
58. Tartagni, M.; Crescentini, M.; Rossi, M.; Morgan, H.; Sangiorgi, E. An AC and phase nanowire sensing for site-binding detection. In Proceedings of the IEEE International Electron Device Meeting, San Francisco, CA, USA, 15–17 December 2014; pp. 31.2.1–31.2.4.

Permissions

All chapters in this book were first published in Biosensors, by MDPI; hereby published with permission under the Creative Commons Attribution License or equivalent. Every chapter published in this book has been scrutinized by our experts. Their significance has been extensively debated. The topics covered herein carry significant findings which will fuel the growth of the discipline. They may even be implemented as practical applications or may be referred to as a beginning point for another development.

The contributors of this book come from diverse backgrounds, making this book a truly international effort. This book will bring forth new frontiers with its revolutionizing research information and detailed analysis of the nascent developments around the world.

We would like to thank all the contributing authors for lending their expertise to make the book truly unique. They have played a crucial role in the development of this book. Without their invaluable contributions this book wouldn't have been possible. They have made vital efforts to compile up to date information on the varied aspects of this subject to make this book a valuable addition to the collection of many professionals and students.

This book was conceptualized with the vision of imparting up-to-date information and advanced data in this field. To ensure the same, a matchless editorial board was set up. Every individual on the board went through rigorous rounds of assessment to prove their worth. After which they invested a large part of their time researching and compiling the most relevant data for our readers.

The editorial board has been involved in producing this book since its inception. They have spent rigorous hours researching and exploring the diverse topics which have resulted in the successful publishing of this book. They have passed on their knowledge of decades through this book. To expedite this challenging task, the publisher supported the team at every step. A small team of assistant editors was also appointed to further simplify the editing procedure and attain best results for the readers.

Apart from the editorial board, the designing team has also invested a significant amount of their time in understanding the subject and creating the most relevant covers. They scrutinized every image to scout for the most suitable representation of the subject and create an appropriate cover for the book.

The publishing team has been an ardent support to the editorial, designing and production team. Their endless efforts to recruit the best for this project, has resulted in the accomplishment of this book. They are a veteran in the field of academics and their pool of knowledge is as vast as their experience in printing. Their expertise and guidance has proved useful at every step. Their uncompromising quality standards have made this book an exceptional effort. Their encouragement from time to time has been an inspiration for everyone.

The publisher and the editorial board hope that this book will prove to be a valuable piece of knowledge for researchers, students, practitioners and scholars across the globe.

List of Contributors

Wei Zheng, Remko van den Hurk and Stephane Evoy
Department of Electrical and Computer Engineering, University of Alberta, Edmonton, Alberta, AB T6G 2V4, Canada

Yong Cao, Rongbing Du and Mark T. McDermott
Department of Chemistry and National Institute for Nanotechnology, University of Alberta, Edmonton, Alberta, AB T6G 2G2, Canada

Xuejun Sun
Department of Experimental Oncology, Cross Cancer Institute, University of Alberta, Edmonton, Alberta, AB T6G 1Z2, Canada

Yiyu Wang
Department of Chemical and Materials Engineering, University of Alberta, Edmonton, Alberta, AB T6G 1H9, Canada

Daniel Schaffhauser, Miyuki Tabata, Tatsuro Goda and Yuji Miyahara
Institute of Biomaterials & Bioengineering, Tokyo Medical and Dental University, Bldg 21-4-403B, 2-3-10 Kanda-Surugadai, Chiyoda, Tokyo 101-0062, Japan

Michael Fine
Department of Physiology, UT Southwestern Medical Center, 5323 Harry Hines Blvd., Dallas, TX 75390, USA

Carla Duarte
INESC-MN Instituto de Engenharia de Sistemas e Computadores – Microsistemas e Nanotecnologias, Rua Alves Redol 9, 1000-029 Lisbon, Portugal
CIISA at Faculdade de Medicina Veterinária, Universidade de Lisboa, Av. da Universidade Técnica, 1300-477 Lisbon, Portugal

Tiago Costa and Moisés Piedade
INESC-ID Instituto de Engenharia de Sistemas e Computadores – Investigação e Desenvolvimento, Rua Alves Redol 9, 1000-029 Lisbon, Portugal

Carla Carneiro and Ricardo Bexiga
CIISA at Faculdade de Medicina Veterinária, Universidade de Lisboa, Av. da Universidade Técnica, 1300-477 Lisbon, Portugal

Rita Soares
INESC-MN Instituto de Engenharia de Sistemas e Computadores – Microsistemas e Nanotecnologias, Rua Alves Redol 9, 1000-029 Lisbon, Portugal

Andrei Jitariu
INESC-MN Instituto de Engenharia de Sistemas e Computadores – Microsistemas e Nanotecnologias, Rua Alves Redol 9, 1000-029 Lisbon, Portugal
Visiting from the National Institute of Research and Development for Technical Physics, 47 Mangeron Blvd, Iasi 700050, Romania

Susana Cardoso
INESC-MN Instituto de Engenharia de Sistemas e Computadores – Microsistemas e Nanotecnologias, Rua Alves Redol 9, 1000-029 Lisbon, Portugal
Instituto Superior Técnico, Physics Department, Av. Rovisco Pais, 1049-001 Lisbon, Portugal

Paulo Freitas
INESC-MN Instituto de Engenharia de Sistemas e Computadores – Microsistemas e Nanotecnologias, Rua Alves Redol 9, 1000-029 Lisbon, Portugal
International Iberian Nanotechnology Laboratory (INL), Av. Mestre José Veiga, 4715-330 Braga, Portugal

Yunqing Du and Wenjun Zhang
Interdisciplinary Engineering Program, College of Engineering, Northeastern University, 360 Huntington Ave, 400 SN, Boston, MA 02115, USA

Ming L. Wang
Interdisciplinary Engineering Program, College of Engineering, Northeastern University, 360 Huntington Ave, 400 SN, Boston, MA 02115, USA
Civil and Environmental Engineering, and Bioengineering Department, Northeastern University, 360 Huntington Ave, 429 SN, Boston, MA 02115, USA

Michael Polanco and Sebastian Bawab
Department of Mechanical and Aerospace Engineering, Old Dominion University, Norfolk, VA 23529, USA

Hargsoon Yoon
Department of Engineering, Center for Materials Research, Norfolk State University, Norfolk, VA 23504, USA

Maysam Z. Pedram, Amir Shamloo and Aria Alasty
Department of Mechanical Engineering, Sharif University of Technology, Tehran, PO Box: 11365-11155, Iran

Ebrahim Ghafar-Zadeh
Department of Electrical Engineering, York University, Toronto, ON M3J1P3, Canada

Manuel Kasper and Ferry Kienberger
Keysight Technologies Austria GmbH, Keysight Labs Linz, Gruberstrasse 40, 4020 Linz, Austria

Lukas Traxler and Andreas Ebner
Johannes Kepler University Linz, Biophysics Institute, Gruberstrasse 40, 4020 Linz, Austria

Jasmina Salopek
Faculty of Science, Department of Chemistry, Division of Physical Chemistry University of Zagreb, Horvatovac 102a, 10000 Zagreb, Croatia

Herwig Grabmayr
Johannes Kepler University Linz, Biophysics Institute, Gruberstrasse 40, 4020 Linz, Austria
University of Applied Sciences Upper Austria, School of Engineering, Stelzhamerstrasse 23, 4600Wels, Austria

Mauro Tomassetti, Giorgia Conta and Luigi Campanella
Department of Chemistry, Sapienza University of Rome, P.le Aldo Moro 5, 00185 Rome, Italy

Gabriele Favero, Gabriella Sanzò, Franco Mazzei and Riccarda Antiochia
Department of Chemistry and Drug Technologies, Sapienza University of Rome, P.le Aldo Moro 5, 00185 Rome, Italy

O. Tolga Gül
Department of Physics and Astronomy, University of California at Irvine, Irvine, CA 92697, USA
Department of Physics, Polatlı Faculty of Science and Arts, Gazi University, Polatlı 06900, Turkey

Kaitlin M. Pugliese
Department of Chemistry, University of California at Irvine, Irvine, CA 92697, USA

Yongki Choi
Department of Physics and Astronomy, University of California at Irvine, Irvine, CA 92697, USA
Department of Physics, North Dakota State University, Fargo, ND 58108, USA

Patrick C. Sims, Deng Pan, Arith J. Rajapakse and Philip G. Collins
Department of Physics and Astronomy, University of California at Irvine, Irvine, CA 92697, USA

Gregory A. Weiss
Department of Chemistry, University of California at Irvine, Irvine, CA 92697, USA
Department of Molecular Biology and Biochemistry, University of California at Irvine, Irvine, CA 92697, USA

G. Denise Hammond, Adam L. Vojta, Sheila A. Grant and Heather K. Hunt
Department of Bioengineering, University of Missouri, Columbia, MO 65211, USA

Ciril Reiner-Rozman, Caroline Kotlowski and Wolfgang Knoll
Center for Electrochemical Surface Technology (CEST),Wiener Neustadt 2700, Austria
AIT Austrian Institute of Technology, Wien 1220, Austria

Erik Steen Redeker
Maastricht Science Programme, Maastricht University, Maastricht 6200 MD, The Netherlands

Peter Adriaensens
Biomolecule Design Group, Institute for Materials Research (IMO), Hasselt University, Diepenbeek BE-3590, Belgium

Wanda Guedens and Tom Vranken
Biomolecule Design Group, Institute for Materials Research (IMO), Hasselt University, Diepenbeek BE-3590, Belgium
Faculty of Food Technology and Biotechnology, Can Tho University of Technology, Can Tho 900000, Vietnam

Katrijn Vanschoenbeek and Luc Michiels
Immunology and Biochemistry, Biomedical Research Institute (Biomed) and School of Life Sciences, Transnationale Universiteit Limburg, Hasselt University, Diepenbeek BE-3590, Belgium
Design Group, Institute for Materials Research (IMO), Hasselt University, Diepenbeek BE-3590, Belgium
Applied and Analytical Chemistry, Institute for Materials Research (IMO), Hasselt University, Diepenbeek BE-3590, Belgium

Bohari Noor Aini, Shafiquzzaman Siddiquee and Kamaruzaman Ampon
Biotechnology Research Institute, Universiti Malaysia Sabah, Jln UMS, 88400 Kota Kinabalu, Sabah, Malaysia

Nor Monica Ahmad
School of Chemistry and Environment, Faculty of Applied Science, UiTM Kuala Pilah, 72 000 Negeri Sembilan, Malaysia
Department of Chemistry, Faculty of Science, Universiti Putra Malaysia, 43400 Serdang, Selangor, Malaysia

Jaafar Abdullah and Nor Azah Yusof
Department of Chemistry, Faculty of Science, Universiti Putra Malaysia, 43400 Serdang, Selangor, Malaysia

Ahmad Hazri Ab Rashid and Samsulida Abd Rahman
Industrial Biotechnology Research Centre, SIRIM Berhad, 1, Persiaran Dato' Menteri, P.O. Box 7035, Section 2, 40700 Shah Alam, Selangor, Malaysia

Md. Rakibul Hasan
Nanotechnology & Catalysis Research Centre, Institute of Postgraduate Studies, University of Malaya, 50603 Kuala Lumpur, Malaysia

Francesca Malvano and Donatella Albanese
Department of Industrial Engineering, University of Salerno, 84084 Fisciano SA, Italy

Alessio Crescitelli and Emanuela Esposito
Institute for Microelectronics and Microsystems of the National Council of Research (CNR), 80131 Napoli, Italy

Roberto Pilloton
Institute of Atmospheric Pollution Research of the National Council of Research (CNR), 00015 Roma, Italy

Enrico Accastelli and Carlotta Guiducci
Institute of Bioengineering, École Polytechnique Fédérale de Lausanne (EPFL), 1015 Lausanne, Switzerland

Paolo Scarbolo, Pierpaolo Palestri and Luca Selmi
DIEGM, Università degli Studi di Udine, 33100 Udine, Italy

Thomas Ernst
Laboratoire d'Électronique et de Technologie de l'Information (LETI), Commissariat à l'Énergie Atomique et aux Énergies Alternatives (CEA), 38054 Grenoble Cedex 9, France

Index